Passport to a Healthy Pregnancy

Dr Gita Arjun is an eminent obstetrician and gynaecologist with a career spanning forty-one years. She is a staunch advocate for women's health and wellness. She started her practice in 1981, and was one of the first obstetricians in India to encourage husbands to be in the labour room. *Passport to a Healthy Pregnancy* was first published in 2009 and has been essential reading for new parents ever since. Dr Arjun lives and works in Chennai.

Passport to a Healthy

Pregnancy

Dr Gita Arjun

Online reviews

'Wow. I was looking for a good pregnancy book and this is the one'.

'Highly recommended book for both working and at-home pregnant women…'

'It made our visits to the doctor so meaningful and interesting, otherwise we would have been stumped by various medical terms and phrases…'

'Lots of photos/illustration to help in understanding…'

'…very relevant for Indian readers.'

'… though we also had some books by foreign authors on pregnancy, this book explains each and every concept very beautifully. In fact this book walks you through it in great detail…'

'As a rst time expecting mother in a new city, far away from family and friends, I was anxious at the beginning of my pregnancy. Consequently, I purchased almost every pregnancy book I could get my hands on. By far, this book was my favourite. The author very clearly explains what is myth and what isn't and the scienti c principles behind the same, which I really appreciated. The book was clear, straightforward and with a surprisingly large amount of detail. I'm letting all my friends and family know about this one. Must read!'

'I'm going to recommend to my friends to buy it'.

'Was able to avoid a caesarean for my wife, based on this book, which details when to go for caesarean. Thus, my wife normally delivered a healthy baby girl. Thanks to the author for her great, momentous e ort to arise awareness in beautifully crafted simple language…'

'This book is really good for rst time parents-to-be.'

'…just buy this book—it will pamper you'.

'Content is super awesome. It has answers to all doubts and questions that will arise during pregnancy.'

'This book provides complete 360 degree information on all the relevant topics right from preparing for pregnancy till newborn baby care'.

'My daughter and I relied on this book to get us through my daughter's pregnancy. It has been an amazing support.'

'Thank you Dr. Gita Arjun, for a wonderful book and for your effort in educating pregnant couples! And more importantly clearing misconceptions (through old wives' tales).'

'As an expectant mother, I was earlier worried about very small symptoms like coughs and cramps because I was afraid it might harm the baby. But after reading the book, I realized that many of the symptoms which I thought were problems are actually normal conditions during pregnancy and I was much calmer and more informed about what changes I was undergoing after reading this book'.

'Most amazing and helpful pregnancy guide till delivery and beyond that…'

'It's a best buy especially when it is purchased right at the start of pregnancy...'

'Awesome book. Covers the minutest details during pregnancy. Highly recommended.'

'One of the best books that me and my wife have read. Covers almost everything under the sun including topics like role of father, twins, planning for next child, various precautions…'

'Each and every word mentioned in this book is true and very knowledgeable. People who are planning for baby MUST buy. Special thanks to the author for this wonderful book…'

'…loved the Indian touch in this book. Some of the things in the book are specifically relevant to Indian mothers…'

First published by westland ltd in 2009

Revised and updated edition published by Westland Publications Private Limited in 2017

Published by Westland Books, a division of Nasadiya Technologies Private Limited, in 2022

No. 269/2B, First Floor, 'Irai Arul', Vimalraj Street, Nethaji Nagar, Alapakkam Main Road, Maduravoyal, Chennai 600095

Westland and the Westland logo are the trademarks of Nasadiya Technologies Private Limited, or its affiliates.

ISBN: 9789395073141

10 9 8 7 6 5 4 3 2

Typeset by Malvika Mehra, Art Works

Printed at Thomson Press (India) Ltd

Dedicated to the women in my life

Dr E V Kalyani, who by her surgical skills made possible my very existence

Vanajakshi Padmanabhan, my mother, who in her own gentle way
taught me to be fearless

Padma Rajagopalan, my mother-in-law, who with immense generosity
gave me the freedom to succeed

Dr T Tharabai and Dr S Neela, my aunts and brilliant obstetricians,
who have been my lifelong role models

And to all the women who have allowed me the
privilege and honour of sharing their joy during their pregnancies.
They taught me the true meaning of courage and resilience,
because that is what it takes to be a mother

For Arjun, the friend of my youth and sunset years,
Ashvin, Kavita and Sruti who have added sparkle to my life,
And Aisha, without whom my life would be leached of all its colours.

How to read this book

You might just want to know the basic details of a pregnancy. Or you may be one of those who like to know everything in great detail. This book will give you exactly what you want.

Just the basics? Read the preliminary chapters and the week-by-week development of the pregnancy. Definitely prepare yourself for labour and delivery by reading the section devoted to that. You can stay away from chapters that make you nervous.

More details? You can get all the information you want by diving into the relevant chapters that impact your pregnancy. If you have a problem that has arisen in pregnancy, this book will make it easier to understand what is happening to you.

You just want answers to common doubts? Look at the boxes with real-life situations and queries raised by mothers and their partners.

Is something somebody has said to you a fact or a myth? The old wives' tales will lay your fears to rest.

Go ahead and enjoy your pregnancy, armed with facts and empowered with knowledge!

Contents

Introduction

You are planning for a pregnancy, or have just discovered that you are pregnant! Your happiness spills over into every aspect of your life. You want to know everything that is happening inside, every change and transformation that will slowly but surely turn you into a parent, in a few short months.

Passport to a Healthy Pregnancy is just the book for you. It has been written with the modern young Indian couple in mind: the couple that is involved, committed and totally invested in bringing a healthy baby into the world. This second edition has been revised, updated and modified to meet your demand for more knowledge, and will empower you to navigate your pregnancy with greater confidence.

Being pregnant is a life-altering event that every woman looks forward to. It is a time of great joy, even as a new life is unfolding within you. With technology and an array of investigations available to the modern obstetrician today, pregnancy has been made safer for mother and child. At the same time, nothing can replace the empathy and compassion that a pregnant woman requires and expects from her family, friends and obstetrician.

Fathers-to-be are definitely more involved in the pregnancy than ever before. Indian husbands are actively taking the responsibility of steering their wives through a comfortable and supported pregnancy. They are there for their wives and involve themselves throughout pregnancy, and even at the crucial moment of delivery. *Passport to a Healthy Pregnancy* has a chapter defining the role of husbands in helping their wives through pregnancy and delivery.

For some couples, pregnancy can be tinged with worry and plagued with anxiety. Sometimes, a pregnancy does not follow the normal, expected path. Things can go wrong, but it is always better to be informed about any such reasons than be blissfully ignorant. *Passport to a Healthy Pregnancy* helps you understand what causes complications, and occasional mishaps, in a pregnancy. This knowledge will help you withstand unexpected setbacks, be they minor or major, and help you move on.

Worries in pregnancy arise due to the lack of knowledge about pregnancy or, worse still, due to misinformation, myths and misplaced beliefs. *Passport to a Healthy Pregnancy* will place all the facts before you and help you proceed through your pregnancy with confidence. We want you to enjoy every moment of your pregnancy, armed with correct facts, specific information and essential details.

It has been an honour and privilege to help thousands of pregnant couples during the course of my career. I have been allowed into their lives and have shared their joy, their tears, their deepest feelings, their hopes and their despair.

Come, learn about your pregnancy and prepare yourself for a great experience—you deserve to have a wonderful, healthy pregnancy!

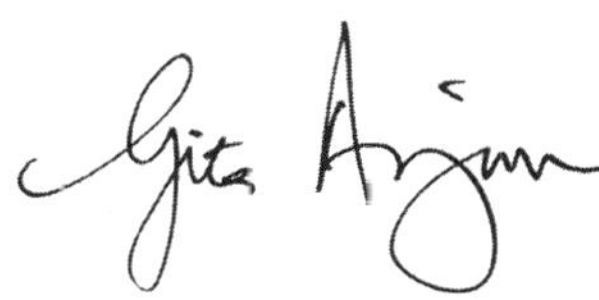

Dr Gita Arjun

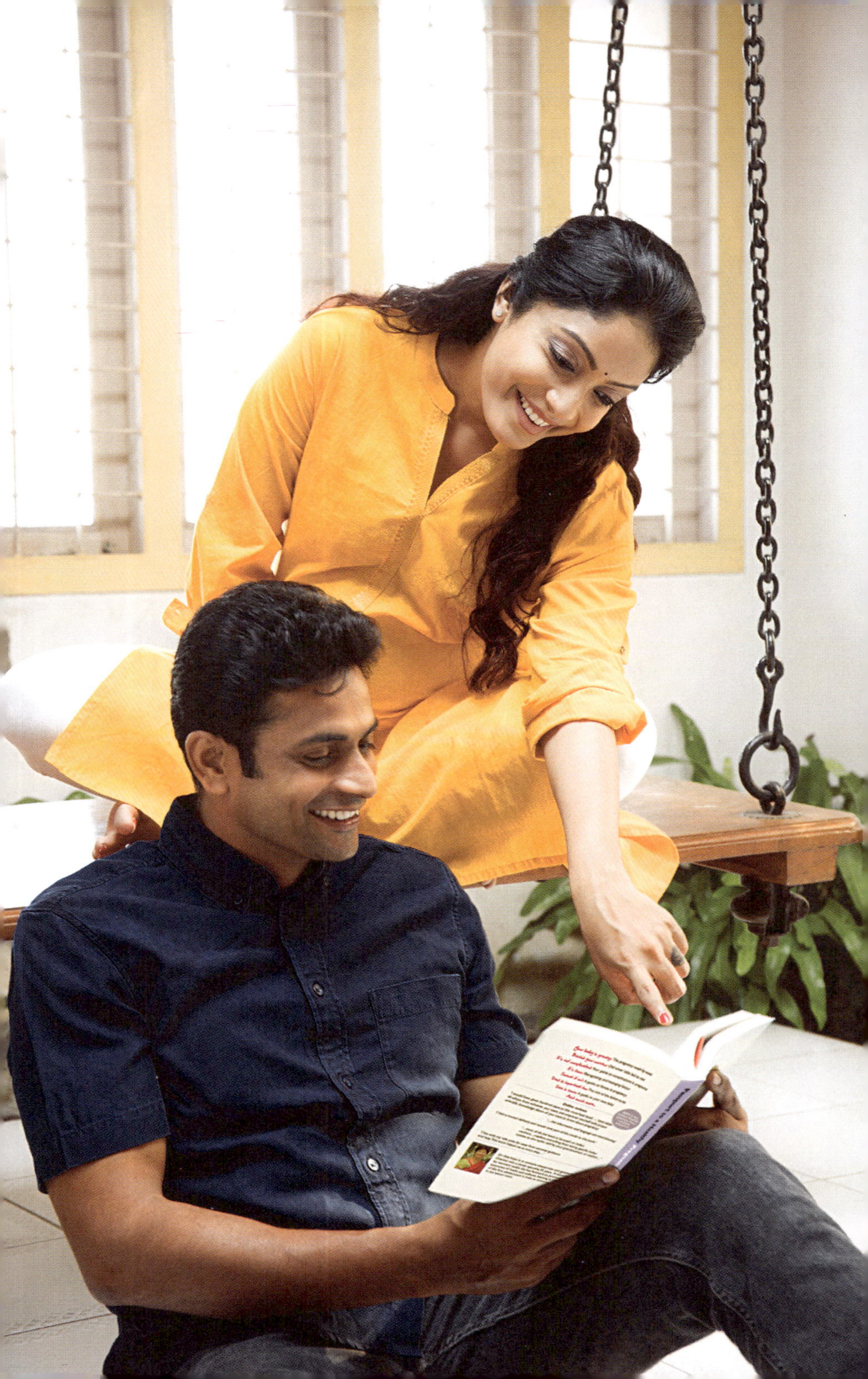

Knowing your pregnancy

CHAPTER 1

Preparing for pregnancy: pre-pregnancy counselling

Smita and her husband are busy professionals who chose to postpone their pregnancy and not have children immediately after marriage. Now they are ready for a baby, and have scheduled an appointment with an obstetrician for pre-pregnancy counselling (also called preconceptional care). Smita and her husband have made the right choice in seeking pre-pregnancy counselling.

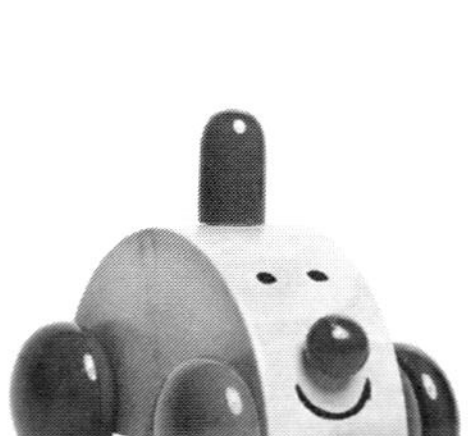

1

Preparing for pregnancy: pre-pregnancy counselling

Would you consider running a marathon without first checking out that you are fit? A pregnancy is as strenuous (if not more!) than a marathon. It would be prudent to go ahead with a pregnancy only after ensuring that you are at your healthiest best, physically and emotionally.

Basically, pre-pregnancy counselling is a checklist for couples to make sure that they have a good outcome with their pregnancy. Becoming a parent is a major decision. It brings with it its own uncertainties and apprehensions. The goal is to check for any potential risks to you and your baby during pregnancy and to address any medical issues you may have before you get pregnant.

Why is pre-pregnancy counselling important?

Planning your pregnancy can help you make sensible choices that will benefit both you and your baby. Most often, women do not realize they are

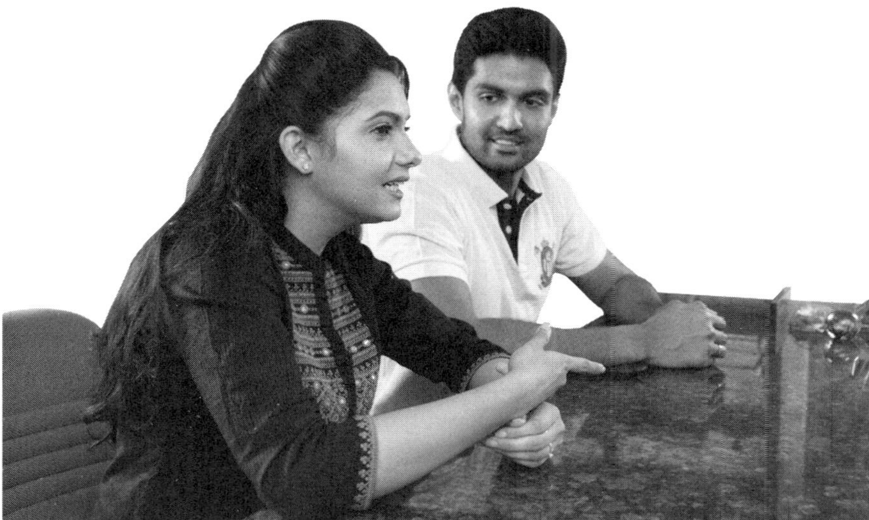

pregnant until several weeks after they have conceived. The early weeks of foetal growth are crucial, because it is during this period that your health can impact the baby.

During a preconceptional visit, your obstetrician will try to identify conditions that may pose risks to you or the baby you are planning to have. Keeping fit, eating healthy and avoiding certain things that could be harmful to the baby are the first steps to a healthy pregnancy.

Previous medical problems

If you have medical problems prior to pregnancy, it is important to seek your doctor's advice before proceeding with a pregnancy, to protect both you and your baby.

Diabetes

Ensuring tight control of blood sugar levels at the time of conception is essential to avoid the risk of a miscarriage and to avoid birth defects in the baby. It is important to maintain the haemoglobin A1C (a test to assess blood sugar control) less than 6.5%. If you are on tablets for diabetes, your doctor may switch you to insulin (see **Chapter 38**, *Diabetes in pregnancy*).

High blood pressure

It is important to make sure that high blood pressure is well under control before attempting pregnancy. Some medications for high blood pressure are not safe in pregnancy and must be changed to those that are safe (see **Chapter 37**, *High blood pressure in pregnancy*).

Anaemia

Anaemia due to iron deficiency is common in Indian women. Your doctor will check your haemoglobin levels and if necessary, start you on iron and folic acid supplementation.

Asthma

A high level of control is essential during pregnancy. Check with your doctor about the medications that are safe when you are trying for a pregnancy. Inhalers, by and large, are safe because the medications do not get absorbed into the blood stream (see **Chapter 46**, *Medical disorders in pregnancy*).

Hypothyroidism

If your thyroid is functioning less than it should be, you are normally placed on thyroid hormone tablets. It is essential to check your levels before you get pregnant. Your low thyroid hormone levels can affect the baby's brain development, so it is absolutely essential to adjust your medication before pregnancy (see **Chapter 46**, *Medical disorders in pregnancy*).

Epilepsy

It is safe for most epileptics on medications to try for a pregnancy. Most anti-epileptic drugs have the potential to cause birth defects although the risk is reduced if a single drug is used.

> **Devi asked:** I have been an epileptic for 10 years. I am on an anti-epileptic drug. My friend said that I should stop the medicine, otherwise I will have an abnormal baby. Should I do that?
>
> **My answer:** Please do not stop your medicine. Stopping the medicine is very unsafe for your health.
>
> Though there is risk of a birth defect with anti-epileptic drugs, the risk is very small. It is essential to discuss with your physician which drug is safer when you are trying for a pregnancy. When you have your ultrasound during pregnancy, they will look carefully to see if there is any birth defect.

Problems in previous pregnancies

Some problems that occurred in a past pregnancy may occur again. If there has been more than one miscarriage, a previous baby with a birth defect or a baby that died before birth or soon after birth, the obstetrician may suggest studies to find out the cause. It is important to keep all the records of previous pregnancies and show them to your obstetrician.

Family health history

Diabetes and high blood pressure are common conditions that may run in families. Even if you do not have these conditions, it is important for the doctor to know if there is a family history because these conditions may present for the first time in pregnancy.

Some genetic conditions such as intellectual disability, cystic fibrosis, thalassaemia and muscular dystrophy, may run in a family. If there is a history of such a condition, then genetic counselling might be offered to help the couple find out the chances of having a child with that problem.

Optimizing pre-pregnancy health

Being overweight can lead to high blood pressure or diabetes in pregnancy. Women who are obese (BMI 30 kg/m^2 or more) have a greater chance of facing problems for the baby as well as for themselves.

Being underweight (BMI 20 kg/m^2 or less) too can cause problems in pregnancy. It may increase the chances of giving birth to a low birth weight baby, which can often face problems during labour and after birth.

Reaching a healthy weight before pregnancy

It helps to plan your diet with the help of a nutritionist. An average woman needs about 2,000 calories per day. Eat plenty of fruits, vegetables and whole-grains such as channa and rajma every day. Consume enough dairy products. If you already are on a balanced diet, it is easy to make changes during pregnancy to get the extra calories and nutrients you need. Also ensure you get at least 30 minutes of brisk walking, 4–5 days a week.

Keeping fit

Good health depends on a balanced diet combined with exercise. Keeping fit and doing regular exercise even before you conceive, can improve your chances of having a comfortable and active pregnancy. Get into the habit of a brisk walk everyday. Check with your doctor on how active you can be after you get pregnant.

Vitamins and minerals

Folic acid

Starting folic acid supplementation 1–3 months before a planned pregnancy is important for the development of the baby's brain and spinal cord and preventing certain birth defects.

Iron

Iron keeps the mother from developing anaemia during pregnancy. It is a good idea to have a blood test to rule out anaemia. If the haemoglobin levels are low, then an iron supplement (combined with B-complex vitamins) should be taken for three months or more to ensure that the iron stores in the body are replenished and maintained.

Preventing infections

Rubella (or German measles) is a viral infection that can cause severe abnormalities in the baby, especially if it occurs in the first three months of pregnancy. A woman planning to get pregnant should either be tested to see if she already has immunity or should directly be vaccinated against Rubella. It is important to avoid pregnancy for 1–3 months after the vaccination.

Viral hepatitis: It is useful to be vaccinated against Hepatitis B. If you already have had Hepatitis B, inform your obstetrician so that she can take the appropriate steps to ensure your baby does not get affected.

Pre-pregnancy checklist and benefits

Intervention	Proven health benefit
Folic acid supplementation (400 mcg) Higher dose (4 mg) for women • On anti-epileptic drugs • Who are obese • With a previous baby with neural tube defect	Reduces occurrence of neural tube defects by two-thirds
Hepatitis B vaccination for at-risk women	Prevents transmission of infection to the infant
Rubella vaccination	Protects against congenital Rubella syndrome
Optimizing weight in overweight and obese women	Reaching a healthy weight before pregnancy reduces the risks of neural tube defects, preterm delivery, diabetes, caesarean section, and high blood pressure that are associated with obesity
Smoking cessation	Completing smoking cessation before pregnancy can prevent smoking- associated preterm birth, low birth weight
Eliminating alcohol use	Eliminating alcohol before and during pregnancy prevents foetal alcohol syndrome and other alcohol-related birth defects

Planning for insurance and maternity leave

Insurance

Does your insurance cover pregnancy and complications that might arise from it? If it does not, then make sure that you obtain proper insurance. Pregnancy and delivery can be expensive, particularly when an unexpected complication springs up. Make sure that you have your finances in order to handle a pregnancy and childbirth.

Maternity leave

It is a good idea to find out how much maternity leave is allowed by your employer. This will help plan for family support after the delivery.

CHAPTER 2

How pregnancy happens

Sadhana and Girish are excited about the pregnancy. Their baby! They can't believe that a life is growing inside her. How miraculous that their love has created a new being. They are curious about how their baby was conceived and how she is developing in the womb.

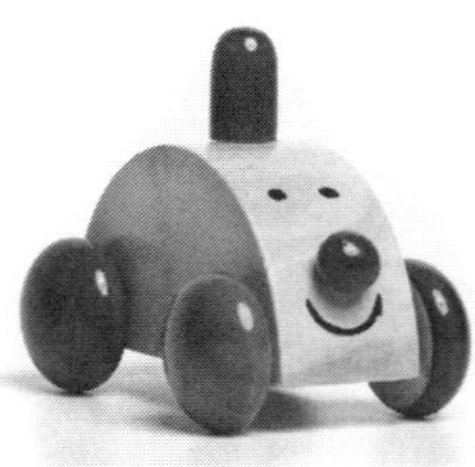

2

How pregnancy happens

Once a month, in most women, an egg is released from one of your ovaries. During intercourse, semen is deposited in the vagina. Though semen contains millions of sperms, only 200–400 of the sperms swim from the vagina into the cervix (mouth of the uterus). Through the cervix the sperms then enter the uterine cavity. The uterus has two small openings into which the Fallopian tubes connect. The sperms find their way through the openings into the Fallopian tubes. It is in the Fallopian tube that one sperm hits the lucky jackpot and gets to fertilize the egg!

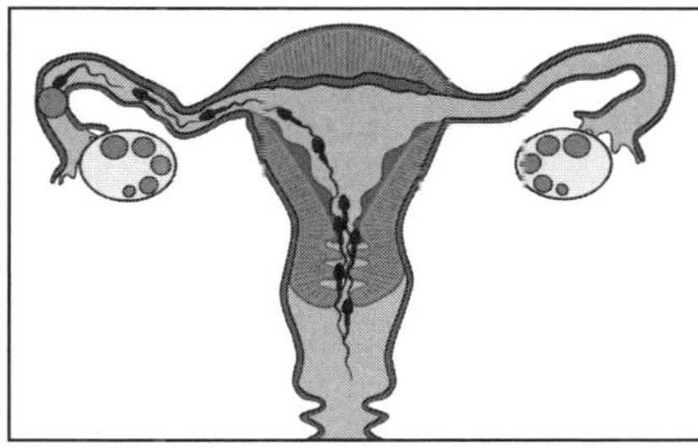

The path of the sperm from the vagina to the egg: though millions of sperm are deposited in the vagina, only a few hundred make the journey through the uterus and into the Fallopian tube. Only one sperm will fertilize the egg.

9 months or 10 months?

You grew up hearing that a human pregnancy lasts 9 months. That's what your mother and grandmother say. That's what the stories and songs say. But your doctor says it is 10 months or 40 weeks (280 days). Why this confusion?

Doctors and nurses count your pregnancy from the first day of your last period. So the counting starts even before your baby was conceived. A human pregnancy is considered full term at 280 days after the first day of your last period. 28 days = 4 weeks = 1 month. Therefore 280 days = 10 months!

You may have been used to counting pregnancy in months. However your doctor will talk about your pregnancy in weeks and as the pregnancy progresses, you will get used to it. Not only your obstetrician but also your ultrasound report will refer to your pregnancy in weeks. A normal pregnancy usually lasts 280 days or 40 weeks. 12 weeks is 3 months, 16 weeks is 4 months, 20 weeks is 5 months—you get the idea!

In the normal course of events, several sperms gain access to the ovum. However, as soon as one sperm penetrates and fertilizes the egg, enzymes are produced so that all the other sperms are immobilized.

The process of fertilization

The phenomenon of fertilization happens without any external sign. When the life force held within the sperm bonds with the life force enclosed within the egg, you will be quite unaware of it. Your little one started its life without your even knowing it!

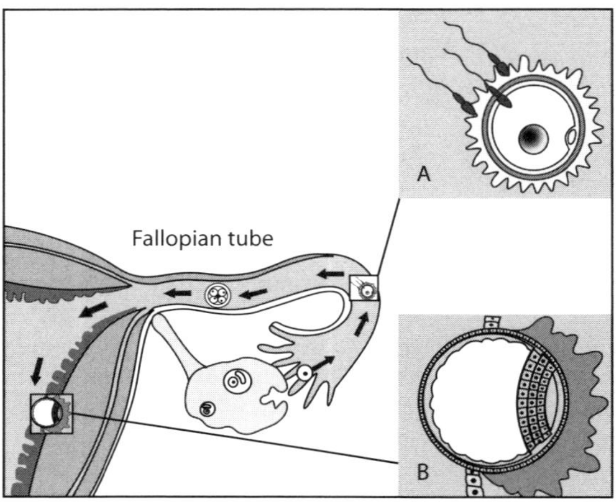

Fertilization of the egg happens in the Fallopian tube (A). It takes 3–5 days for the fertilized egg to reach the uterine cavity. About a week after fertilization, the baby starts burrowing into the uterine wall (B)

During the cycle that you conceived, an egg (ovum) was released from one of your ovaries, about 12–14 days before the next menstrual period. The process is called **ovulation**. Your Fallopian tubes have finger like projections (fimbriae) that picked up the egg and transported it into the funnel-shaped end of the tube.

Some women may have an indication that they are ovulating. There could be a slight ache in the lower part of the abdomen. A few women spot at the time of ovulation. The most common symptom that you might notice is an increase in the normal vaginal discharge. This happens because, at ovulation, the mucus in the cervix becomes thin and watery, helping the entry of sperm into the uterus.

What happens if fertilization does not occur?

If fertilization does not occur, the egg disintegrates and is passed out of the uterus with the next menstrual period.

Gina asked: We have been married for a year. We have now decided to go ahead with a pregnancy. Do we need to time intercourse to conceive? I have received all sorts of advice on the best days of the cycle to conceive.

My answer: Remember that countless women have conceived without timing their intercourse. And you have just started trying for a pregnancy. If you have regular periods, you need not worry about timing intercourse. If you have intercourse more frequently around the middle of the cycle, then your chances of conceiving are 80 per cent.

Many apps are available now that track your periods and the most fertile part of your monthly cycle. These apps may be useful when you are attempting a pregnancy. These apps are also useful for women with mildly irregular periods (35–45 day cycles). Since they also track your period, you may get a quick heads up when your period is delayed. This may prompt you to do a pregnancy test.

If you have very irregular periods (45–120 days apart), you may need to regularize your periods. Exercising, eating healthy and losing a little weight (if you need to) can help regulate your periods. Your doctor will help you with medications if needed. You might then be given instructions on how to time intercourse to coincide with ovulation.

What happened after fertilization?

Once fertilization occurred, the fertilized egg (**zygote**) divided repeatedly and went from being 2-celled to a 16-celled solid ball. It rolled along the Fallopian tube towards the uterus (propelled by tiny hair-like cilia lining the Fallopian tube). The zygote would have entered the uterus 3–5 days after fertilization.

In the uterus, the cells continued to divide, becoming a hollow ball of cells called a **blastocyst.**

Development of the blastocyst

Within a week of fertilization, the blastocyst burrowed into the lining of the uterus and started growing there. This is called *implantation*. The ball of cells (that will become the little one you will cuddle in a few months) snuggled into the uterine lining around the 20th to 24th day of your menstrual cycle. This is where it started its long journey of growth and development.

At this point, the blastocyst divides into two parts: the inner cells develop into the **embryo**, and the outer cells burrow into the wall of the uterus and develop into the **placenta.**

The wall of the blastocyst becomes the outer layer of membranes called *chorion*, surrounding the embryo. An inner layer of membranes (*amnion*) develops, forming the **amniotic sac**. The amniotic sac is filled with a clear fluid called **amniotic fluid** and expands to envelop the developing embryo, which floats within it.

How your uterus prepared for implantation

In preparation for receiving the fertilized egg, the uterine lining (*endometrium*) became thick and spongy because of the hormones being produced in the first half of the menstrual cycle. There is a small window of about four days when the lining of the uterus is receptive to the blastocyst and allows the blastocyst to adhere and burrow into the uterine lining.

If a pregnancy does not occur during that cycle, the thickened lining is shed as menstrual blood. If a pregnancy does occur, you miss your period.

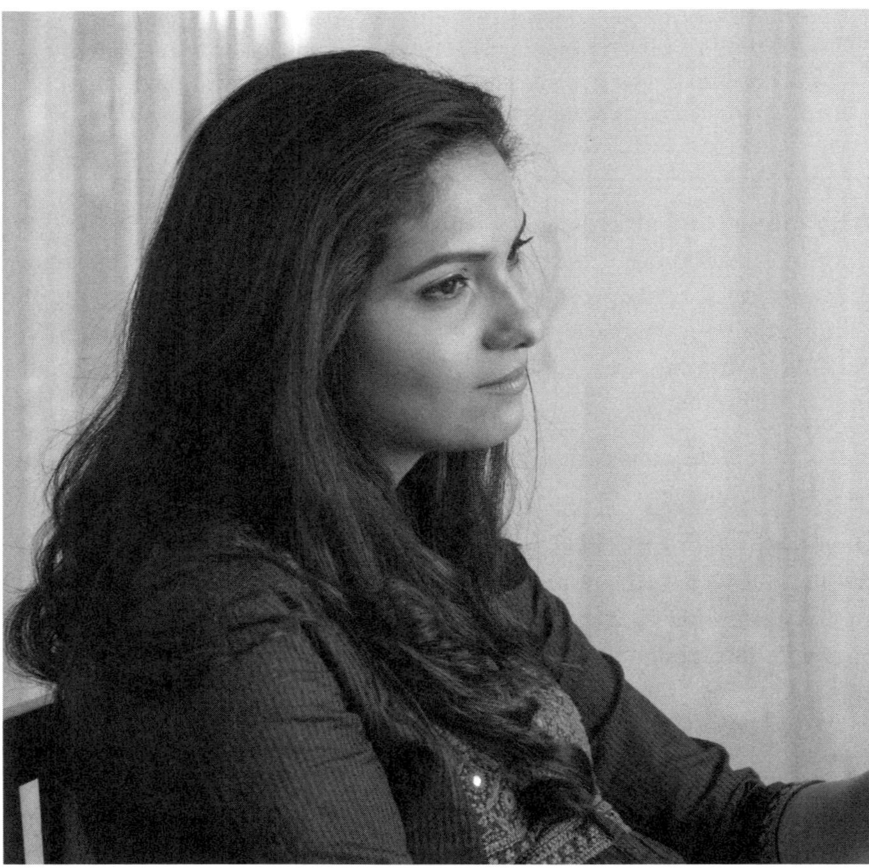

A timeline for conception in a woman with 28–30 day cycles

Day 1 of menstrual cycle	Your period started
Day 12–14 of cycle	You ovulated (released an egg)
Day 13–15 of cycle	**You have conceived!**
Day 17–20 of cycle	Your little one is a solid 16-celled ball (zygote) and has reached the uterus
Day 21–24 of cycle	Now she (or he!) is a little hollow ball of cells (blastocyst) and has started burrowing into the uterus. Implantation has occurred
Day 22–28 of cycle	The placenta has formed. You and your baby have now truly connected!

Development of the placenta

The placenta is an amazing organ. It develops just for this one pregnancy and is the vital link between you and your baby: it nurtures your baby by transferring nutrients and oxygen from your blood stream into the baby's umbilical cord. It also removes the waste products from the baby.

As the placenta develops, it extends tiny finger-like projections (*villi*) into the wall of the uterus. The projections branch and re-branch in a complicated tree-like arrangement. This arrangement greatly increases the area of contact between the wall of the uterus and the placenta. The villi are constantly in contact with the mother's blood so that nutrients and waste materials can be exchanged. As the baby grows, the placenta also grows. At delivery, the placenta weighs about 500 grams.

One of the important functions of the placenta is the production of several hormones that help maintain the pregnancy. This includes large quantities of estrogen and progesterone.

Why are estrogen and progesterone important for your pregnancy?

These two hormones are essential for the pregnancy to continue normally.

Estrogen

- Increases the quantity of blood flowing through your uterus. This makes sure that your baby is getting all the nutrition it requires
- Gets your breasts ready to produce milk once the baby is born
- Is essential for starting the process of labour

Progesterone

- Maintains the pregnancy in the uterus
- Keeps the uterus quiescent and prevents contractions till it is time for labour to start

The placenta also produces **human chorionic gonadotropin** (hCG), the quintessential pregnancy hormone. Once pregnancy occurs, hCG prevents the ovaries from releasing more eggs. It also stimulates the ovaries to produce the hormones, estrogen and progesterone continuously.

Human chorionic gonadotropin (hCG) for confirming pregnancy

Human chorionic gonadotropin (hCG) is known as the pregnancy hormone. Since hCG can only be present in your body during pregnancy, this placental hormone is used for the pregnancy test. The presence of hCG in urine or blood confirms that you are pregnant. It can be detected as early as 8–10 days after fertilization (see **Chapter 3**, *Am I pregnant?*).

Boy or girl?

Your egg carries a single X chromosome (your egg has no say in the matter when it comes to having a boy or a girl!). Your partner produces sperm that could carry either a single X chromosome or a single Y chromosome. If your egg is fertilized by an X sperm, you will have a girl. If the egg is fertilized by a Y sperm, you will have a boy.

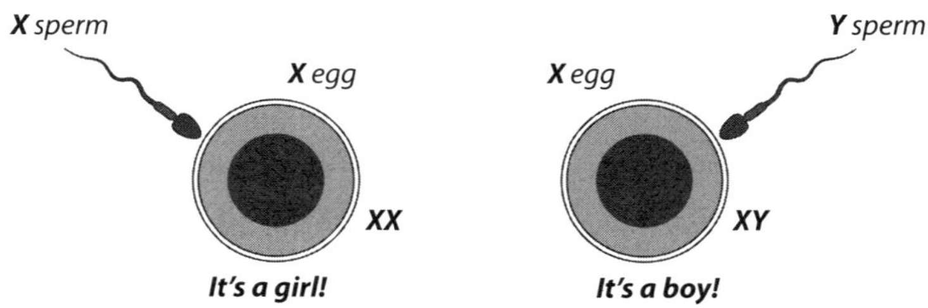

The week-by-week development of the baby is described in detail in **Chapters 6, 7** and **8**. Enjoy reading, and following your baby as she grows and becomes your little bundle of joy!

Your baby from 6 to 12 weeks

By the end of 6 weeks	• All major systems and organs begin to form • The embryo looks like a tadpole • The neural tube (which becomes the brain and spinal cord), the digestive system, the heart and circulatory system begin to form • The beginnings of the eyes and ears are developing • Tiny limb buds appear (which will develop into arms and legs) • The heart starts beating
By the end of 8 weeks	• All major body systems continue to develop and function, including the circulatory, nervous, digestive and urinary systems • The embryo takes on a human shape, although the head is larger in proportion to the rest of the body • The mouth develops tooth buds (which will become baby teeth) • The eyes, nose, mouth and ears become more distinct • The arms and legs are clearly visible • The fingers and toes are still webbed but can be clearly distinguished • The main organs continue to develop • The bones begin to develop and the nose and jaws rapidly develop • The embryo is in constant motion but these movements cannot be felt by you
From embryo to foetus	After 10 weeks, the embryo is now referred to as a foetus Although the foetus is only 2.5–3.5 cm long at this point, all major organs and systems have been formed
During weeks 10–12	• The external genital organs are developing • Fingernails and toenails appear • Eyelids are forming • Foetal movement increases • The arms and legs are fully formed • The voice box (larynx) begins to form in the trachea

CHAPTER 3

Am I pregnant?

Stella is excited and overjoyed. She and her husband have been trying for a pregnancy for the past few months. She has just missed her period. Is she really pregnant?

Samhita has irregular periods. She feels tired and is plagued with nausea. Just yesterday, she almost threw up at the smell of fried potatoes, one of her favourite foods. Could she be pregnant?

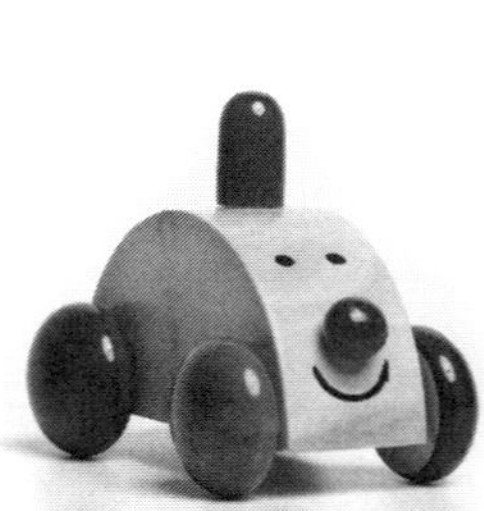

3

Am I pregnant?

One of the most commonly asked questions by women is, 'Am I pregnant?' Even if they have never been pregnant before, most women have heard of the symptoms of early pregnancy. Whenever a woman in the reproductive age group misses a period, pregnancy is the first thought that jumps to mind. The chances of pregnancy increase as the days past the missed period increase.

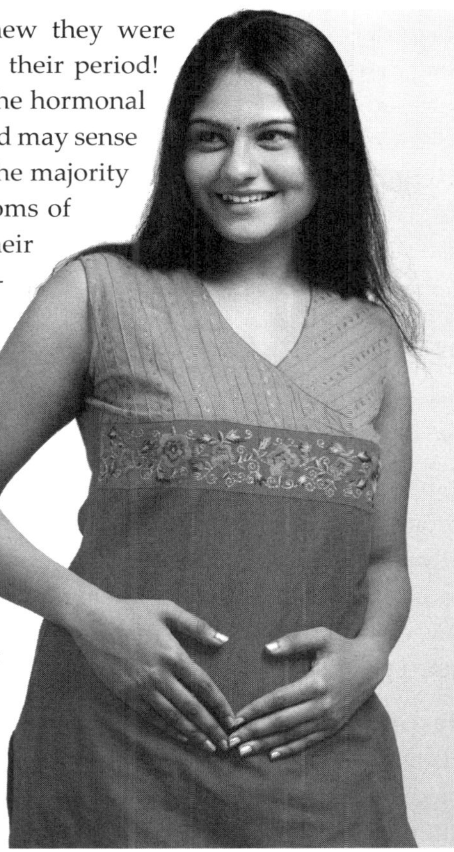

Some women claim that they knew they were pregnant even before they missed their period! They are particularly sensitive to the hormonal changes that occur in pregnancy and may sense that they are pregnant. However, the majority of women start having the symptoms of pregnancy only after they miss their period. One of the earliest symptoms is extreme sleepiness and exhaustion. This can also be accompanied by heavy and sore breasts. The intolerance of the sight and smell of food soon follows. These symptoms are discussed in more detail in **Chapter 4**, *What pregnancy feels like.*

Women who have been pregnant before will recognize the symptoms that occurred in their previous pregnancy. Surprisingly though, some women may have severe symptoms during one pregnancy and hardly any in the next. The fact is that each pregnancy is different and a woman may not have the same symptoms or the same intensity of symptoms during each of her pregnancies.

> Some women may have severe symptoms in one pregnancy and hardly any in the next.

When to suspect a pregnancy

Missing a period

This is one of the most common reasons for suspecting a pregnancy. Women who have regular periods will take this as the first sign of pregnancy. Only a urine or blood pregnancy test, followed by a pelvic exam, can confirm a pregnancy. Occasionally a period can be delayed due to hormonal problems, even in the absence of pregnancy. If you are trying for a pregnancy, keep track of your periods. Mark the first day of your period on a calendar, as that is what determines the due date of the pregnancy.

Why is a period missed?

Every month, signals from the brain cause the hormone estrogen to be released from the ovary. **Estrogen** acts on the lining of the uterus (endometrium). The endometrium responds by getting thicker and spongier in anticipation of a pregnancy. The uterus literally 'lines the nest' to receive the baby. Most women produce an egg around the middle of the cycle, usually between the 11th and 16th day (see **Chapter 1**, *How pregnancy happens*). Following this, the ovary produces the hormone **progesterone**. When the egg does not get fertilized in that cycle, the level of progesterone drops and the lining of the uterus is shed, leading to menstruation. In fact, the menstrual period has been described as 'the bloody tears of a disappointed uterus'!

When fertilization occurs, the levels of progesterone and estrogen rise dramatically and the lining of the uterus continues to get thicker to receive the embryo. In this case, the period is missed. The ovary stops producing further eggs for the duration of the pregnancy.

> The first day of the last period is used to calculate the due date of delivery.

Testing for pregnancy

Human chorionic gonadotrophin (hCG) is a hormone secreted by the placenta during pregnancy. It can be detected both in the urine and blood soon after fertilization. Detection of hCG forms the basis for pregnancy tests.

Urine pregnancy tests

Testing the urine is the commonest method for diagnosing pregnancy in a lab and also is the preferred method for home pregnancy testing. These tests measure the levels of hCG in your urine. The amount of hormone each test can detect varies widely. The home pregnancy kits commonly available in the market will measure as low as 25–50 mIU/ ml of hCG, which can be found in urine between the 4th and 5th weeks of pregnancy.

First morning urine will always contain the highest concentration of hCG. However, most tests do not require that you use first morning urine. Wait four hours after you last urinated to take the test. This will allow hCG to build up in your urine.

These tests are usually accurate but sometimes a false result can be obtained. A negative test that then turns out to be a pregnancy is usually the result of the test being performed too early. A false-positive test is a test where the test comes out positive even when you are not pregnant. Talk to your doctor if you have questions about your pregnancy tests.

Home pregnancy tests

> A home pregnancy test is most accurate 6 weeks after the last period.

For the past several years, it has become convenient for women to perform a home pregnancy test to confirm or rule out a pregnancy. Pregnancy kits usually will indicate pregnancy with coloured lines or dots. If there is no change in colour, or only a very faint change in colour, then the pregnancy test is negative. If the dot or line changes colour, it indicates a positive pregnancy test.

When should you perform the home pregnancy test?

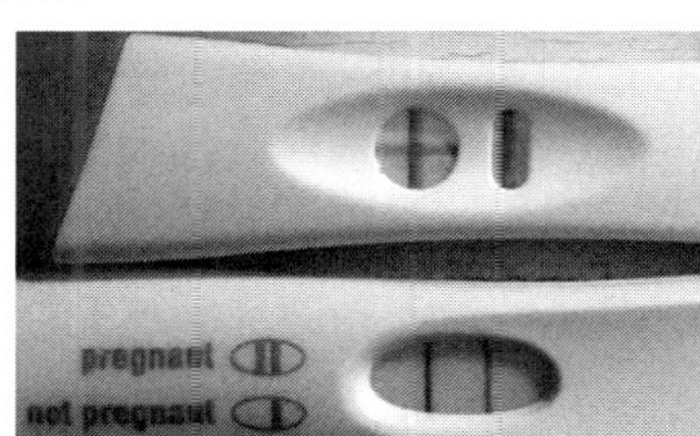

In your hurry to check and see if you are pregnant, you may be tempted to do the pregnancy test within a day or two of missing your period. However, a pregnancy test done so soon may come back negative even though you actually are pregnant. This is because the level of the pregnancy hormone in the urine may not be high enough to show up on the home pregnancy kit. To be absolutely sure, you should perform the test at least a week after your missed period. For example, if you were expecting your period on the 1st of February, you may still get a negative result if you do the test on the 3rd or 4th of February. However, if you do the test between the 8th and 10th of February, the chances of getting a positive test are much higher, if you are pregnant.

For women with irregular periods

If you have irregular periods, when should you suspect a pregnancy and when should you do a home pregnancy test? Wait till your period is delayed more than your longest cycle. For example, if you get your periods every 45–50 days, wait till 60 days and do the test. Of course, you can do the test earlier if you are having definite symptoms of pregnancy. If your test says you are not pregnant, but you still think you may be pregnant, wait a few more days and take another pregnancy test.

Were you on birth control pills? You may have a few irregular cycles after you go off the pills. It may take 3–4 months for you to get back to your regular cycles. You should do a pregnancy test if your period is delayed for more than 45 days after stopping the pills.

How should you do the home pregnancy test?

You can directly pass urine on the pregnancy stick or you can collect urine in a small, clean container and dip the stick into the urine. Wait for the time specified on the kit and then check the lines or dots that are supposed to appear. If the line or dot is very faint, repeat the test after 4–5 days. If it is still faint, then check with your doctor whether you really are pregnant or not.

Rani asked: I missed my period last month. When I did my home pregnancy test, the line on it was very faint. I felt very sleepy, had painful breasts and mild nausea. One week later I got my normal period and all my symptoms disappeared. Was I pregnant? Did I have a miscarriage?

My answer: If you are used to having regular periods, the home pregnancy test usually turns positive within 1 week after your missed period. Having symptoms of pregnancy with a pregnancy test that is not definitely positive and then having a normal period is suggestive of a 'chemical pregnancy'. This just means that there may have been a slight elevation in the pregnancy hormone without an actual established pregnancy. This does not count as a miscarriage.

The one other complication that you must keep in mind is an *ectopic pregnancy*. This is a pregnancy that does not happen inside the uterus but commonly occurs in the Fallopian tube (tubal pregnancy). In such cases, the urine pregnancy test may be faintly positive. In such a situation, if you also develop severe pain in the lower part of the abdomen, you should see your obstetrician immediately to rule out a tubal pregnancy.

Blood pregnancy tests

A blood pregnancy test is the most sensitive method of confirming a pregnancy. It is not done routinely. In women who have irregular periods or in women undergoing fertility treatment, your doctor might ask for a blood test to confirm the pregnancy. Occasionally it may be done to determine if the pregnancy is growing normally. A blood test for hCG levels is also very useful in the diagnosis and management of a tubal pregnancy (where the pregnancy is growing abnormally in the Fallopian tube instead of the uterus).

In early pregnancy, if all is well with the pregnancy, the level of hCG in the blood will double every 2 days. The level in the blood peaks between 60–80 days of pregnancy. The levels of hCG in your urine and blood will be different.

The amount of hormone each pregnant woman produces may vary but usually falls within a certain range. The level of hCG in the blood is maximum in the 3rd month and then gradually decreases. It reaches the lowest level on the completion of the 4th month and is maintained at that same level for the rest of the pregnancy.

Levels of hCG in the blood

Weeks from last menstrual period	(mIU/ml)
5th week (1 week after missed period)	200–7000
6th week	200–32,000
7th week	3000–160,000
8–12 weeks	32,000–210,000
13–16 weeks	9000–210,000
16–29 weeks (second trimester)	1,400–51,000
29–41 weeks (third trimester)	940–60,000
4–6 weeks after delivery	nonpregnant levels (<5)

Calculating the estimated date of delivery (EDD)

A normal pregnancy usually lasts 280 days (40 weeks). 37–40 weeks of pregnancy is called a 'term' or 'full-term' pregnancy.

The due date is based on the assumption that the conception occurred exactly 2 weeks after the first day of the last period. This is the time ovulation occurs in women with regular periods. Obviously, this calculation only applies to women who have 28–30 day cycles! The method used by

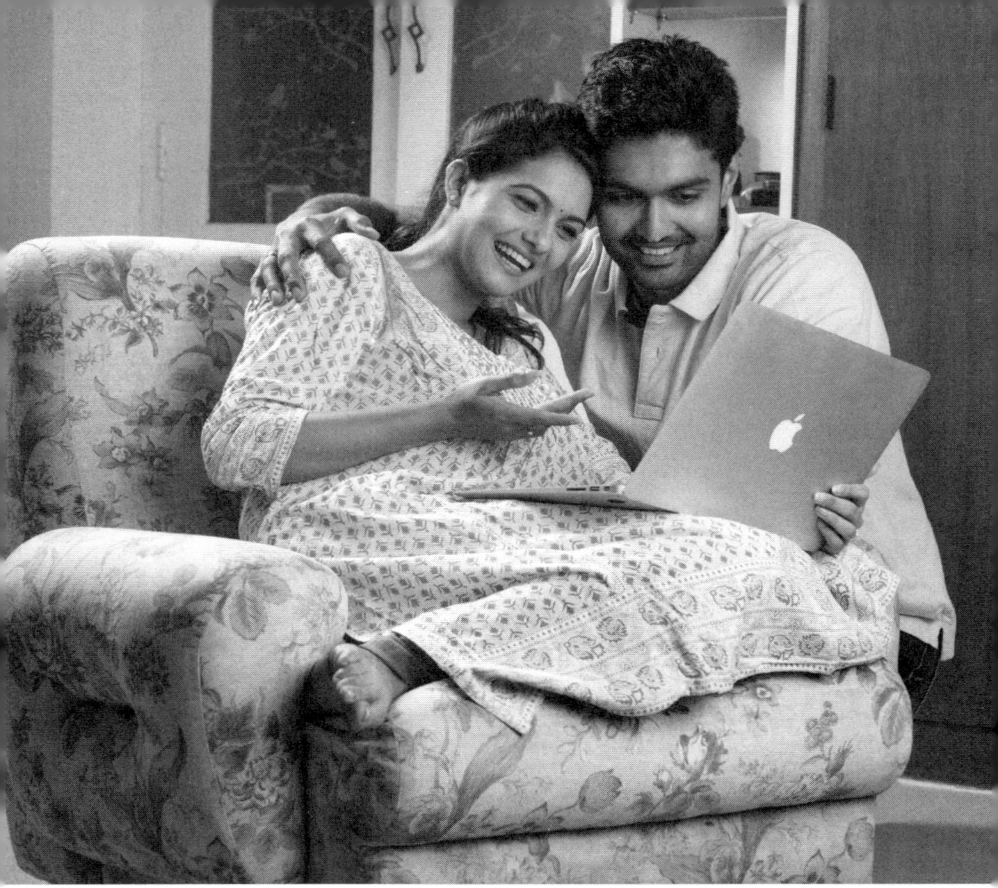

obstetricians around the world is to add 7 days and subtract 3 months from the date of the first day of the last menstrual period.

> **Formula for calculating due date: 1st day of last period + 7 days minus 3 months**
>
> Example: 1st day of last period: June 1, 2017
>
> June 1 + 7 days = June 8
>
> June 8 – 3 months = March 8
>
> Therefore, your due date is March 8, 2018

What about women with irregular periods?

If your periods are irregular, it usually means that you do not ovulate regularly. This means that it might be difficult to calculate when you actually conceived. In such a case, an ultrasound scan may be used to calculate the due date. With the scan it is easy to determine the age of the foetus in weeks and the doctor will then give you an EDD based on that (see **Chapter 13**, *Ultrasound scans in pregnancy*).

Will I deliver on my due date?

Did you know that only 5 per cent of women deliver exactly on their calculated due date? Most will deliver just before or after the EDD. Remember that it is called *estimated* date of delivery (EDD), not exact date of delivery! So you and your husband definitely need not get hung up on that date. It is just an indication about your expected time of delivery. In case of a pregnancy complication, your doctor uses that date to determine the exact age of your baby and whether it is safe for the baby to be delivered.

The importance of knowing the EDD

Knowing the EDD is very important for you and your doctor. EDD determines which week of pregnancy you are in and helps in

- Deciding the timing of investigations, since many tests are done at specific weeks of pregnancy. For example, first trimester screening for Down syndrome is done between 11–14 weeks of pregnancy
- Calculating whether you are preterm or postterm
- Timing of interventions
- Monitoring the growth of your little one

Using technology to track periods and fertility

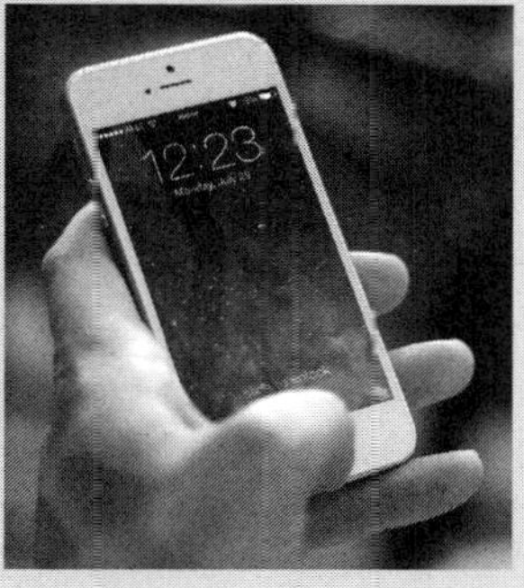

Many apps are available now that track your periods and the most fertile part of your monthly cycle. These apps may be useful when you are attempting a pregnancy. Since they also track your period, you may get a quick heads up when your period is delayed. This may prompt you to do a pregnancy test.

A word of caution: Though these apps also tell you the time of the cycle when your chances of pregnancy are low, do NOT depend on that to avoid a pregnancy. The chance of pregnancy may be low but is definitely not impossible. If you are absolutely sure you do not want a pregnancy, use birth control; do not depend on the app to prevent a pregnancy.

CHAPTER 4

What pregnancy feels like

Sarita has been trying for months to get pregnant and her pregnancy test has just come back positive. But guess what? She feels let down. She knows she should be super excited but she only feels exhausted and miserable. She wakes up in the morning with a headache, her breasts are painful and she doesn't even want to look at food.
Isn't pregnancy supposed to be a happy and joyful event? Why does she feel like this?

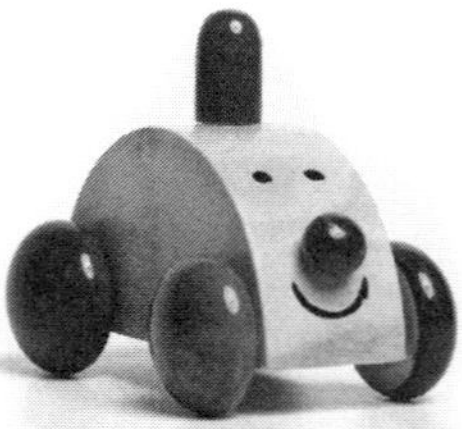

4

What pregnancy feels like

Pregnancy is quite a challenge for your body. Within a short time, your blood stream is inundated with vast quantities of hormones that bring about drastic transformations. Each trimester is associated with its own set of changes. You may not experience each and every symptom. The intensity of symptoms also differs from woman to woman and from pregnancy to pregnancy.

Missing a period is the first and most fundamental symptom of a pregnancy (see **Chapter 3**, *Am I pregnant?*).

> Do you have a friend, or a sister-in- law, or a colleague who sailed through pregnancy without any problem and without suffering from all the symptoms that you are feeling? Do you feel envious and want to know how they did it? Or are you one of those who have felt totally comfortable through most of your pregnancy? Just remember, that's fine too. Some women just get lucky and may not have all the symptoms listed here.

Swollen, tender, or sore breasts and/ or nipples

This is one of the earliest symptoms of pregnancy. The breasts and/or nipples are often particularly painful during a first pregnancy. Some women may start experiencing this around the time of the missed period.

After the second month, the breasts start increasing in size and delicate veins may become visible just beneath the skin. The nipples can become considerably larger, darker and can be very sore. Usually this discomfort disappears in a few weeks. In the third trimester, the areola (the dark area around the nipple) will become broader and much darker. There are several tiny glands called sebaceous glands scattered throughout the areola. These become more prominent as pregnancy progresses and form tiny bumps on the areola.

Close to delivery, some women may start having a watery or milky discharge from the nipples. This is nothing to be alarmed about. It is just the breast preparing itself to feed the little one when the time comes.

Why are the breasts tender and sore?

The reason breasts and/ or nipples are often tender, swollen or sore during early pregnancy is because of the response to the pregnancy hormone, hCG. There is also an increased production of estrogen and progesterone. The breasts undergo changes to prepare for breastfeeding. The milk-producing glands within the breasts respond to the hormones and start enlarging. After a few weeks, the immediate response to the hormones settles down and the breasts feel less painful.

> As the breasts enlarge in response to the hormonal changes and in preparation for lactation, you might find that your bra size changes. You may go up one size. Make sure to get bras that are well fitting and give you good support.

Exhaustion or unusual tiredness

It is normal for a woman to feel extremely fatigued during the first 2–3 months of pregnancy. There is an intense desire to sleep, and waking up seems to be a difficult proposition. This can become difficult and frustrating, especially for working women or for women who have to take care of another child. You will just not be able to find any energy to do your normal chores. It is not unusual to wake up groggy, lethargic and exhausted even after a good night's sleep.

Be kind to yourself

It is important to rest whenever possible. Learn to listen to your body and allow some periods of rest during the day. Don't overwhelm yourself with too many chores. Have family and friends help out by sending you food. Too tired to cook? Order out. Try to have early nights and get your full quota of sleep. Your husband can take your older child (or children) out for a few hours, so you have some respite and peace.

Relax! These symptoms only last for the first 2–3 months of pregnancy. Once your body gets used to the tremendous metabolic changes caused by hormones, these symptoms will subside. Soon you will feel energetic and after completing the fourth month, some women actually say they 'don't feel pregnant anymore!'

Why do you feel tired and exhausted?

These symptoms are caused by the hormone progesterone, which is produced in large amounts. This hormone can make a woman feel tired and intensely sleepy. In some cases, the tiredness may be compounded by the stress of daily chores. If a woman has to go to work, she might also have to cook in the morning. If this is not your first pregnancy, you may feel constantly exhausted because your other child/children also need your attention.

> A husband who pitches in and allows his wife to sleep in a little longer, is worth his weight in gold!

Dizziness and feeling faint

Dizziness or feeling faint is such a common symptom in pregnancy. Though it can be worse during the first trimester, it can hit you anytime in pregnancy. Most often it happens when you are standing for a long time. It can also happen when you get up suddenly from a sitting or lying position.

What causes dizziness during pregnancy?

The hormone progesterone is again the culprit. It causes the blood vessels to relax and increases the blood flow to the baby (which is a good thing). However, this also results in pooling of blood in your legs. When this happens, the blood pressure drops a little, especially if you have been standing for a long time. The blood flow to your brain temporarily decreases, causing dizziness.

> **Ridhima asked:** I am doing my postgraduate training in surgery. I am two months pregnant and find it very difficult standing in the operation theatre for a long time. In fact I fainted one day. How do I prevent dizziness and fainting?
>
> **My answer:** If possible, scrub on short cases. If you have to scrub on a long case, keep moving your feet and calf muscles so that the circulation in your legs is good. This will prevent pooling of blood in your legs. This advice is for anyone who has to stand for a long period of time at work or at home.
>
> Make sure you hydrate yourself well. Eat frequent small meals so that your sugar levels don't drop. Get up slowly from either sitting or lying down so that your blood pressure doesn't fall from the change in posture.
>
> Anytime you feel like you are going to faint, sit down and put your head between your knees. Take slow deep breaths and try to get some fresh air. If you are at home when this happens, it is best to lie down for a few minutes with your feet raised on a pillow or cushion.

Low blood sugar levels are the result of metabolic changes in early pregnancy and can lead to dizziness.

Lying on your back in the last three or four months of pregnancy may cause sudden dizziness, because the weight of the uterus and baby press on the vena cava that carries blood to your brain. This cutting off of blood supply to your brain can cause dizziness and is called *supine hypotension*.

Nausea and vomiting

Ask anyone what is the commonest symptom of pregnancy and they will immediately say: vomiting! Nausea, with or without vomiting, is most common in the first three months of pregnancy. Unfortunately, some women experience this symptom almost throughout their pregnancy. Most women become oversensitive to smells and almost anything can trigger nausea and vomiting.

Did you know that women who have nausea and vomiting have a less chance of miscarriage?

Common triggers for nausea and vomiting:

- Coffee
- Milk products
- Spicy and strong smelling foods
- Non-vegetarian dishes
- Brushing teeth
- Iron supplements

Is it really *morning sickness?* It should really be called 'anytime sickness' because in 80 per cent of women, the nausea lasts throughout the day. Typically, the nausea starts around six weeks of the pregnancy (or about two weeks after the missed period). Some women start experiencing nausea just a few days after missing the period. The symptoms may continue until about 12–14 weeks of the pregnancy. However, morning sickness may start later than six weeks and may continue until 16–20 weeks of the pregnancy. About 90 per cent of women will have relief by 20 weeks (the 5th month).

Uma asked: My grandmother says I should not take tablets prescribed for vomiting because it may affect the baby. Is that true?

My answer: If the nausea and vomiting are causing distress, we prescribe medications that will control the vomiting. In fact taking these tablets will prevent the problem escalating to hyperemesis that may lead to hospitalization. The commonly used drugs are doxylamine and meclizine. They may cause sleepiness and dry mouth. These are absolutely safe in pregnancy and can be used without any fear. Vitamin B6 (pyridoxine) is also sometimes prescribed to control nausea.

Occasionally, some women may find a recurrence of the nausea in the last one or two months of pregnancy. This is usually due to increased acidity and the pressure of the growing baby on the stomach. Morning sickness may make you feel constantly nauseous, or occur as bouts of nausea at different times of the day. As for the vomiting, some women may vomit almost continuously, whereas some may vomit without warning, usually in response to a particular smell.

Increased salivation can occur by itself but it is usually associated with nausea and vomiting in early pregnancy. Some women also complain of bitter or metallic tasting saliva.

Most women will suffer partial or complete suppression of appetite because of the nausea, and will not gain weight initially and may even lose weight. This is quite normal, though you and your husband might feel anxious that the baby is not getting enough nutrition. Actually, the foetus is not at all affected by your lack of appetite and poor intake of food. The pregnancy will only be affected if you have intractable vomiting and lose 4–5 kilos, which can happen with *hyperemesis gravidarum.*

What is hyperemesis gravidarum?

When the vomiting becomes uncontrollable, a woman might get dehydrated and require hospitalization. This intractable vomiting is called hyperemesis gravidarum. There can be excessive loss of weight associated with hyperemesis gravidarum.

What causes nausea and vomiting?

The most common reason for this symptom is the rapid rise in *estrogen* and *human chorionic gonadotrophin* (hCG), produced in large quantities in pregnancy. Since women carrying twins or triplets produce higher levels of these hormones, they can experience more severe morning sickness.

Ginger containing foods like ginger tea, ginger rasam and ginger candy have been shown in scientific studies to help in mild nausea and vomiting.

The nausea and vomiting can be aggravated by the increased acidity and low blood sugar that results from poor intake of food. Eating small quantities of food at frequent intervals can improve the symptoms. Dry, bland, non-oily food is better than spicy, oily food. Salt biscuits, dry toast and bland food like idlis will be better tolerated.

Persistent emotional stress can often be accompanied by nausea and vomiting. This can make the situation even more difficult to deal with. The nausea may continue until after the pregnancy progresses beyond a certain point in time, or even until your baby is born. Sharing your fears with people you trust or seeking professional advice may be helpful.

Lower abdominal discomfort and cramping

Lower abdominal discomfort and cramping, similar to cramping during periods, occurs during early pregnancy. This happens because the uterus starts expanding as the baby grows. This discomfort can continue for the first few months and can get worse on getting up after sitting down for a while, or on turning from side to side while lying down. You may worry that this may indicate that there is something wrong, but this pain is normal and does not need you to be at bed rest. If the pain occurs or worsens on walking briskly for a while, just rest for a few minutes and then continue walking.

> In early pregnancy, mild lower abdominal discomfort is common and does not signal an impending miscarriage. You need to see your doctor if the pain is unbearable or is accompanied by bleeding.

Later on in pregnancy, some women experience pain on one or both sides of the lower abdomen. This is because of the stretching of the *round ligaments* that hold the uterus in position. Lying on the side of the pain relieves the stretching of the round ligament and therefore, will offer respite from the pain.

Frequent urination

In early pregnancy, there will be a frequent urge to pass urine. The bladder seems to fill up in no time at all and you may find yourself running to the bathroom very frequently. This usually eases off around 16 weeks but don't be surprised if this feeling recurs in the last few weeks of pregnancy.

What causes frequent urination?

The growing uterus pressing against the bladder causes this problem. This symptom is worse in early and late pregnancy. Sometimes, you may lose a few drops of urine on sneezing or coughing. This will usually disappear a few months after delivery.

Headaches

Headaches can be quite a problem during pregnancy. They are often intense and occur usually in the early months of pregnancy. Though some of these

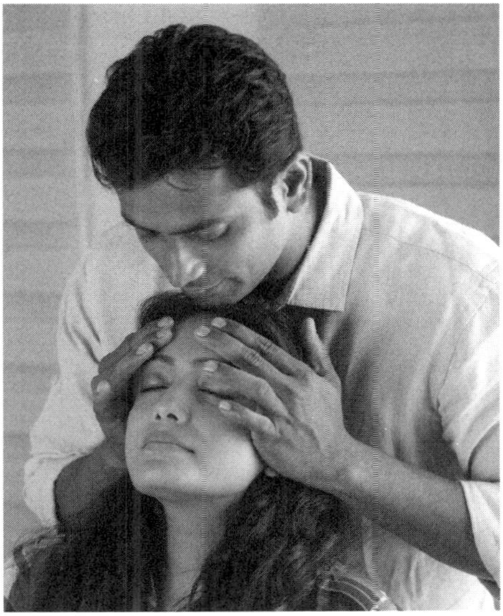

headaches can be caused by eye strain or sinusitis, the vast majority have no known cause. Paracetamol can be taken for the headaches and will not harm the baby. Women who suffer from migraine may find the condition aggravated in pregnancy because of the rise in the levels of estrogen.

Other symptoms

Mood swings are common in early pregnancy. Due to the sudden and huge increase of pregnancy hormones, women will face emotional ups and downs. It is common for a pregnant woman to burst into tears or get angry and upset for no apparent reason. This may leave her husband and family bewildered and a little concerned, but this phase is usually short-lived. Once the body gets used to the surge of hormones, the emotional roller-coaster ride ends and stability usually returns. Husbands and partners, do read how to deal with this in **Chapter 9**. *The role of the father-to-be.*

> **Stretch marks**
>
> **Padma asked:** Is there any way I can prevent stretch marks?
>
> **My answer:** Stretch marks occur when the growing uterus stretches the skin over the abdomen. Some women may also get stretch marks over the thighs. There are no specific ways of preventing these marks. Do not waste money on creams and lotions that falsely promise to prevent stretch marks. Just apply moisturizer daily to the skin—this will keep the skin supple and reduce the chances of getting these marks.

Feeling feverish and cold in the first few weeks of the pregnancy may have you reaching for the thermometer. However, your temperature will be normal. This symptom will usually subside by the fourth month.

Constipation is a result of poor intake of food and fluids in the early weeks. Many women find that they cannot tolerate fluids, even water, due to the nausea. Even if you had normal bowel habits before pregnancy, you might find yourself having hard stools. This can lead to pain while passing stools and even bleeding. Increasing the intake of fluids and a reasonable amount of exercise will resolve the problem. If the nausea does not allow the increase in fluids, your obstetrician might prescribe a mild laxative. Later on, the intake of iron supplements can also aggravate constipation. Make sure you take enough fluids, fresh fruits and raw vegetables (as in salads) to relieve this problem.

Haemorrhoids (or piles) are swollen veins of the rectum that can cause discomfort, itching and pain. They most often appear during the third trimester. Constipation, combined with increased pressure on the rectum by the growing uterus, is the main cause for these. They will usually disappear after the baby is born.

Increased vaginal discharge results from increased mucus discharge from the cervix. It can be uncomfortable but is a normal and common symptom in early pregnancy. You need treatment only if the increased vaginal discharge is associated with itching or burning. When those symptoms are present, then you might have a vaginal infection. This will require treatment with antibiotics and local applications (see **Chapter 42**, *Vaginal discharge and itching*).

Low back pain

The majority of women will face back problems at some time or another during pregnancy.

Back pain may start even in early pregnancy but mostly gets aggravated as the baby grows and your uterus becomes larger.

Hormones released during pregnancy **loosen up the ligaments** in your low back and in the groin area. This affects the support for your back and can result in back pain. Your **centre of gravity also shifts** due to the change in your posture because of the enlarging uterus. This puts a lot of stress on your low back. If your daily routine involves **long periods of standing**, there can be more pressure on your low back.

Things to avoid

- Don't bend over to pick up something from the floor. Instead, squat down to pick it up
- Don't wear high heels. Flat slippers also are not comfortable. Short platform heels (1 inch or 2.5 cm) provide support and are more comfortable

Pain medication like paracetamol (and massages from your husband!) can certainly relieve some of the pain.

Two simple exercises can relieve low back pain.

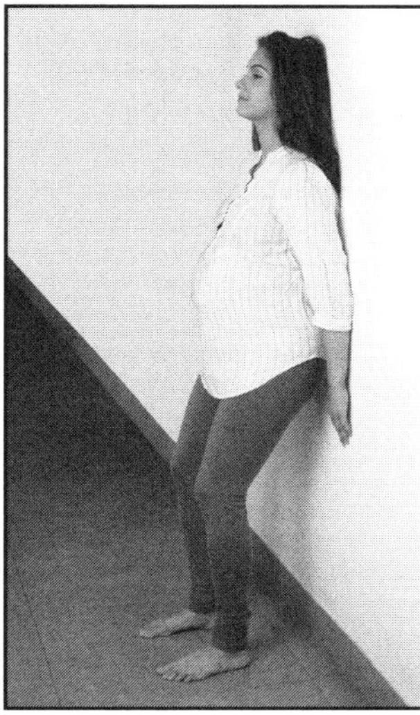

Left: *Stand up straight with your back against a wall, your feet about shoulder-width apart. Then push the small of your back against the wall. Hold for several seconds, and then return to the starting position. Gradually work up to 10 repetitions.*

Below: *Rest comfortably on a soft mat with a small pillow under the head. Place your feet on the chair with the knees well supported. This helps straighten your lower back.*

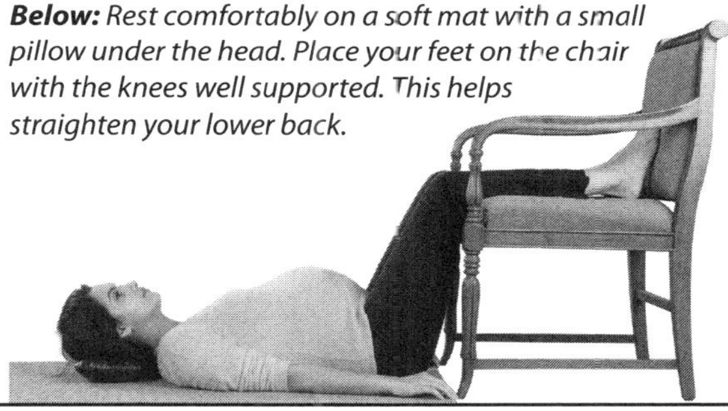

Old wives' tales

- If the foetus has a lot of hair, you will have increased vomiting—**not true!**
- If you don't eat well in the first three months of pregnancy, the baby will not grow—**false!**
- You should be under complete bed rest in the first three months of pregnancy—**not true!**
- You should not climb stairs in the first three months of pregnancy—**false!**
- You should not eat papayas, mangoes or pineapples because they may cause a miscarriage—**false!**

CHAPTER 5

A visit to your obstetrician

Sabeeha is excited. She suspects she is pregnant. She and her husband have fixed an appointment with an obstetrician. She has doubts and questions that she hopes her obstetrician will clear. She has also received advice (mostly unasked for!) from friends and relatives. She hopes her obstetrician is sympathetic and kind, and will allay her fears.

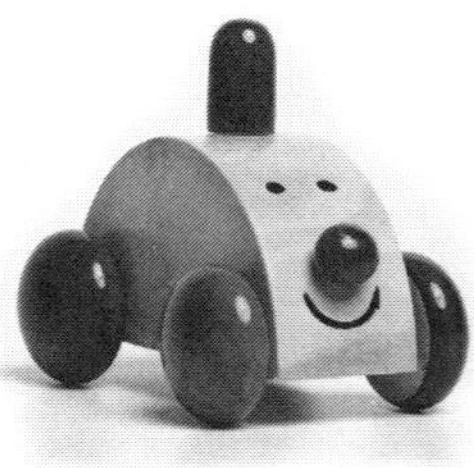

5

A visit to your obstetrician

Choosing the right obstetrician is a very important step towards ensuring the best for you and your unborn baby. Check with your family and friends. Go on online forums. Does the doctor have a sympathetic attitude towards you and your concerns? It is understandable that the busy doctor might have a short period of time to spend with you but does she engage with you during that time? The most important reason to choose a doctor is the comfort level you have with entrusting your health and your little one's health in her hands.

Choosing the hospital is also very important. Are you particular about having a painless delivery? Then check if the hospital provides epidural analgesia. Do you want your husband in the labour room with you? Check the hospital's policy on this.

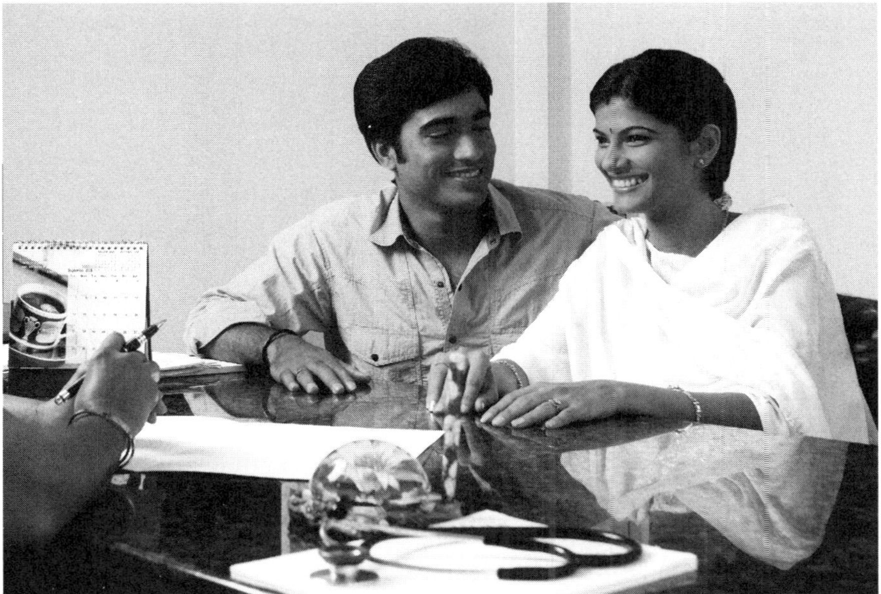

The best way to ensure that you will have a normal vaginal delivery is to ask for the caesarean section rates for the hospital or obstetrician you are consulting. It is important to know that caesarean section rates may vary from hospital to hospital. On an average, an overall rate of 25 per cent is acceptable.

Making the best use of your visit to the obstetrician

- Write down any information you think is important for the obstetrician to know
- Take along your records from a previous pregnancy, if you have had one
- Don't forget to take your medical records if you have had any medical problem or surgery in the past
- Take along any medicines that you are on so that the doctor can tell you if it is safe for you to continue them
- Jot down any questions and doubts you have so that you can have them cleared

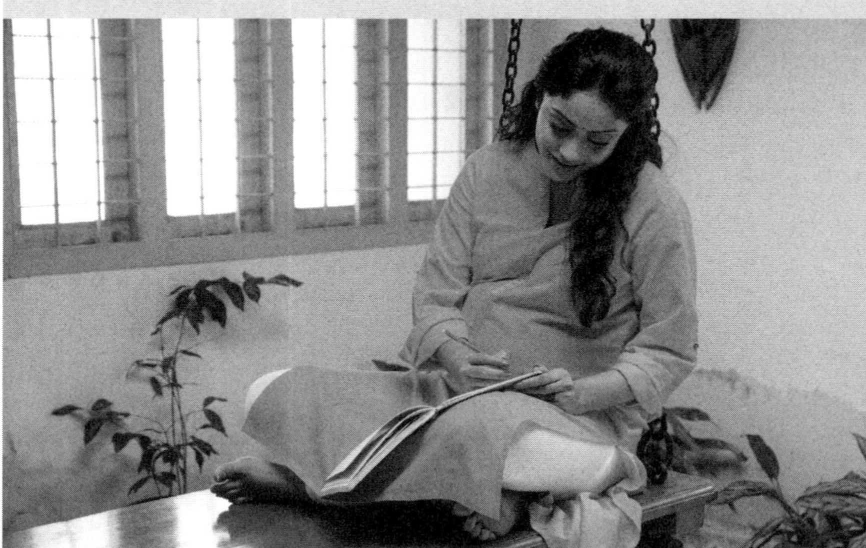

The first visit

Your first visit to the obstetrician is an important milestone in your pregnancy. I am sure you are excited and, at the same time, a little nervous. Don't worry! All couples have mixed emotions when they schedule their first visit. 'Am I really pregnant?' 'Will the baby be alright?' 'Will my pregnancy proceed smoothly?' These are just a few of the questions that will run through your mind.

It is during the first visit that your pregnancy will be confirmed. Usually this visit should be scheduled about 6–8 weeks after your last period. This is the ideal time for your obstetrician to confirm that you are pregnant.

It is in the first visit that you will get instructions on what you should or should not eat, your activity level (how much physical work you can carry out), what exercises you can do and what iron and vitamin supplements you will require. Make sure you get your doubts cleared.

Do I need to see the doctor sooner than 6–8 weeks?

Some women might need to see the doctor sooner than 6–8 weeks. You might need an earlier appointment if:

- You already have a medical condition, for example, diabetes, high blood pressure, epilepsy or asthma
- You have had problems with a pregnancy in the past
- You are having bleeding, abdominal pain or severe nausea and vomiting
- You are taking medication that you are worried might affect the baby

In your nervousness and excitement, you may tend to forget your questions and doubts about the pregnancy. Make sure you jot down any queries you have so that you can have them answered.

What happens during the first visit?

The first visit is usually the longest. This is when you are registered for your delivery. You will be asked several questions relating to your periods, your medical history and your family history.

Your obstetrician will calculate the expected date of delivery from the date of your last period. She will ask if you have any symptoms such as nausea or vomiting, breast tenderness, frequent urination and excess sleepiness. This will help her in confirming your pregnancy. If you have some symptoms that might be alarming, for example spotting or bleeding from the birth passage, she might perform an ultrasound examination to confirm that the pregnancy is healthy.

Gravida and para

Gravida refers to the number of times you have been pregnant. *Para* refers to the number of times you have delivered a baby anytime after the 7th month.

If this is your first pregnancy, you are called a *primigravida*. A *multigravida* is one who has been pregnant more than once. A *primipara* is a woman who has delivered a child once. A *multipara* is one who has delivered more than once.

Do you have any medical problems?

If you have any medical conditions for which you are already on medications, let your obstetrician know at the first visit. Conditions such as asthma, epilepsy, hypothyroidism or hyperthyroidism, diabetes and hypertension might require modification of your medications. At the same time, make sure you do not abruptly stop your medications just because you are pregnant. Always check with your doctor before stopping any medication. The other thing you must not do is to increase or decrease the dosage without consulting the doctor.

Kamini has a condition called hypothyroidism. Her thyroid gland does not function well and does not produce the thyroid hormone (see **Chapter 46**, *Medical disorders in pregnancy*). She has been taking thyroid hormone tablets for the past two years. When she told her family that she was pregnant, her aunt told her to stop taking the hormone tablets immediately!

This is absolutely the wrong thing to do. Kamini must not stop taking the tablets. The thyroid hormone is essential for Kamini's body to function normally. If she does not take the tablets, she will be hypothyroid and that condition can be detrimental to the baby, especially to its brain growth.

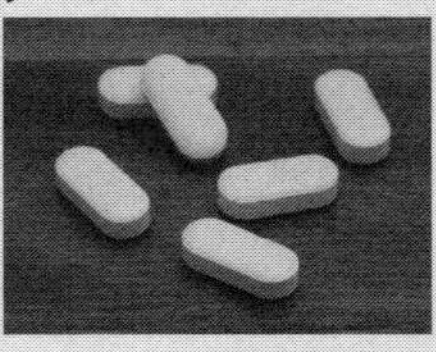

Before stopping any medication, do check with your obstetrician.

If you have had any previous illnesses like hepatitis (jaundice), kidney or heart conditions, do inform your doctor.

Have you had surgery in the past?

Do let your obstetrician know about any surgery you may have had. If it was major surgery, take your surgical discharge summary with you.

Does anyone in your family have medical problems?

You will be asked about your family's medical history. The emphasis will be on the presence of diabetes, hypertension and hereditary conditions. If you have any family history that worries you, this is the time to discuss it. Your family medical history will let your obstetrician know if you should be tested for certain conditions during the pregnancy.

What happened during your past pregnancy/ pregnancies?

If you have been pregnant before, your obstetrician will ask you about the number of times you have been pregnant, any miscarriages you may have had, and the details of the type of delivery you had.

Some questions you may be asked at your first visit

- What is the pattern of your periods?
- When was your last menstrual period?
- What type of birth control have you used?
- Have you been pregnant before?
- Have you ever had a miscarriage?
- Have you ever had an induced abortion?
- If you have had a baby before:
  - What did the baby weigh at birth?
  - How long did labour last?
  - Was it a normal vaginal delivery?
  - Was it a caesarean delivery? If so, what was the reason for doing it?
  - Were there any problems during or immediately after the delivery?
  - Did the baby have any birth defect?
- Is there a history of birth defects in your family?
- Is there a history of diabetes or hypertension in your family?
- Do you take any medicines on a regular basis?
- Do you have any allergies or health problems?
- Have you been exposed to any infections?

Confirmation of pregnancy

Your obstetrician will then confirm the pregnancy. She may perform an examination to determine the size of your uterus. This will tell her how pregnant you are.

Examination of the uterine size

The first visit usually involves assessment of the uterine size to determine if the pregnancy corresponds to the dates that you have given. If you are less than three months pregnant, your obstetrician may do an internal examination and feel the size of the uterus. If your uterus is enlarged and soft, she will confirm that you are pregnant. Though the internal examination may be uncomfortable and embarrassing, try to relax as much as you can. Taking slow deep breaths helps relax your muscles. You can insist on privacy and a sheet to maintain your modesty.

After the third month of pregnancy, your doctor will be able to feel the uterus by gently pressing on your abdomen. This is because, after the third month of pregnancy, your doctor can feel the uterus in the lower part of the abdomen.

Madhu asked: Will I miscarry if my doctor does an internal examination? Or if I have a vaginal ultrasound scan? Can't the pregnancy be confirmed just with a pregnancy test?

My answer: Of course, a pregnancy can be confirmed with a pregnancy test. However, the internal examination at the first check-up gives the doctor a lot of information and will NOT lead to a miscarriage. It tells her whether the size of the uterus corresponds to the estimated pregnancy week. It gives information about the length of the cervix (mouth of the uterus) that might impact on your delivery. It also reveals if there is any other issue like a large fibroid or ovarian cyst.

If the doctor cannot confirm the pregnancy with an internal examination, she might have to perform a vaginal ultrasound scan. A vaginal ultrasound scan will in no way affect your pregnancy. It will give accurate information about your pregnancy.

Some doctors may skip the internal examination completely and proceed directly to an ultrasound scan.

Listening for the baby's heartbeat

If you have completed 3 months of pregnancy, the doctor can use a special hand-held Doppler device to hear the baby's heartbeat. You and you husband can hear it too! For me, it has always been a very special moment when the couple listens to the baby's heartbeat for the first time. If a regular stethoscope is used, then the heartbeat can be heard only from the fifth month onwards.

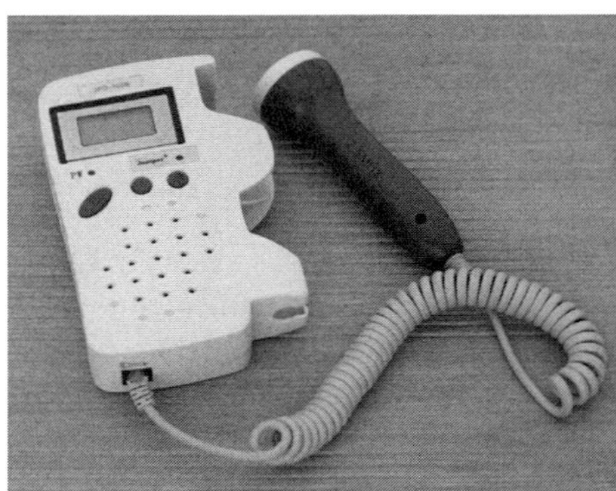

Hand-held Doppler device

Ultrasound scan to confirm pregnancy

Sometimes, your obstetrician will perform an ultrasound examination to confirm the pregnancy. This will tell her the exact age of the foetus and will also show the heartbeat of the baby. (See **Chapter 12**, *Ultrasound scans in pregnancy*). The first sight of your tiny little baby and its rapidly beating heart can be so exciting!

Preliminary blood tests

At the first visit, you will have to undergo a few blood tests:

- **A complete blood count**.

  Haematocrit and **haemoglobin** values indicate whether you are anaemic or not. Low values indicate anaemia. You will be given iron and multi-vitamin supplements to maintain your haemoglobin levels throughout pregnancy. If you are anaemic, the iron tablets will normalize the red blood count. Along with checking for anaemia, the white blood cell and platelet counts are also checked.

- **Blood group** and **Rh typing:** Your **blood group** can be A, B, AB, or O. Your **blood type** can be Rh positive or Rh negative. If you have the *Rh antigen*, you are Rh positive. If your blood lacks the antigen, you are considered to be Rh negative. 85 per cent of Indian women are Rh positive.

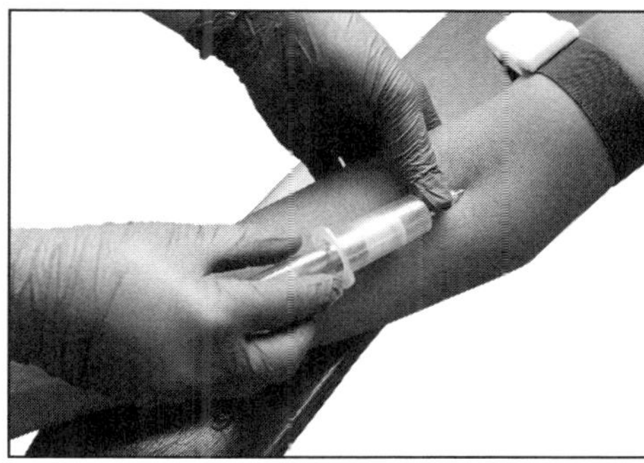

  Rh antibodies: If you are Rh negative and your partner is Rh positive, you will be checked for Rh antibodies with each pregnancy. This is done with a simple blood test called indirect Coomb's test (ICT). If you have Rh antibodies it can affect the baby (see **Chapter 39**, *Rh factor and your pregnancy*).

- **Hepatitis B virus:** This virus is present in the blood of infected individuals. If you have it, you can pass it to your baby and this can affect her. After the baby is born, she will be given an immunoglobulin injection and a course of vaccines against the virus. This will protect her for life.

- **VDRL** or **RPR** are tests for syphilis, a highly infectious disease caused by bacteria. Though rare, it can cause abnormalities in the baby.

- **Human immunodeficiency virus (HIV):**

  HIV is a virus that attacks certain cells of the body's immune system and causes AIDS (acquired immune deficiency syndrome). If the mother has HIV, there is a chance that it can be passed to the baby.

  It is important to be tested for HIV in pregnancy. If the mother has it, it is important to make sure that the infection does not pass on to the baby.

During pregnancy and delivery, the mother can be given medication to help reduce the risk of transmission to the baby and to protect him.

Repeat visits

Usual schedule for antenatal visits in an uncomplicated pregnancy

- Every month from confirmation of pregnancy till 32 weeks
- Every two weeks till 36 weeks
- Every week from 36 weeks till delivery

If there is any complication in the pregnancy, you might be asked to come for more frequent visits.

At each repeat visit:

- Your uterine growth will be checked and the baby's heart beat will be listened to
- Your weight will be recorded
- Your blood pressure will be taken
- A urine test will be done for protein and sugar

Checking your weight

Your weight will be recorded at every check-up. It is normal to gain ½ to 1 kg during each month of your pregnancy. If you start out with a normal weight, a weight gain of about 10 to 12 kgs is considered normal for the entire pregnancy. If your weight gain is poor, the size of the baby may be small. If you gain too much weight, it increases the risk of developing complications like diabetes in pregnancy, high blood pressure, premature birth and caesarean section. The other problem with gaining too much weight in pregnancy is that you will struggle to shed the extra kilos after delivery.

Vimala asked: My husband wants me to have a chubby baby. He is making sure that I eat badam (almonds) and drink 3–4 glasses of milk so that the baby puts on weight. Please tell me how to make sure the baby is not underweight at birth.

My answer: Your baby's weight depends on many things, including your own weight. However, you should hope to deliver a baby with a normal weight, not an overweight baby. A 'chubby', overweight baby may actually cause problems during delivery. The aim of a proper, healthy diet is to maintain your health as well as to provide proper nutrition for the baby (see **Chapter 10**, *Eating Healthy in Pregnancy*).

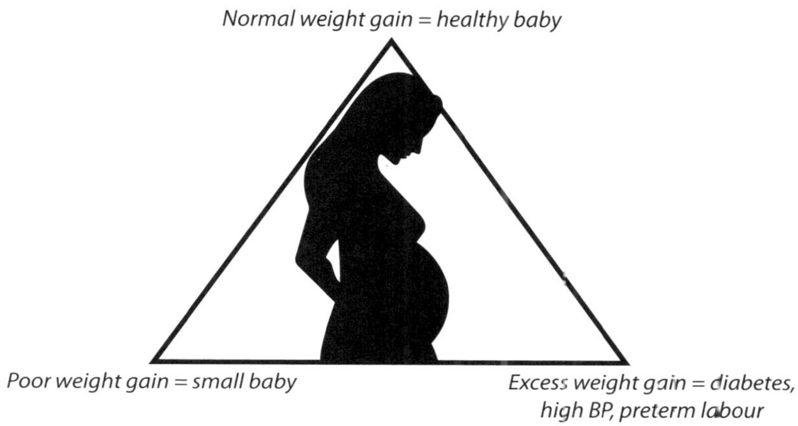

Checking your blood pressure

During every visit, your blood pressure (BP) will be checked. The obstetrician looks for an abnormal rise in the blood pressure. A healthy Indian woman can have a blood pressure ranging between 90/60 mm of Hg and 120/80 mm of Hg.

'Low' blood pressure?

It is very common for young Indian women to have a blood pressure of 90/70 or 100/70. This is absolutely normal. Unlike high blood pressure, there is no disease known as 'low blood pressure' in a healthy woman who is otherwise normal.

High blood pressure is diagnosed when the blood pressure is 140/90 mm of Hg or higher, when checked at least 4 hours apart. If one reading of the BP is high, the doctor will check it again after a few hours to confirm it.

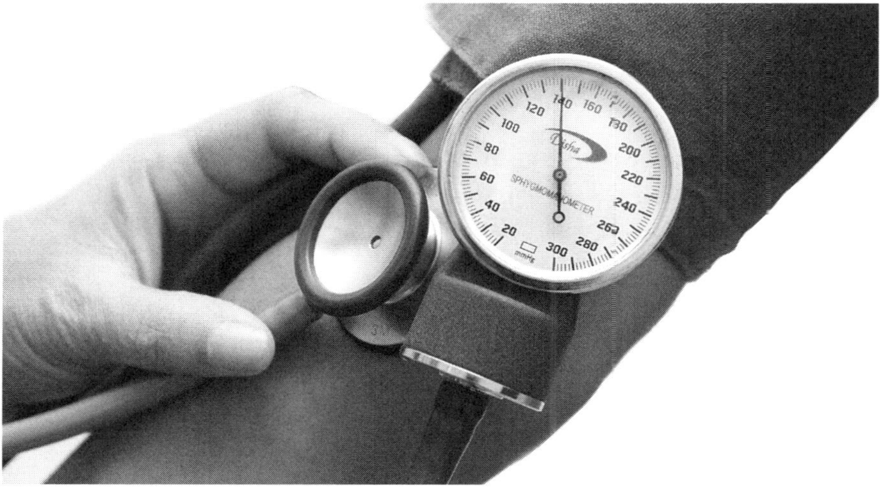

Urine test

At each antenatal visit, you will be asked to give a sample of your urine for testing.

- Urine is tested for **sugar** and **protein (albumin)**. Although the presence of sugar in the urine may be normal in pregnancy, it could be the first sign of diabetes. A blood test will be done to check your blood sugar levels
- Protein in the urine may be present as a complication of high blood pressure that occurs in late pregnancy (see **Chapter 37**, *High blood pressure in pregnancy*)
- Urine may also be tested if you have signs of urinary infection (see **Chapter 44**, *Urinary tract infection in pregnancy*)

Special tests during pregnancy

Testing for diabetes

Indians have a high risk for diabetes in pregnancy so you will be screened with a blood test at the first visit. If the test is normal, your doctor will test you again for diabetes between 24 and 28 weeks of pregnancy. This test is important for all women since diabetes is particularly common in Indians (see **Chapter 38**, *Diabetes in pregnancy*).

Testing for Down syndrome

Down syndrome is the commonest cause of intellectual disability (or learning disability) in humans. It is caused by the presence of an extra **chromosome 21** in the baby. Since a baby with Down syndrome can be born to a woman of any age, all women should ideally undergo testing for it (see **Chapter 14**, *Screening tests in pregnancy*).

Ultrasound scans during your pregnancy

Ultrasound scans are a very important part of your regular check-ups during pregnancy (see **Chapter 13**, *Ultrasound scans in pregnancy*).

First trimester

An ultrasound examination may be done in the first trimester to confirm the presence of a pregnancy, the size of the foetus and the number of babies present. The most important ultrasound scan in the first trimester is recommended at 11–14 weeks. This is done as part of Down syndrome screening, as mentioned earlier.

Second trimester

In the second trimester, a scan is done between 18–22 weeks to look for any abnormalities in the baby (see **Chapter 13**, *Ultrasound scans in pregnancy*).

Third trimester

An ultrasound examination might be repeated in the third trimester.

Tetanus toxoid immunization

The baby is born with no immunity to any infection. Tetanus is a dreaded, though extremely rare infection that the baby can acquire at birth. During your pregnancy, you will be immunized with two doses of tetanus toxoid, six weeks apart, so that you can temporarily pass on your immunity to the baby. Some doctors may give the tetanus vaccine every month, for three months. After the baby is born, he will receive permanent immunization against tetanus along with other immunizations.

You will receive your tetanus toxoid injections any time after the third month. Some doctors may give it later in pregnancy.

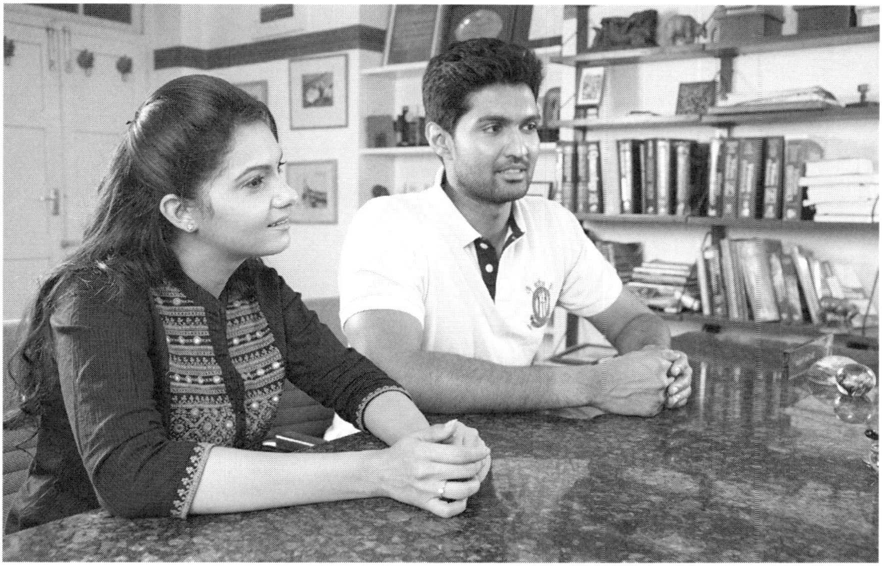

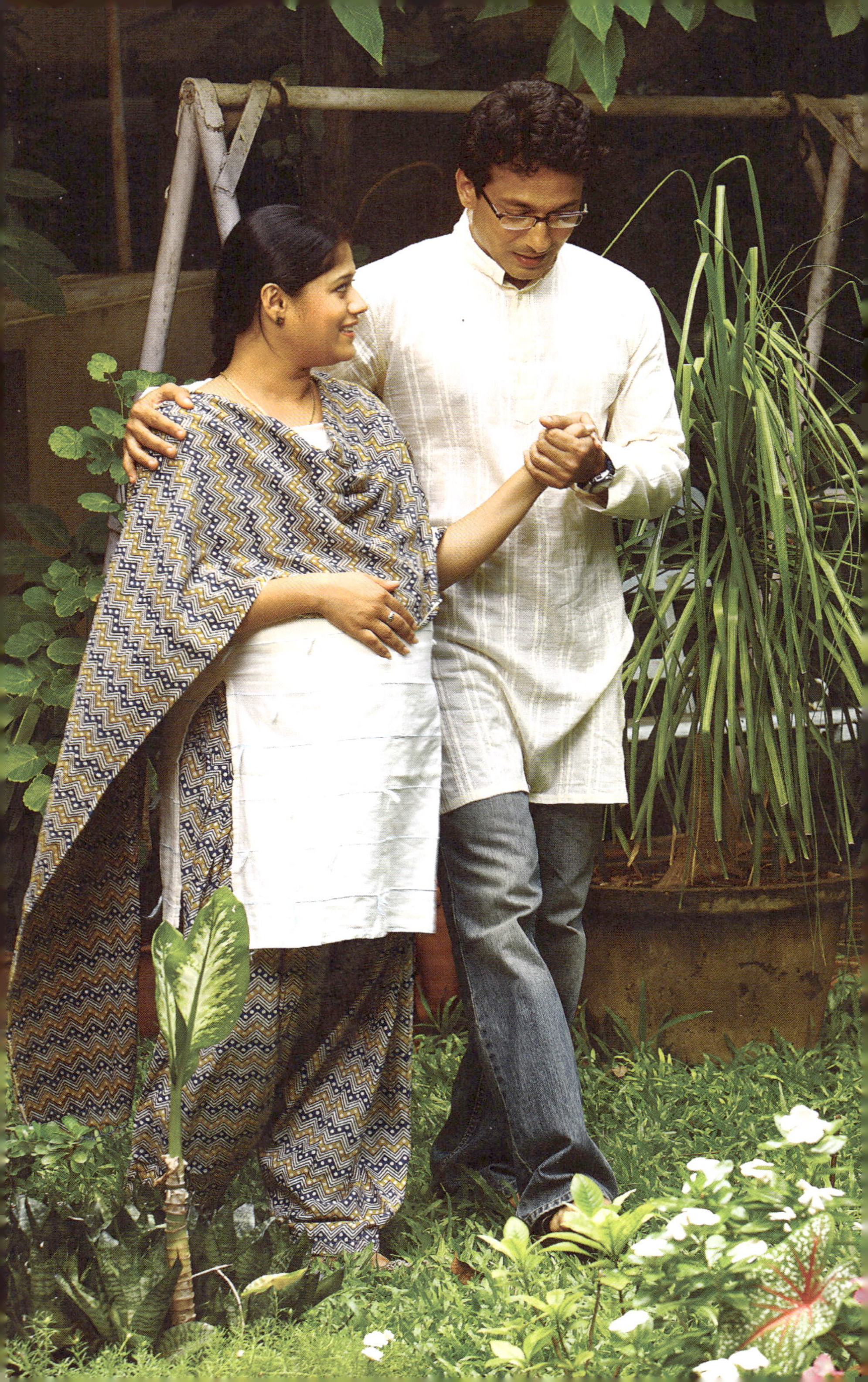

Weekly guide to pregnancy

CHAPTER 6

The first trimester (0-13 weeks)

A new life has found a home in your womb. Your little one is growing and developing day by day. It is a time filled with changes. You are amazed at how rapidly your body is adapting itself to provide a safe environment for this new being. Your body is also preparing itself to nourish and nurture this baby after he is born.

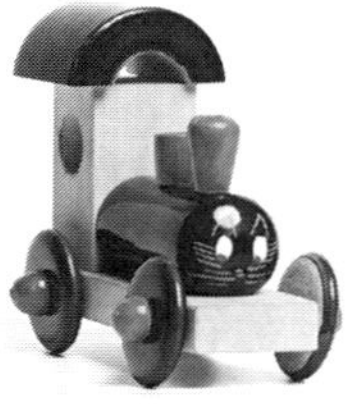

6

The first trimester

The day you and your partner found out that you were pregnant must have been one of the most exciting days in your life! I am sure you are absolutely thrilled about this miracle taking place in your body. To be equipped to take care of yourself, along with the growing baby inside you, you need to be aware of all the alterations and adaptations that your body is undergoing.

The most dramatic changes and development of your baby occur during the first trimester. During the first 10 weeks, the growing baby is called an **embryo**. After completing 10 weeks, the baby is called a **foetus**. Your baby develops rapidly and by the end of the first trimester, it measures an average of 6–7 cm in length, which is roughly the length of your index finger!

Week-by-week changes in mother and baby

Let us look at what happens to both you and your baby. This way you will understand and be able to cope with the sometimes drastic changes that are occurring. We will discuss the changes happening simultaneously in your body and the baby within you. We will count from the first day of the last period. We start counting the weeks of the pregnancy from the first day of the last period because it is impossible to pinpoint the day ovulation and conception actually occur. Most women will remember the first day of their last period.

The first trimester	0–13 weeks
The second trimester	14–27 weeks
The third trimester	28–40 weeks
Gestational age	Weeks are counted from the first day of the last period
Conceptional age	Weeks are counted from the age of conception. Thus conceptional age will be two weeks less than the gestational age

In this book, we will use only gestational age i.e., the weeks starting from the first day of the last period

When is the baby conceived?

If you have regular periods, the baby is usually conceived 11–15 days from the start of the period. So, though we count the number of weeks of the pregnancy from day 1 of your cycle, the pregnancy is actually forming from day 11–15 of the cycle.

In you have very irregular periods, with no definite cycle, gestational age may have to be calculated by performing an ultrasound scan once pregnancy is suspected. This would be the most accurate way of calculating when your baby is due.

What if you conceived with in-vitro fertilization (IVF or 'test tube baby')? The day the embryo is transferred into your uterus is considered the day of conception. Your due date will be calculated by adding 38 weeks to the date of transfer.

Week 1

Mother: You started your period on the first day of this week. This will be the last period you will have for at least the next nine or ten months. After the baby is born, breastfeeding will delay your periods even more. Though it is difficult to predict when your periods will resume, most breastfeeding women may not have a period for 6–9 months after the delivery.

If this month you are trying for a pregnancy, it is a good idea to note the first day of your periods on a calendar or a diary.

- If you have regular periods (28–30 days cycles) you should try to have intercourse from the 11th to the 15th day of the cycle (counting the day the period started as the first day). You will most probably ovulate in that time frame.
- If your periods are irregular with cycles that go beyond 45 days, your doctor may suggest that you have intercourse after the 14th day of your cycle, since your ovulation also will occur much later than in a person with regular periods. She may also advise the use of an ovulation kit that may help you pinpoint ovulation.
- If you are planning to become pregnant, now is the time to improve your diet and add vitamin supplements such as folic acid and iron.

Week 2

Mother: Preparing for conception

- Your last period is now over. Your uterus is lined with a new thickened layer of cells that will cushion, support and nourish your soon-to-be-conceived baby.

- An egg is growing in one of your ovaries. Soon it will ripen, reach the right size and be released from the ovary. This is called ovulation.
- There is a surge in the estrogen levels accompanying ovulation. The middle of the cycle, when ovulation occurs, is a good time for most women. Many women find that they are at their peak level of energy and creativity during this time.

Week 3

Mother: Congratulations! You are pregnant.

- Ovulation and conception occurred sometime during this week. One of your ovaries ripened and released an egg (ovum). Pulled in by the finger-like projections of the Fallopian tube, it began its journey toward the uterus.
- During intercourse, the partner usually ejaculates anywhere from 60 to 100 million sperm. Some of those sperm can live up to five days.
- Only about 200 sperm will actually make it through the uterus and into the correct Fallopian tube, eventually encountering the ovum.
- Sometime between 12 and 24 hours after you ovulated, a sperm would have penetrated the outer layers of the ovum. That's when the miracle of life happened and you conceived.
- Your progesterone levels will start increasing this week. High levels of progesterone keep the uterus quiescent, making it less likely to cramp. This helps the pregnancy to continue. That is why progesterone is often called the *hormone of pregnancy*.
- Over the next seven days, the fertilized egg will move down the Fallopian tube to the uterus. Once it reaches the uterine cavity, the embryo, which is a ball of cells by now, will burrow into the lining of the uterus. You may experience a little bloody spotting at the time of this implantation. This is called *implantation bleed*. Some women may mistake this for a period.

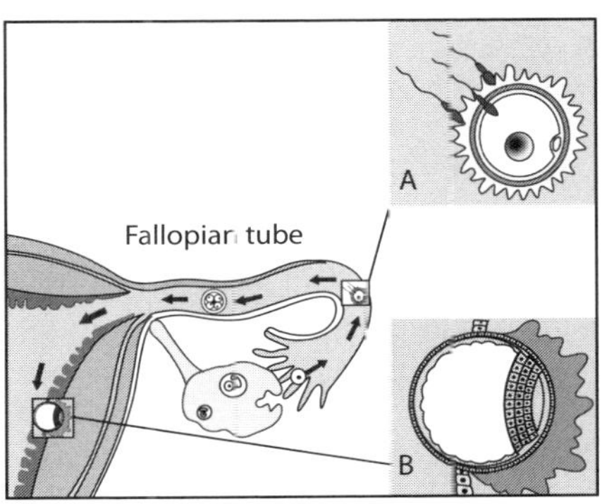

The process of fertilization (A) and implantation (B)

Week 4

Baby:

- Although you are as yet unaware that you are pregnant, your baby is already undergoing great changes. The fertilized egg is now a quickly growing ball of cells called a *blastocyst*. It is embedded more deeply in the uterine wall and the amniotic cavity is being formed. The group of cells that will make up the placenta is being organized and circulatory networks containing maternal blood are being formed.

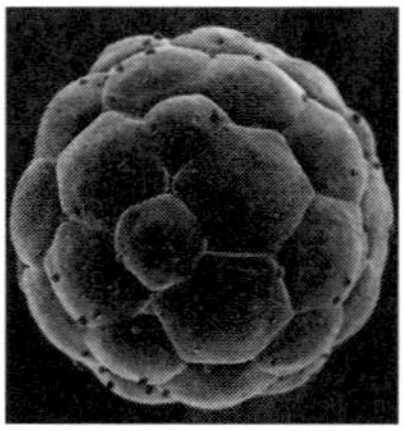

Blastocyst

- Three layers of cells are forming within the blastocyst. The *ectoderm* will form the nervous system, hair and skin of your baby. The *endoderm* will become the lining of the gastrointestinal tract, and various organs such as thyroid, liver and pancreas. The *mesoderm* will develop into the skeleton, connective tissues, blood systems, urogenital system and most of the muscles.

Mother:

- If you have been trying for a pregnancy, you should avoid any over-the-counter medication at this point because some medications can be harmful to the developing embryo. If you need to take any medication, tell your doctor that you might be pregnant. Let your doctor give you a medicine that is safe for the baby.
- Some women notice a metallic taste in their mouth, though no one knows the reason for this. It may probably be caused by the surge in hormonal levels.

Week 5

Baby:

- Your baby is now an embryo with a little tail at the end of its developing spine.
- You know how big your baby is right now? It is 5 mm, which is the size of a whole black pepper!
- In that tiny form, the spinal column, brain and heart have begun to develop.

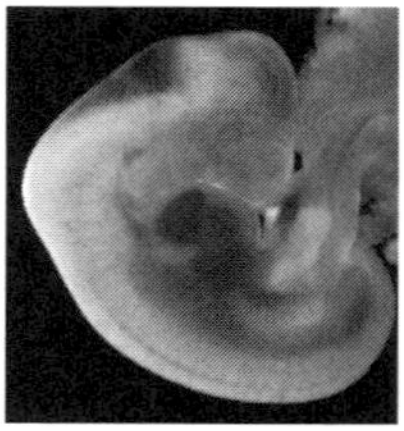

Tadpole-like embryo

Mother: Am I pregnant?

- Your period is delayed and you are starting to wonder if you are pregnant. A pregnancy test can be positive at this point. A home pregnancy kit can be used. Don't be surprised if the pregnancy test comes back negative. It will turn positive only when the hCG level reaches a certain threshold. If it is negative the first time, you can repeat the test again after a few days (see **Chapter 3**, *Am I pregnant?* for more details on pregnancy tests).

- Your breasts become tender, particularly over the nipples. Due to congestion of blood in your pelvis, you may need to urinate more frequently than usual. Also, you may notice that you feel tired and sleepy. This is not surprising since your body is going through several physical and chemical changes.
- You may begin to experience nausea or vomiting. Many women feel this only in the morning, but some may have to deal with it all day long.

The pregnancy test

Most chemical tests for pregnancy detect the presence of the **beta-subunit of human chorionic gonadotropin (hCG)**. A urine test can detect a pregnancy as early as the 4th–5th week from the first day of the last menstrual period. In most cases, the test is sensitive enough to detect pregnancy even on the day of the missed period. In some women though, the levels of hCG are not detectable so early. It is, in fact, advisable to wait a week after missing your period, before you perform the test. This will help avoid a falsely negative test.

Home pregnancy kits are easy to use and most require you to hold the strip in the urine stream. A specific change in colour in the line or dot will indicate a pregnancy (see **Chapter 3**, *Am I pregnant*?).

Blood tests are more sensitive and may be ordered by your doctor if you have undergone treatment for infertility or if there is a doubt that the pregnancy may not be growing normally.

Week 6

Baby:

By week 6, the baby is as big as your little fingernail or a pomegranate seed. She has buds where her arms and legs will be and her head has the beginnings of eyes, ears and a mouth.

Her heart has begun to beat. On an ultrasound, you can clearly make out the beating of the heart.

Mother:

- Your baby has been growing inside you for one month now though you may not find any physical changes. You might just find yourself sleepy and unusually tired.

When should you schedule your first appointment?

Once your pregnancy test comes back positive, and you are having the symptoms of pregnancy, it might be prudent to decide who is going to deliver your baby. Check with your family and friends and find an obstetrician who has a reputation for a high rate of vaginal deliveries.

In your anxiety to confirm the pregnancy, don't rush to a doctor as soon as your pregnancy test comes back as positive. It is difficult to confirm a pregnancy by physical examination or ultrasound scan before 6 weeks. Schedule an appointment for at least 6 weeks past your last period.

- Occasionally, some women may feel dizzy or faint if they stand up for a long time. For many years, Indian movies have used the fainting of a woman as a clue to the fact that she is pregnant!
- You may suddenly find an aversion to common smells. Cooking might become impossible as the smell of frying, or for that matter, any smell in the kitchen may set off nausea. Many women develop an aversion to milk and milk products.

Sumana asked: Do I need any hormonal tablets or injections to keep my baby safe?

My answer: The growing pregnancy releases a huge amount of hormones into your blood stream. This is enough to keep your baby growing well. There is no need for hormonal tablets or injections in the first three months. Research over many years has proven that they are of no benefit. If the pregnancy is normal, it will continue without any external hormonal 'support'. If it is an abnormal pregnancy, it will miscarry in spite of tablets and injections. Some doctors may prescribe hormonal tablets and injections in women who have had previous miscarriages. However, this treatment is controversial.

Women who conceive after IVF ('test tube baby') will require hormonal support till the placenta takes over hormone production. This is usually till the 12th–16th week of pregnancy.

Week 7

Baby:

- The baby is about 1.25 cm long or the size of a pistachio. The baby's heart is now beating regularly at 140–150 beats per minute.
- The arm buds have grown and the hands begin to develop.
- The brain, intestines, pituitary gland and pancreas are growing.

- The baby's face is developing rapidly. The nasal pits form, the ears and lenses of the eyes are developing.

Mother:

- You will still be feeling tired. However, your body is slowly adjusting to the huge surge of hormones.
- You may start developing pimples on the face, chest and back. These are due to changing hormone levels.
- Your appetite will be poor, though there are women who feel hungry all the time! In fact, it is not unusual to lose weight at this point.
- Some women will find it difficult to drink any liquids, including water. Constipation can be a problem because of the poor intake of food and fluids.
- You will definitely not be 'showing'. The baby and your uterus have not grown enough to be visible abdominally.

Mala asked: I am two months pregnant. I travel an hour by bus to work I have been told that I may miscarry because of this. Is it safe for me to travel by bus?

My answer: You can travel by any vehicle: two-wheelers, autos, buses or cars. The bumps on the roads cannot cause a miscarriage. You can even travel by train or air. If you have any bleeding in early pregnancy, you may be asked to rest for a short while and avoid travelling for a week. Once the bleeding stops and your doctor has made sure that the baby is doing well, she will ask you to resume your travelling again.

Week 8

Baby:

- The baby is now about 10,000 times bigger than what he was at conception but is still only about 2.0 cm long. That's as big as a rajma bean!

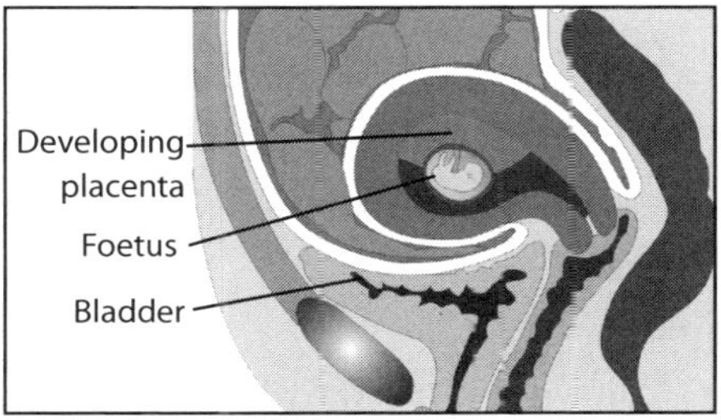

Your baby at 8 weeks

- This is the week that the baby responds to signals from the brain and differentiates into a boy or girl. This means that the gonads will either become testes (a boy) or ovaries (a girl).

- The eyes are formed and covered by a fold of skin, though the eyelid will not open as yet.
- The arms and legs are growing longer and the arms are bent at the elbow.
- The tip of the nose is visible and teeth are forming under the baby's gums.
- Your baby has started moving inside the uterus but you cannot feel the movements yet.

Padmini asked: Is it okay for me to have sex in the first few months of pregnancy? I have discomfort and quite frankly, I feel so exhausted that I am not even interested.

My answer: It is quite common for some women to feel less interested in sex because of the nausea and tiredness. On the other hand, some women may actually have a greater interest in sex. However, there is no physical reason to avoid intercourse. It will not cause any harm to the pregnancy. You might have some lower abdominal pain during sex or orgasm but this will in no way affect the baby. It is only if you have had any bleeding in early pregnancy that you might be advised to avoid intercourse for two weeks.

Mother:

- You are now two months pregnant! When your obstetrician does an internal examination, she will feel the enlargement of the uterus.
- The breasts get larger and heavier, and may still be painful when touched.
- The nipples may be darker and the little bumps around the edge of the areola are more pronounced.
- You may feel the need to urinate more frequently as the growing uterus puts pressure on the bladder.
- Some mothers develop acidity that causes heartburn.
- Do not be surprised if you have recurrent headaches. This is quite common in early pregnancy. It is quite safe to take paracetamol to relieve the ache.

Week 9

Baby:

- Your grape-sized little one is transforming day by day. Bones and cartilage are beginning to form.
- The umbilical cord and placenta are forming and growing.
- The fingers have formed but are webbed.

Mother:

- Your appetite might improve but do not be surprised if the nausea persists for another month or so.
- You might still lose weight but in most women, the weight will stabilize. Some may even gain a little weight.
- Due to hormonal changes, the gums become softer and thicker. You might bleed from your gums while brushing your teeth. Be sure to use a soft toothbrush.

Should you stop sleeping on your stomach now?

Not at all. You baby is just a tiny being, the size of a grape. She is also well-cushioned by the amniotic fluid surrounding her. There is no way she feels any pressure. In another three or four months you will start finding it uncomfortable sleeping on your stomach because your baby bump will get in the way. So, you can sleep on your stomach as long as you are able to. Your baby will be just fine! You can also turn from side to side while lying down. When you get up from a lying posture, make it a point to turn to your side and then get up (this saves you from spraining your back as the pregnancy progresses).

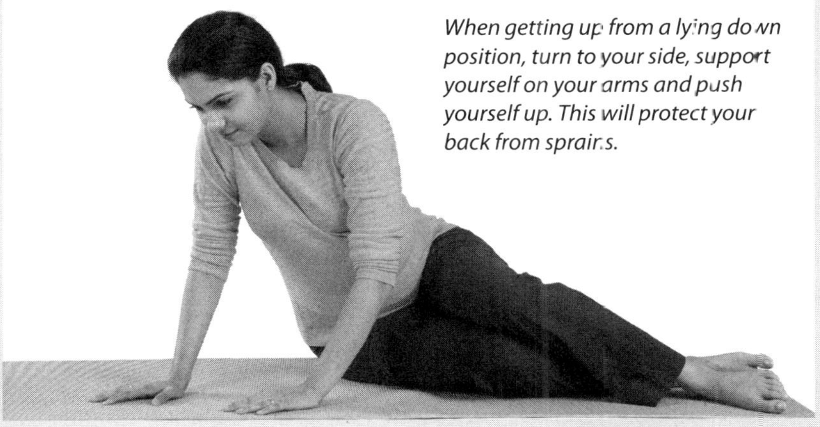

When getting up from a lying down position, turn to your side, support yourself on your arms and push yourself up. This will protect your back from sprains.

Week 10

Baby:

- This week, your baby graduates from being an embryo to a foetus!
- Most of the joints are formed—shoulders, elbows, wrist, hands and fingers, knees, ankles, feet and toes.
- All of the organs are there, but not fully formed or functional.

Mother:

- You will have mood swings because of the surge in hormone levels. You might swing from happiness to crying to anger in minutes. Your husband and family have to be prepared for this!
- If you are feeling a little more energetic, start going for walks. This will make you feel healthy and fit and is a good practice to follow throughout pregnancy.
- You may feel breathless. This may cause you to take deep breaths and sigh a lot. This is an effect of the increased levels of progesterone in your blood. The breathlessness will reduce at the end of the first trimester but will come back in the third trimester.

Week 11

Baby:

- Nails are just starting to develop on your baby's little fingers.
- The length of the baby will probably double this week.
- The irises of the eyes are developing now.

Mother:

- You may still suffer the effects of morning sickness, but it will soon disappear. Your energy levels will start going up, though you may still want to take naps at the oddest times.
- You might be advised to have your first ultrasound scan to assess the growth of the baby. The thickness of the skin over the baby's neck (nuchal translucency) is measured during this scan. This provides information about the health of the baby (see **Chapter 12**, *Ultrasound scans in pregnancy*).

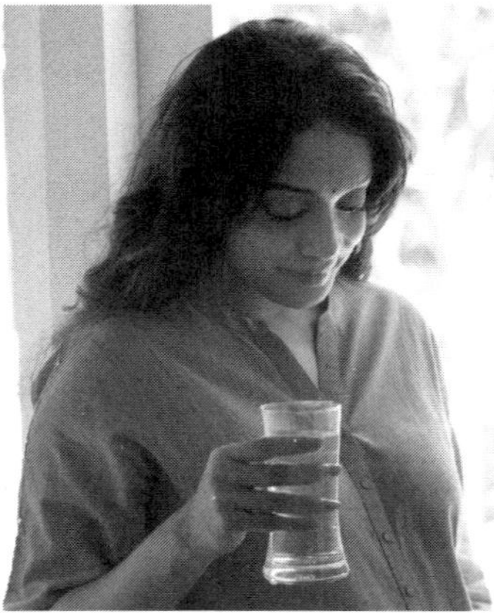

Eating and drinking in the first three months

Your appetite may be very poor. Eat small quantities and frequently. Avoid oily and spiced food. Salt biscuits/crackers help in suppressing the nausea. Bland foods such as dry toast and idlis are well tolerated. Drink plenty of fluids. Remember, this too shall pass! See **Chapter 10**, *Eating healthy in pregnancy*.

Week 12

Baby:

- The baby is about 6 cm long, fully formed and looks like a human being. The size of a tomato, he would fit in the palm of your hand!
- The beginnings of hair are seen on the scalp.
- Skin and nails have developed.
- The webbed hands and feet separate into fingers and toes.
- The baby's chest rises and falls as he practices breathing movements.
- With kidneys fully functioning, the baby can swallow amniotic fluid and excrete it as urine.
- The amniotic fluid is completely replaced every three hours, so the baby's environment stays fresh.

Activity in the first three months

- Keep up your usual level of activity. Lie down or sleep when you feel very tired but don't spend the day in bed!
- You can carry on all normal housework but avoid lifting anything very heavy. You might sprain your back
- You can carry your older child, if you have one, but see if you can pick her up from a chair or have somebody hand her to you
- If you have a job, there is no need to take leave of absence from work.
- You can climb up and down stairs any number of times
- If you have had any spotting or bleeding, your obstetrician might advise you to restrict your activities for a few days or weeks

Mother:

- This is the turnaround week—your tiredness and exhaustion will slowly be replaced with a sense of well-being.
- Your uterus just about fills your pelvis. If you press your fingers into your lower abdomen, just above the pubic bone, you may be able to feel it. Your obstetrician will be able to feel the top of the uterus abdominally.
- A hand-held Doppler device may be used to hear the baby's heartbeat. The first time you hear the baby's heartbeat is an amazing milestone! Make sure that your husband is there to hear the heartbeat with you. It will sound like a rushing train because the baby's heartbeat is very fast at this stage.

- As the uterus grows, it will shift upwards a bit and will not press on your bladder as much as before.
- The placenta will take over the production of hormones from the corpus luteum of the ovary.

Week 13

Baby:

- Your baby continues to grow and is almost 8 cm long. He weighs about 25 grams.
- The vocal cords begin to develop.
- All the twenty baby teeth are formed and waiting beneath the gums until well after birth. However, every once in a while a baby is born with one or two teeth already showing.
- The baby's bone marrow, liver and spleen have taken over the production of red blood cells.
- Initially, the eyes on the foetus are on the sides of the head, but this week, they move to the front and appear closer together (to begin the makings of the face). The ears also move to the proper position on either side of the head.

Mother:

- As the uterus grows and is stretched by the baby inside, you will start to feel some heaviness and a mild ache in your lower abdomen. You might find it uncomfortable when you get up after sitting down. When you turn from one side to the other while lying down, there may be a pulling sensation in the lowest part of your abdomen. Walking fast may also cause this heaviness or discomfort. This feeling increases over the following few weeks. There is no need to worry. This is a very common feeling.
- The veins on your breasts are probably much more noticeable and your nipples will become darker in colour.

First trimester screening for Down syndrome

This screening test is done between 11 and 14 weeks of pregnancy. It combines the results of a special ultrasound test called *nuchal translucency* screening and *blood tests* (PAPP-A and hCG) to look for signs of Down syndrome, trisomy 18, and heart defects. If this test is available to you, it might be a good idea to have it done (see **Chapter 14**, *Screening tests in pregnancy*).

The role of the father-to-be

The first trimester can be a roller coaster ride for the father-to-be. You may feel helpless as you see your wife tired and exhausted, nauseous and unable to eat. If she does not eat, will the baby's development be affected? Do not worry; the baby does not require more than what your wife is able to eat. Once her appetite is back to normal, she can start eating nutritious food.

You may also be filled with anxiety about your ability to handle the pregnancy and its demands on your feelings. Your wife might be emotionally labile, with mood swings which leave you bewildered and sometimes, upset.

How can you help?

Just being there for her is an enormous mood elevator for a new mother-to-be. With words and deeds, let her know you are delighted that she is pregnant. Help her out with housework because she may find it hard to do all the household chores, especially during the first trimester when she seems tired all the time.

Make sure you go to all her antenatal check-ups. This will allow you to clear your doubts too. Knowing what is happening with her pregnancy will enable you to be a supportive and comforting husband.

Old wives' tales

- Having intercourse in the first trimester will cause a miscarriage. **Not true!** If you have had any spotting or bleeding in the first trimester, your obstetrician might ask you to avoid intercourse for a period of time.
- Avoid bumpy rides—it might lead to a miscarriage. **Not true!**
- Do not climb stairs in the first few months because it can lead to a miscarriage. **Not true!**
- Do not cross your legs when you sit—you may cause pressure on the baby and that may lead to a miscarriage. **Not true!**

CHAPTER 7

The second trimester (14-27 weeks)

Sagarika is feeling so much better! The queasiness in the early mornings is almost gone. She actually feels her energy coming back. She now feels she may start enjoying her pregnancy. Her husband is relieved because she is slowly developing an appetite again. Both of them are excited because they know that they will feel the baby move in this trimester. They can't wait!

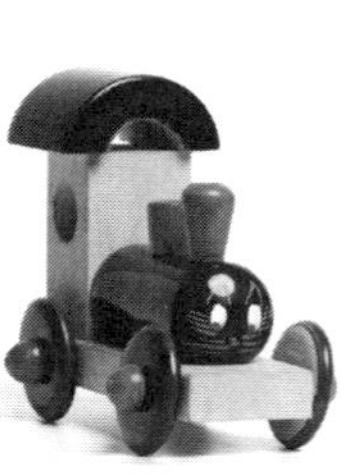

7

The second trimester

The first trimester has come to an end. You are feeling great and the nausea has eased up. You and your husband may have heard the baby's heartbeat when you visited your obstetrician. Let us move on to the second trimester.

Most women consider this stage of pregnancy the easiest to deal with. Energy levels are rising and the intense sleepiness of the first three months is letting up.

Week 14

Baby:

- Your baby is about 7.5 cm long and the weight has tripled to about 45 grams.
- She is moving actively inside your womb but it will be too early for you to feel anything yet.
- The facial features become more defined and the baby looks so much more human! The facial muscles become active and the baby is able to smile, frown and wrinkle her forehead.
- The baby's neck becomes well defined.
- Reflexes begin to operate. She will start opening and closing her fists.
- The external genitalia have clearly differentiated into that of a boy or a girl.
- Whorls start developing on the fingertips and will in time become the future fingerprints.

Mother:

- Having made it through the first three months, your risk of miscarriage is very low.
- You might start developing acidity, leading to heartburn. Your doctor will prescribe antacids to relieve it. The Indian habit of eating dinner very

late, well after 9 pm, is probably the worst thing for your heartburn. Eat dinner early. This will ensure that you have a gap of at least an hour-and-a-half or two hours between dinner and lying down. This will decrease the chance of reflux and heartburn.

- Your breasts are heavy but the tenderness should have subsided by now. Some women find that they may have to change their bra size to one size larger.
- Constipation can still be a problem. Start adding more fibre to your diet e.g., leafy greens, raw vegetable salads, and roughage-rich vegetables like carrots and cabbage. Make sure you drink plenty of fluids.
- You may just about start 'showing'. Many first-time mothers are concerned that they are not showing yet. Remember that in the first pregnancy, you may not start showing till after another month or so. Loose Indian clothing also hides a pregnancy fairly well till 5 months.
- If your interest in sex had decreased in the first three months, you might find that your desire for sex returns now.

Week 15

Baby:

- Your baby is about 10 cm long. It is approximately the size of an apple!
- Colourless eyebrows and eyelashes have now appeared.
- The baby's heart is beating well and the blood circulation is fine.
- The hair on the top of the head is starting to show up more.
- Skin formation is progressing, but the skin is still thin (you can even see small blood vessels forming underneath).
- At this point, the baby is exploring everything and sometimes, on ultrasound, can even be seen sucking his thumb!

Mother:

- The heaviness in the lower abdomen is likely to increase. The top of your uterus (the fundus) is now halfway between your pubic bone and umbilicus. It can be easily felt and your obstetrician will be able to assess if the uterus is growing normally.
- Have the palms of your hands started looking red and feeling warm? This is because of the increased blood circulation.
- From the 15th week onwards, you can undergo the quadruple or triple screen test for Down syndrome, if the screening was not done in the first trimester.

Second trimester screening for Down syndrome

The quadruple screening test for Down syndrome is done between 15 and 20 weeks of pregnancy. It combines an ultrasound with blood tests for estriol, hCG, alphafoetoprotein and inhibin. If this test is not available, a triple screening test may be done.

Week 16

Baby:

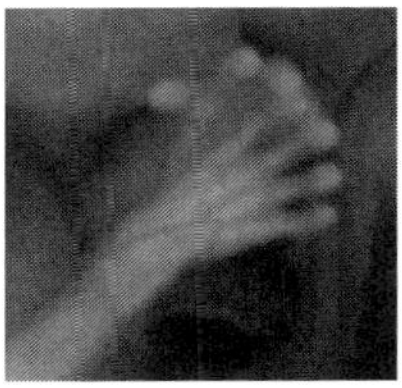

The baby's hands

- Your baby is about 11 cm long and the average weight is about 100 grams.
- The head is erect.
- The limbs are well developed.
- The baby's eyes are moving though the eyelids are still not open.
- The skin is getting thicker and is less transparent.

Mother:

- If you have had a baby before, you might start feeling the slightest of flutters as your baby starts moving. First-time mothers have to be patient for at least another two to four weeks to start feeling the baby's early movements.
- You may notice more changes in your skin. Some women may develop irregular brown patches, called the 'mask of pregnancy' (chloasma) on their face or neck.
- Look for the linea nigra, a dark line of pigmentation running from the top to the bottom, in the midline of your abdomen. This may develop even later in pregnancy.
- Sleeping on your stomach might start becoming uncomfortable. You can still sleep on your back, but you can start learning to sleep on your sides so that later on in pregnancy, you will be more comfortable in that position.
- The placenta is now fully formed and functional.

Week 17

Baby:

- The baby will start making purposeful movements.
- Fat starts getting deposited under the baby's skin.

Mother:

- Now that your appetite is back, you start gaining weight.
- Your energy levels are back to normal so this is the time to start a regular antenatal exercise programme and stick to it.
- If you have not started your iron supplementation, this is a good time to do it. You will be able to tolerate iron much better than in the first trimester.

Week 18

Baby:

- In two weeks, your baby's weight has doubled to 200 grams.
- The ears stand out from the head.
- The baby's bones are growing harder and stronger.
- The kidneys are producing 7–14 ml of urine every day.
- Meconium, a greenish substance, is beginning to accumulate in the bowel. It is made up of undigested debris from the amniotic fluid and various secretions of the digestive tract. This will come out in the early days after birth as the baby's first few bowel movements.
- The placenta transfers nutrients and oxygen from your blood to the baby via the umbilical cord.
- The baby is beginning to be covered in a white, waxy substance called vernix. This protects the baby's delicate skin from getting wrinkled because of constantly being immersed in amniotic fluid.

Mother:

- You still feel good. Your energy levels are high.
- Many women get worried because they do not seem to have symptoms of pregnancy anymore: the nausea is gone, the appetite is healthy and you have become used to the weight of the uterus so there is no abdominal discomfort. Don't worry; this is the good time of pregnancy, so enjoy it!
- The uterus is not big enough yet to cause any discomfort though you may continue to feel the weight in the lower abdomen, especially when you sit down and get up.
- Have you started thinking of a name for the baby? Pick a boy's name and a girl's name so that you will be ready when the baby is born.

Week 19

Baby:

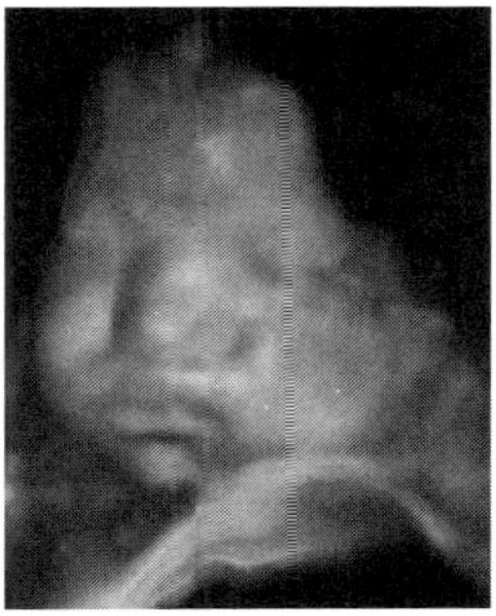

3D ultrasound image of baby's face at 19 weeks

- If your baby is a little girl, millions of undeveloped eggs will start forming in the ovaries. By the time she is born, she will have about a million undeveloped eggs in her ovaries.
- Buds for permanent teeth start forming behind the buds for baby teeth.
- The baby's toenails grow but not as rapidly as the fingernails.
- You will feel the baby move more often. However, don't be surprised if the baby does not seem to be moving all the time—she will be sleeping a lot.

Mother:

- Your lower abdomen starts to get fuller. If this is your first pregnancy, this is when all your friends can easily notice that you are pregnant!
- This is a good time to start applying moisturizers over the abdominal skin. As the skin stretches due to the growing uterus, moisturizing the skin helps to minimize stretch marks.

Week 20

Week 20 or the 5th month of pregnancy is an important milestone. You have reached the midpoint of your pregnancy. Five months over and five more to go!

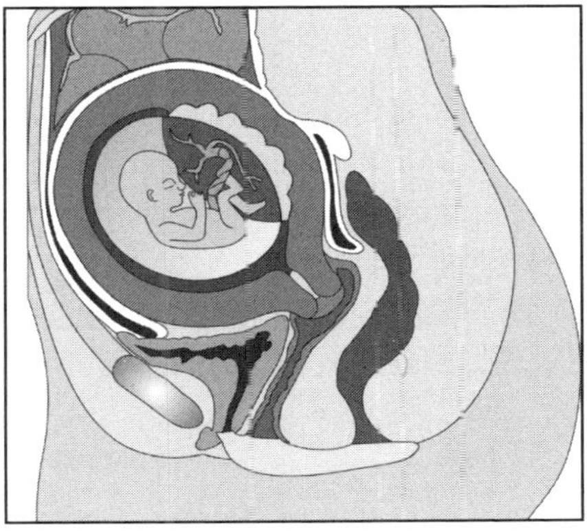

Your baby at 20 weeks

Baby:

- Your baby weighs approximately 320 grams, the size of a mango!
- If the baby is a girl, her uterus has started developing.
- Your baby's heart is beating at a rate of 120 to 160 beats per minute.

Mother:

- The top of the uterus reaches the level of your umbilicus.
- Your umbilicus might start looking a little protuberant and as the pregnancy progresses, may protrude quite a bit.

- Right from the very beginning of pregnancy, you might have noticed increased vaginal discharge. The discharge might get more pronounced now. This is very normal and not of any concern. However, contact your obstetrician if itching or burning accompanies the discharge. That is indicative of an infection and will require treatment (see **Chapter 45**, *Vaginal discharge and itching*).

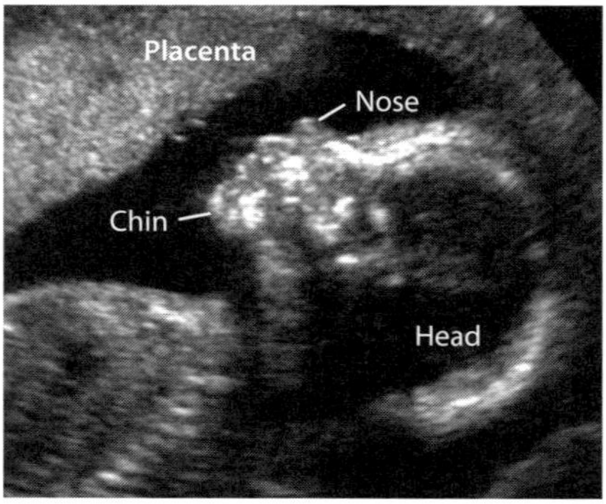

Ultrasound image of baby at 20 weeks showing profile

> **Bharathi asked:** I am a teacher. I have just completed my 5th month. I notice that at the end of the day my feet get a little swollen. Should I be worried?
>
> **My answer:** If your feet start to get a little puffy, there is nothing to be concerned about. This is due to the water retention that is part of pregnancy and is called oedema of pregnancy. As the pregnancy progresses, you will retain more and more water in your body and the feet will get more swollen. As a teacher your day involves standing for long periods of time and that will aggravate the problem. This may also affect working women who have to sit at a desk all day. Try putting your feet up when you get home. Elevate your feet with pillows when you sleep. You will find that your feet will be fine in the morning.

Week 21

Baby:

- Your baby is quite active now. However, you won't be feeling him move all the time. Don't worry if he sleeps for long periods of time. His movements will be felt vigorously one day and may be mild another day.
- The baby's bone marrow starts making blood cells. The baby's liver and spleen were producing the blood cells prior to this.

Ultrasound scan at 20–22 weeks

This scan is extremely important to have. The baby has grown big enough to visualize all of her organs. If there is an abnormality, it can be recognized in this scan. The growth of the baby and the position of the placenta are also determined (see **Chapter 13**, *Ultrasound scans in pregnancy*).

Mother:

- For the past few weeks, you might have asked your husband to feel the baby's movements by placing his hands on your abdomen. Now, he will be able to feel the baby move really well, without having to pretend he does!
- Be as active as you can. Keep up the daily walking and don't forget to do your prenatal exercises.

Week 22

Baby:

- Your baby weighs about 460 grams and is about 25 cm long.
- There is a downy layer of hair on the skin, called lanugo. This will disappear before the baby is born or soon after birth.
- Taste buds are starting to form on your baby's tongue.
- The brain and nerve endings can process the sensation of touch. Your baby may experiment by feeling his or her face or anything else within reach.
- For boys, this week the testes begin their descent from the abdomen into the scrotum.

Mother:

- You may feel the effects of the change in your centre of gravity. Your gait will change when you walk.
- You may be more comfortable with a slight platform heel on your footwear, rather than completely flat footwear. Avoid wearing high heels because you may lose you balance and hurt yourself.

Week 23

Baby:

- Your baby weighs about 500 grams (half a kilo) and is about the size of a medium papaya!
- The pancreas is developing well and begins to produce insulin. Insulin is the hormone that maintains normal sugar levels in the blood stream.
- The bones in the little one's middle ear are hardening now and the baby can hear muffled sounds. In fact, she can hear the rhythmic beat of your heart! Some mothers notice that the baby may be startled by a sudden loud noise and may settle down to gentle movements on hearing soothing music!

Mother:

- The baby's movements are quite obvious now. Sometimes it feels like he is playing football in there!
- Your may develop a sharp pulling pain on either or both sides of the lower abdomen. This is due to the stretching of the round ligaments. The round ligaments are attached from the top of the uterus to the sides of the lower abdomen. They help in holding the uterus up. Lying down and resting on the same side as the pain can relieve *round ligament pain*.
- When you sit for a long time, your lower ribs may ache as the uterus pushes against them. Try to lean back when you sit, so that the uterus does not push directly into the ribs.

> **Sunanda asked:** I have developed painful piles in the 6th month of my pregnancy. Is this common?
>
> **My answer:** In pregnancy, it is common to develop haemorrhoids (piles). Haemorrhoids are swollen veins in the lowest part of your rectum and anus. If they are painful or cause a small amount of bleeding, you can ask your doctor for a stool softener and an ointment to reduce the pain. Constipation may aggravate haemorrhoids, so make sure to drink plenty of fluids and take fibre-rich food.

Week 24

Baby:

- The baby gains weight rapidly and weighs about 630 grams.
- The lungs are developing blood vessels now, preparing them to take over the task of getting oxygen into the blood stream.
- The lungs begin to produce **surfactant**. This substance allows the air sacs in the lungs to inflate and prevents them from collapsing at birth. This substance is the reason why newborn babies can breathe air as soon as they are born.
- Unfortunately, babies have just the opposite of our sleep rhythms. That is why you will find her jumping around at night and keeping you awake, just when you are desperate for a good night's sleep.
- Your baby is developing the ability to suck.
- Don't forget, the baby can hear muffled sounds. Play some music. She can't hear the words but she can definitely listen to the intonation and the rhythm.

Mother:

- Just four more months to go! You look obviously pregnant now.
- Keep exercising, keep fit.
- Anytime from the 24th to the 28th week, you might be asked to undergo a blood test to determine whether you have diabetes in pregnancy.

Week 25

Baby:

- The baby's hands are fully developed. With her sense of touch well developed, she spends her time trying to touch everything!
- The spine has developed completely.

Mother:

- Your face looks rounder. The nose may start changing shape and get a little plumper.
- Your skin may darken in various places: neck, abdomen, and around the mouth. Don't worry, this will fade after the baby is born and your skin colour will return to its normal tone.

Week 26

Baby:

- The baby may weigh about 800 grams.
- The skin is becoming less transparent.
- The baby's brain is now registering brain wave activity for sight and hearing.
- Your baby's body still appears lean.

Mother:

- Have you had your tetanus toxoid injection? If not, make sure you start your immunization schedule now.
- Your back will ache a little more as the lumbar curve gets exaggerated due to the growing uterus. Try this simple exercise to relax your back muscles: Stand with your back against the wall, knees slightly bent. As you inhale, press the small of your back against the wall. Exhale and relax your back.
- Do you feel your abdomen tighten and relax at irregular intervals? These painless contractions are called Braxton-Hicks contractions. They help the uterus prepare for labour and birth.

Stretch marks

Between 75–90 per cent of women develop stretch marks to some degree during pregnancy. Stretch marks are the result of the rapid stretching of the abdominal skin associated with rapid growth of the uterus. They first appear as reddish lines, but tend to gradually fade to a lighter colour. The affected areas appear empty and soft to the touch. Stretch marks may start appearing during the sixth or seventh month. Applying moisturizers on the skin may help reduce the amount of stretch marks. Do not waste money on creams and ointments that promise to prevent stretch marks.

Week 27

This week marks the end of the second trimester.

Baby:

- The baby's lungs, liver and immune system are continuing to mature. At 27 weeks, your baby's length would have tripled or even quadrupled from the length she was when you were 12 weeks pregnant.
- The baby's skin is still wrinkled and red. As more fat gets deposited under the skin, it will start to slowly even out the skin texture.
- Your baby's eyelashes are developing. The hair on the head is getting thicker and more prominent.

Mother:

- You will gain weight more rapidly now. Make sure you do not put on more than one to two kilos per month.
- You may find yourself short of breath at times. That's because the growing baby is pushing your diaphragm upwards and against your ribs. This reduces the space available for the lungs to expand.
- Your baby has plenty of amniotic fluid to swim in—this fluid cushions him well. You will be able to see parts of your baby move around in your abdomen, as he pushes against your body!

The role of the father-to-be

The second trimester is the good part of pregnancy. Your wife feels energetic and is able to carry on all her work. The size of the pregnancy is still manageable and she is not very uncomfortable yet. Her appetite is back to normal.

How can you help?

Make sure your wife gets a healthy, nutritious diet. At the same time, do not get carried away and force her to eat so much that she puts on unnecessary weight. If you insist on overfeeding her, the excess weight gain may leave you, at the end of the pregnancy, with more wife than you bargained for! Remember that the redundant weight put on during a pregnancy is difficult to get rid off and can be the beginning of lifelong obesity.

She may have leg aches and back pains. Help her exercise by taking time to walk with her. You can also help by massaging her legs and low back.

Make sure that she takes her iron and vitamin supplement everyday.

Old wives' tales

- Lifting your arms over your head can cause the umbilical cord to wrap around the baby's neck. **Not true!**
- Turning from side to side while lying down may cause the baby to suffocate or will cause the cord to wrap around the baby's neck. **Not true!** You do not have to sit up first before you change your position while you are lying down.
- Avoid sex and exercise during pregnancy. **Not true!** Unless you have had a complication for which your obstetrician has asked you to avoid intercourse or exercise, there is no need to avoid sex or exercise.
- If you take iron tablets, your baby will be dark. **Not true!** The baby's genes determine the skin colour, not what you eat or ingest.

CHAPTER 8

The third trimester (28-40 weeks)

Shyamala is feeling so good! She knows she has officially entered the third trimester. It is the final stretch. It is exciting and at the same time, she gets twinges of apprehension. How will labour be? Will her baby cooperate and come into the world easily and without problems? She is getting impatient to see the little one who has taken up residence inside her for the last several months.

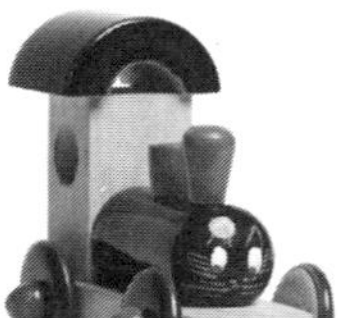

8

The third trimester

It is time to prepare yourself for labour and delivery. It would be wise to start gathering information on the process of labour and delivery. Exercise regularly and keep fit (see **Chapter 11**, *Exercising in pregnancy*). Remember, in a few short months, you will become a mother!

Week 28

Baby:

- Your baby reaches the 1 kilogram (1000 grams) mark!
- His hair is growing thicker and is getting darker.
- The lungs are more mature and if the baby is born now, the lungs are capable of breathing air.
- The baby's eyes are partially open and sensitive to light.
- The surface of the brain, smooth till now, will start developing wrinkles called *sulci* and *gyri*—this is part of the normal development of the brain.

Mother:

- You will feel the baby getting heavier. The lower back starts feeling uncomfortable, especially at the end of the day.
- You may lose a few drops of urine when you cough or sneeze This is quite normal in pregnancy. Make sure you learn Kegel's exercises to make your pelvic muscles supple and strong.
- Have you been tested for diabetes in pregnancy? If not, you should be getting the test done now.
- If you are Rh negative and your husband is Rh positive, your obstetrician may suggest that you take an injection now to prevent any problems for the baby. The injection at this stage is optional but if your baby is born as Rh positive, you definitely need to take the injection after birth (see **Chapter 39**, *The Rh factor: how it can affect pregnancy*).

Kegel's exercises

Kegel's is a specific type of exercise for the muscles that support the rectum, vagina and the urethra. Pregnant women who perform Kegel's exercises may find they have an easier birth. Strengthening these muscles during pregnancy can help you develop the ability to control your muscles during labour and delivery.

To learn how to contract the right muscles, try to stop the flow of urine when you are urinating. Do this several times. Once you know how to squeeze the muscles to stop the flow of urine, you know how to contract the right muscles.

You can then start doing these exercises, anytime, anywhere, while you are sitting down. You can squeeze the pelvic muscles at least 20–30 repetitions at a time, at least three times a day. Make sure you empty your bladder before doing the exercises. Check with your obstetrician, if you are not sure how to do them.

Week 29

Baby:

- You will find the baby tucking herself under your ribs. Sometimes, you might experience pain under the ribs on the right side—this is because the baby is pushing against your liver. Just push her away gently.
- You will find plenty of movements and kicks—she is building her muscles by moving around.
- She will now be in the classic 'foetal position': In this position, her back is curved, the head is bowed, and her arms and legs are bent and drawn up to the front of her body.
- The bone marrow has now completely taken over production of red blood cells.

Mother:

- Your breasts may feel heavy. The nipples and the area around them (areolae) become larger and are deeply pigmented. You might feel small bumps on the areolae—this is normal. Some women will notice a clear discharge from the breast. This is common and just a sign that the breasts are getting ready for breastfeeding.
- You may start being bothered by cramping of the calf muscles. It is not unusual to wake up in the night with severe pain when the calf muscle gets stiff and knotted. The best way to relieve the cramping is to grasp

your toes and flex your foot up towards your knee. The pain may seem to get aggravated for a few seconds but then the calf muscle will relax. Your husband can also do this for you.

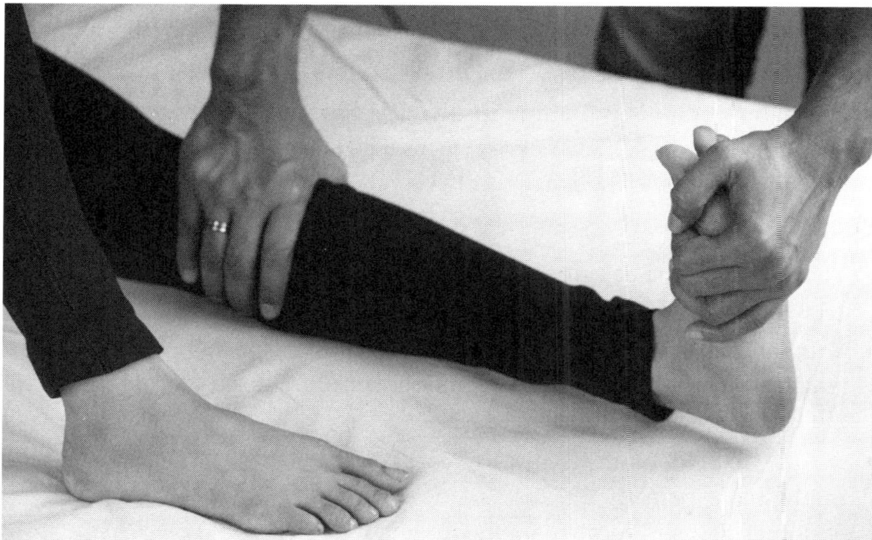

- Acidity and heartburn become more common now. Take an antacid if you need to. Do not lie down for at least 2 hours after a meal.
- Are you regular with your iron supplement? Remember that the iron you get from your diet alone is insufficient to prevent anaemia.
- You may not be able to sleep too well. This is common—your body is preparing itself for the sleepless nights after the baby is born! Make sure you have magazines and books (or your tablet device!) to take to bed so that you have something to do when you are unable to sleep at night.
- You might feel your uterus tightening on and off. When you place your hand on your belly at that time, it may feel very hard. These painless contractions are called Braxton-Hicks contractions and are just preparing your uterus for childbirth.

Supine hypotension

When you lie on your back, the enlarged uterus causes pressure on the large blood vessels (vena cava and aorta) in your body. This causes your blood pressure to fall and you may feel dizzy and nauseous. To avoid this, try to sleep on your sides. If you have back pain and it feels comfortable to sleep on your back, you can do that for short periods of time.

Week 30

Baby:

- Your baby now weighs about 1,250 grams.
- Your baby's skin is getting smooth though some wrinkles still remain.
- The downy hair over the body (lanugo) is starting to disappear.
- The baby's brain is growing rapidly, developing hundreds of billions of new nerve cells. No new nerve cells will be added after birth, though the brain will not reach full size until your child is 5 years old.

Mother:

- Your antenatal check-ups will become more frequent now. You will be seen every two weeks from now on.
- You may start to feel heaviness and discomfort in the vaginal area. When you sit down and get up, there may be a pulling sensation in that area. All this is normal.
- As the weight of the baby increases, you might have pain in the lower sides of the abdomen. This is because the ligaments that hold the uterus in place (called the 'round ligaments') get stretched. You will get relief by lying down on your side, on the same side as the pain.

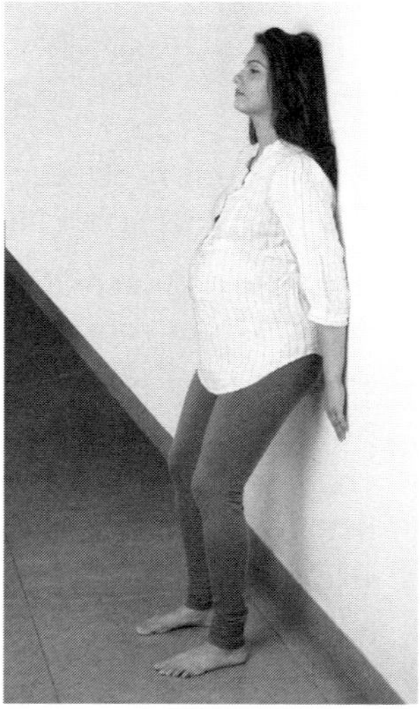

- The nagging low back pain gets worse. This is because of the exaggeration of the normal curve of the lower back. Prenatal exercises will relieve the pain so don't stop your exercises. A quick tip to relieve low back pain: Stand with your back against a wall, your feet about 10–12 inches from the wall. Press the lower part of your back against the wall. Hold for a count of 10. Release and repeat 10 times.

Week 31

Baby:

- As the baby gets more padded with fat, her skin goes from deep red to pink.
- The eyelids open on and off.
- She has plenty of hair on her head.

Water retention

You will retain a large amount of water as your pregnancy progresses. By the time you are ready to deliver, there will be 3.5 litres of water in the baby, placenta and the amniotic fluid around the baby. You will accumulate another 2.5–3 litres in your uterus, breasts and blood. So by the end of a pregnancy, you would have about 6.5 litres of extra water in your body!

Your feet will swell up by the end of the day because there is about one litre of water in your legs. All this fluid gravitates down through the day. After you lie down, the swelling will decrease.

- Do you feel your baby jump when there is a loud noise near you? That is the 'startle reflex' that the baby will continue to have even after he is born. Some babies even respond and move a great deal when they hear music!

Mother:

- Your gait might be getting altered. Your centre of gravity changes because of the protuberant stomach. You may find that you start walking with your legs a little wider apart to keep your balance. Women who have been fairly active and athletic till now may not find it that difficult.
- The hormones produced in pregnancy cause the relaxation of the joints between the bones in your pelvic area. This relaxation will cause you to waddle. The back pain can get worse as the pregnancy progresses.
- Finding a comfortable position to sleep in can be difficult. Try lying on your side with pillows to support the uterus and a pillow between your knees. If you want to sleep on your back, keep one knee or both knees bent. This will relieve the pressure on the low back.

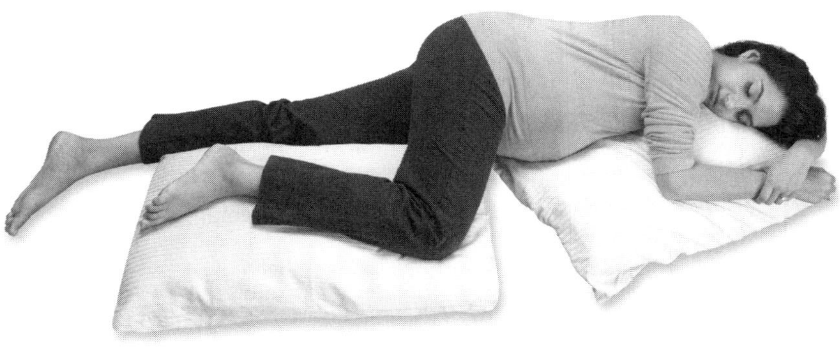

Martina asked: I have itching all over my body. It started over my stomach but now has spread over my arms and legs. I just can't stop scratching!

My answer: Itching after the 7th month is fairly common and is usually mild. Some women have severe, incessant itching and it can be quite disturbing. The rashes may be all over the body but are usually worst over the abdomen and the extremities. This is called PUPPP (pruritic urticarial patches and plaques of pregnancy). It is treated with moisturizers, local steroid creams or if really bad, oral steroid tablets. It does not harm the baby in any way. The most important thing to remember is that scratching makes the condition worse. Apply powder containing boric acid. Moisturizers also help. The good thing is that the rashes and itching disappear after the birth of the baby.

Week 32

Baby:

- Your baby is starting to fill out and probably weighs around 1,700 grams, the size of a watermelon!
- From this point on, your baby's weight will increase faster than the length.
- As your baby continues to grow, her movements will become more frequent and vigorous. Some of your baby's kicks may actually be painful! Quite often, the little one will kick against your bladder and you might get a sudden urge to pass urine.

Mother:

- Getting nervous and anxious? Remember that every mother-to-be, especially a first time one, worries about the baby and the coming labour. Prepare yourself by reading about labour and delivery and by attending labour preparation classes.

Back pain

If you have to stand for a long time, place one foot on a low stool. Sit on chairs with good back support (take a small cushion to office as support for your low back, if you have to sit for a long time at work). Apply a hot water bottle or ice pack to the painful area. Ask your husband to massage your back. Ask your obstetrician whether you can take a paracetamol or ibuprofen tablet for pain relief.

If the back pain is intense and is accompanied by spotting or bleeding or profuse white discharge, contact your obstetrician.

- The baby will still be tumbling around in your uterus. She may not get into a head-down position for another week or two. Sadly for you, your baby loves to be up and partying at night, just when you want to get a good night's sleep!
- If you are carrying twins, your uterus is already as large as if you were full term with a single baby.

Week 33

Baby:

- Iron is being stored in the baby's liver.
- If it is a boy, his testicles have descended partially into the scrotum.
- Your baby may practice breathing by moving her diaphragm in a rhythmic movement. This can actually be seen on an ultrasound scan.
- The waxy layer of vernix covering the skin gets thicker now.

Hiccups

Do you feel repeated, rhythmic taps or thumps in one particular point in your abdomen, lasting for a few minutes? You will wonder why your baby is moving in such a funny manner. Well, that's your baby having hiccups! This is common and she will continue to have them even after she is born.

Mother:

- You might feel breathless most of the time as the uterus pushes your diaphragm up and that, in turn, compresses the lungs.
- You may be urinating more often. As the baby pushes against your bladder, you might get up more often in the night to go to the toilet.
- Pressure on the bowels may cause you to have frequent or irregular bowel movements. Avoid constipation by taking fibre-rich food and drinking plenty of fluids.
- Start planning for what you will need to do when you go into labour. Start buying the things that you need for the newborn baby to avoid the last minute rush. See the section on What to take to the hospital for childbirth in **Chapter 17**, *Preparing to go to the hospital*.

Week 34

Baby:

- Your baby weighs about 2 kilos by now. You can really feel the weight at the lower part of your abdomen and your back will also feel the strain.

- Your baby's nails are long enough to reach to the tip of the fingers or beyond. When she is born, the nails might be long and she might even scratch herself, and may require the first nail trimming soon after birth!
- If you are carrying twins, they will probably be in the position now that they will stay in until birth. A single baby may still change his position, though not so frequently.
- If for any reason your baby is born now, he has a good chance of survival. His lungs are reasonably mature and he may be able to breathe on his own.

Repeat ultrasound scan

Your obstetrician might want another ultrasound scan done around 34 weeks. This is particularly important in women who have diabetes or high blood pressure in pregnancy. In case your doctor suspects that your baby is not growing well enough or is larger than expected, a scan may be ordered. If you have twins, this is a good time to assess whether they are growing well or not.

Mother:

- Do you know how to recognize when labour has started? Read about it in **Chapter 19**, *Labour and delivery*, and attend labour preparation classes.
- Make sure you keep up with your walking and exercise regimen. Keeping fit is particularly important at this point.
- Have you noticed some tingling, numbness, and pain in the hands? These symptoms can be common during pregnancy, especially in the last trimester. This is commonly caused by **carpal tunnel syndrome**, and the symptoms usually go away after pregnancy. The water retention in pregnancy can cause pressure on the nerves in the arm and result in this problem. Resting the joint and a wrist splint will usually reduce the pain and tingling.

Sarayu asked: I am 34 weeks pregnant now. Should I quit work?

My answer: Continue to work for as long as you can. The physical activity is useful for you. Moreover, don't squander away your maternity leave. Save your leave to stay at home after the baby is born and not before.

Week 35

Baby:

> **Preterm or premature labour**
>
> If pains start or the water breaks before 37 weeks, it is called premature or preterm labour. You should be aware of the warning signs. Learn what to look out for in **Chapter 32**, *When the baby comes too early: preterm labour and birth.*

- Your baby is moving into the head-down position. This means that the head will be closest to the birth canal (vagina) and the baby's bottom is near your diaphragm. 95 per cent of babies will get into the head down position before birth. 4 per cent will remain with their bottom closest to the birth canal and they are called breech (see **Chapter 35**, *Breech delivery*). Another 1 per cent will be in other positions that may make it difficult for a normal delivery.
- The character of movements is changing—instead of kicks, the baby will roll and wriggle. This is because, as she continues to grow and fill up the uterus, the space around her is getting cramped.
- The fat deposition all over the body continues and the baby is starting to look plump now.

Mother:

- You are starting to feel tired and want to rest more often.
- The pressure in your pelvic area is increasing. When you walk, you might feel the weight in your vagina. You may need to support yourself when you get up after sitting for a while.
- Do you feel that the front of your thighs are numb? The enlarged uterus is pressing on some nerves in the pelvis and so you lose sensation over the front of the thighs. This will get back to normal a few weeks after delivery.

Week 36

Baby:

- Your baby's face is getting rounder now. With more fat being deposited under the skin, the baby starts to have chubby cheeks. This 'buccal pad' of fat helps the baby suckle at the mother's breast after biirth.
- The baby's head is finding its way into the birth canal.
- The movements are not so vigorous now.

Mother:

- You will start your weekly check-ups now.
- The baby should have got into its final position by now. You will feel the baby's head finding its way into the birth canal.
- Besides examining your abdomen, your obstetrician may start doing a vaginal examination this week or the next week. This is to assess the condition of your cervix and the position of the baby's head.
- Your uterus has grown to 1,000 times its non-pregnant volume.
- It is important to keep checking to see if the baby is moving well. Though the force of the movements will get less, the baby should move for a minimum of 10–20 times during the day.

Counting your baby's kicks

It is a good idea to keep an eye on your baby's movements from 36 weeks onwards. If you have had a stillbirth before, your doctor may advise you to start counting from 34 weeks. A healthy baby will move well, whereas a baby that is experiencing trouble inside the womb, will move very little.

There are many ways to count the baby's kicks but this is the method I recommend:

From the time you wake up in the morning till 12 noon, you should be able to count at least 10 movements. From 12 noon to 6 in the evening you should be able to count at least another 10 movements. You might feel 10 kicks in a very short period or it may take longer if the baby is sleeping. Once you have counted 10 movements, you can stop counting for that half of the day. If you feel the movements have decreased, lie on your side for an hour. If you feel at least three movements in that hour, then your baby is healthy. If you have not, then it is important for you to go and see your obstetrician immediately.

Most babies are much more active from the evening through the night.

How do you monitor your baby's movements if you are a working woman? In that case I recommend that you track the kicks for an hour at a time: for example between 10 and 11 am, 2 and 3 pm and 5 and 6 pm. If you feel at least 3 kicks in each observed hour, the baby is fine.

Week 37

Baby:

- At the end of the 37th week, your little one crosses over from being preterm to being called a 'term baby'. This means that your baby can survive comfortably if born now.

- The waxy white coating over the baby's skin starts decreasing as the baby matures. If the baby is born now, you will still find it over the scalp and in the creases of the joints.
- As the baby occupies more and more space, the movements become less vigorous. Keep counting the movements to ensure the baby is healthy.

Mother:

- Once you have completed 37 weeks of pregnancy, you are considered to be 'full term'. If you deliver your baby before 37 weeks, the baby is considered 'premature'.
- The pressure on your ribs may have eased off considerably now. This is called 'lightening' because the baby's head has dropped into the birth canal. The older women in your house might point out that the abdomen has 'dropped'!
- The mucus or watery discharge from your vagina will increase since the cervix has started to open up a little.
- Learn what the signs of labour are (see **Chapter 19**, *Labour and delivery*).
- Check with your obstetrician what her protocols are for admission to the hospital. If your doctor's clinic is not in the hospital you are going to deliver in, make it a point to visit the hospital. This will give you a sense of familiarity and comfort.
- Have you attended a labour preparation class yet?
- If you are keen on having epidural analgesia, now is a good time to discuss it with your obstetrician. (see **Chapter 22**, *Pain relief in labour and delivery*).

Pranathi asked: The baby seems to have dropped lower in my abdomen. My mother says I will have the baby very soon. Is that true?

My answer: Actually, you cannot predict when labour is going to start just based on when your baby drops into the pelvis. If this is your first pregnancy, the baby's head can drop anywhere from 2–4 weeks before delivery. In women who have already had children, the baby may not drop until labour begins. You may or may not notice a change in the shape of your abdomen. However, you may notice that you are able to breathe much easier and heartburn may ease a bit. On the other hand, the baby's head may press on your bladder and make you want to run to the bathroom more often.

Week 38

Baby:

- The baby has been putting on weight rapidly and now weighs between 2,500–2,900 grams on an average.
- The downy hair over the body (lanugo) is almost gone.
- The baby is plump because of a good deposition of fat under the skin.

Mother:

- You might have frequent false pains. False pains are irregular, more over the low back and do not progress in frequency and intensity. These pains are caused by the thinning out (effacement) and slight opening out (dilatation) of the cervix in preparation for labour. Learn how to differentiate between false pains and real pains in **Chapter 19**, *Labour and delivery*.
- You can be as active as you want to be. You will feel tired more often, so rest whenever you get the time.
- Your obstetrician will do an internal examination to find out how your cervix is preparing for labour and also if the baby's head has dropped into the birth canal. If this is your first baby, the head will usually be in the birth canal by now. If it has not dropped in, do not worry; some babies drop in once labour has started. If you have already had a baby or babies before, the head might not drop in till labour starts.

Week 39

Baby:

- Your baby is preparing for life outside the uterus. He will have plenty of breathing movements—pushing his little chest in and out.
- He might weigh between 2,700–3,000 grams on an average. An Indian baby is considered large if he weighs 3,500 grams or more.

Mother:

- The last weeks are the toughest to get through. Everybody will call to find out if you have delivered the baby yet!
- You might not want to do much since the uterus is so stretched out and you are really uncomfortable.
- Be sure to have all your stuff packed and ready to take to the hospital (see the suggested list of things to take to the hospital in **Chapter 17**, *Preparing to go to the hospital*).

Week 40

Baby:

- Your baby is fully mature to face life outside the womb. All her vital organs are ready to function.
- The baby's bowels are filled with meconium, a greenish black stool that will be the first motion that the baby passes.
- Though most of the lanugo hair is gone, the baby may still be born with downy hair over the forehead, on top of the ears and over the shoulders.
- The waxy coating of vernix on her skin is almost all gone.

Mother:

- The days are dragging! Though you may be a little apprehensive about labour, you wish it would just be over with.
- Remember that most babies are born a week before or after the due date. Only 5 per cent of babies are born on the exact due date.
- Your obstetrician will make sure the baby is doing well inside. She might want to wait till 41 weeks to induce labour (see **Chapter 33**, *When the baby is overdue: the postterm pregnancy*).

Travelling for your delivery

If you are going to your mother's house for delivery, do not postpone travelling till too late. If you are working or your first child is going to school and you want to travel as late as possible, remember that the optimum time to travel would be about six weeks before your due date i.e. 34 weeks. Check with your doctor if there is any condition that may require you to go to your new obstetrician earlier than that. It is in the last six weeks that the majority of complications can occur so it is safer to get to wherever you are going before that. This also gives you enough time to build a rapport with the doctor who is going to deliver you.

The role of the father-to-be

The third trimester can be as stressful for you as it is for her. You might be worried about how she is going to handle labour. The responsibility of having to make sure that she reaches the hospital on time weighs heavily on you. You will need to make all the arrangements at home to ensure smooth admission to the hospital. The reality that a new life with her own demands is entering your life is just about sinking in.

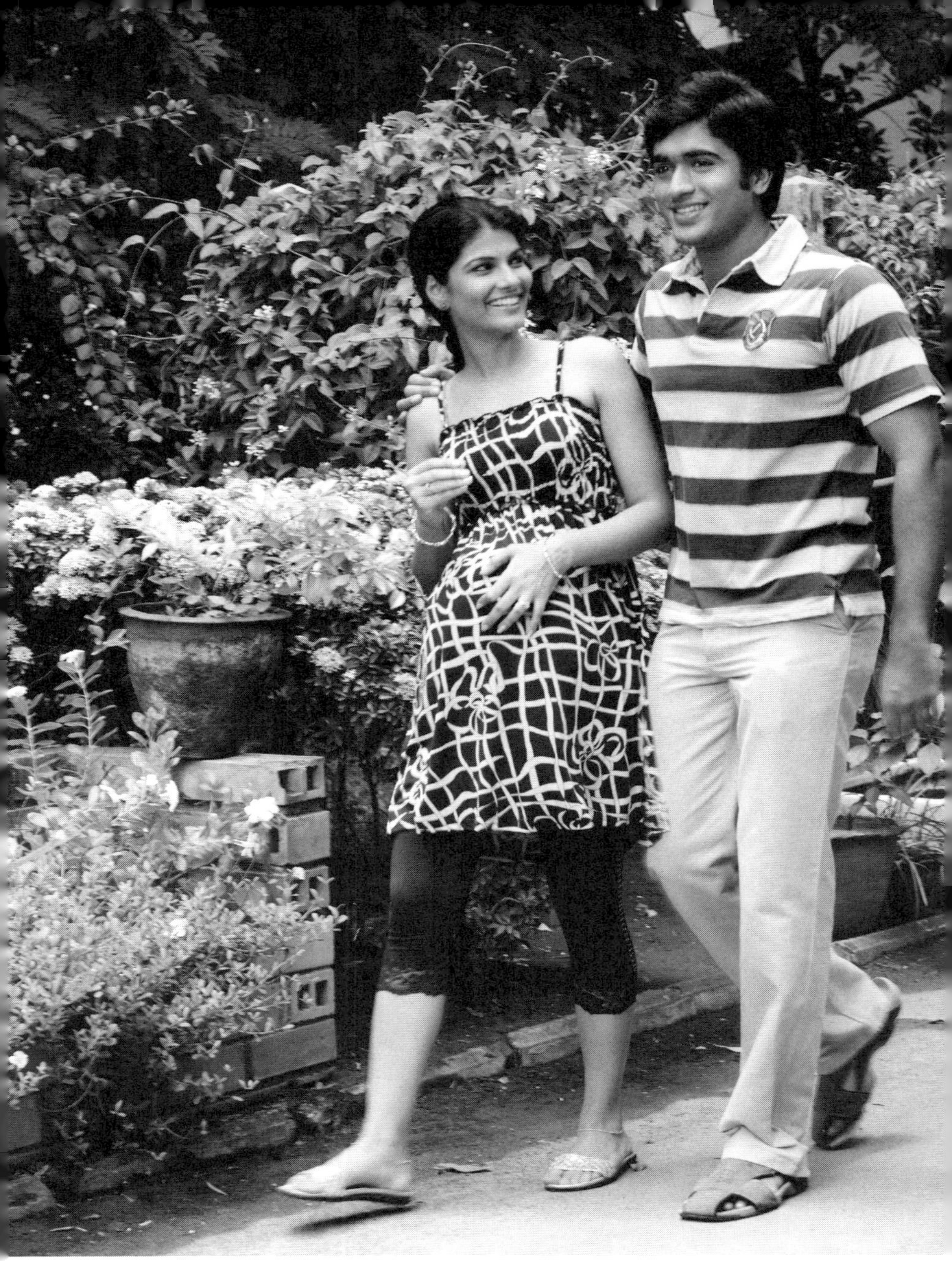

How can you help?

Be prepared for labour by reading about it and also by attending labour preparation classes with your wife. Talk to the obstetrician and request that you should be allowed into the labour room to provide comfort and support during labour. Apart from being there with your wife when she is at her most vulnerable, seeing your baby born before your eyes can be one of the most miraculous experiences in your life.

Be prepared for the eventuality of a caesarean. Nearly 20–25 per cent of pregnant women may end up having a caesarean section. In some hospitals, the rate of caesarean may be much higher. Make sure you have already discussed with your obstetrician what your wife will undergo if she needs a caesarean section. If an elective caesarean section has been planned and blood is being reserved as is usually done, you can make arrangements for blood donors from your circle of friends or relatives.

As a husband, you may have eagerly waited to play a part in the birth of your baby. When you learn that your wife will be undergoing a caesarean section, you may at first feel a little cheated that you are not able to be in the labour room participating in the birth of the baby. Don't worry. There will be plenty of opportunities to participate in the bringing up of your baby.

Bond with your baby

Make sure that you are allowed to hold the baby as soon as possible after birth. This strengthens the bond between you and your newborn. It is important to cuddle your baby so that he can recognize and become familiar with your feel and touch.

Never forget: all babies need their dad as much as they need their mother!

Old wives' tales

- You should not travel in the 'even' months of pregnancy i.e. 6th month or 8th month. **Not true!**
- Avoid sleeping on your back or, always sleep on your left side. **Not true!** For normal, healthy women in an uncomplicated pregnancy, the best position for sleeping is the one that's most comfortable.
- You must have regular intercourse to have a normal vaginal delivery. **Not true!** Though there is no reason to avoid intercourse, you may feel uncomfortable closer to term so you may not want to have sex. This will not prevent you from having a normal vaginal delivery.
- You should eat well when labour starts because you will not be given food for another few hours. **False!** It is very important that you do not eat or drink anything once the water breaks or pains start. Wait for the doctor's instructions.

CHAPTER 9

The role of the father-to-be

Pregnancy is replete with changes. The physical and emotional changes that occur in the pregnant woman can leave her partner bewildered and sometimes a little worried. To truly enjoy the pregnancy, it is important for the father-to-be to have a complete understanding of the process and the innumerable adjustments needed.

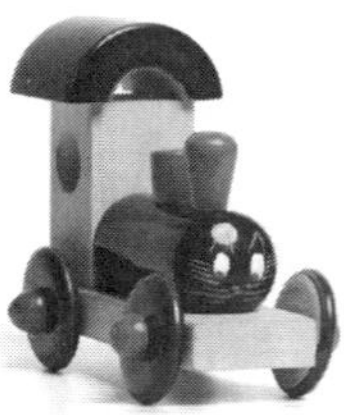

9

The role of the father-to-be

The days are long past when women usually came for their obstetric consultation with only their mother or another female relative. Even a decade or two ago, it was uncommon to see a husband accompany his wife for an antenatal check-up! Nowadays, husbands are very involved with the pregnancy right from the beginning. There is also a commitment and desire to be in the labour room to provide emotional support. Today, the majority of women come for their consultation with their husbands and this is how it should be.

It is heartening to see husbands getting involved right from the time the pregnancy test comes back as positive. They go for antenatal appointments with their wives, and attend classes for labour preparation. At the same time, they may be filled with anxiety about their ability to handle the pregnancy and its demands on their feelings.

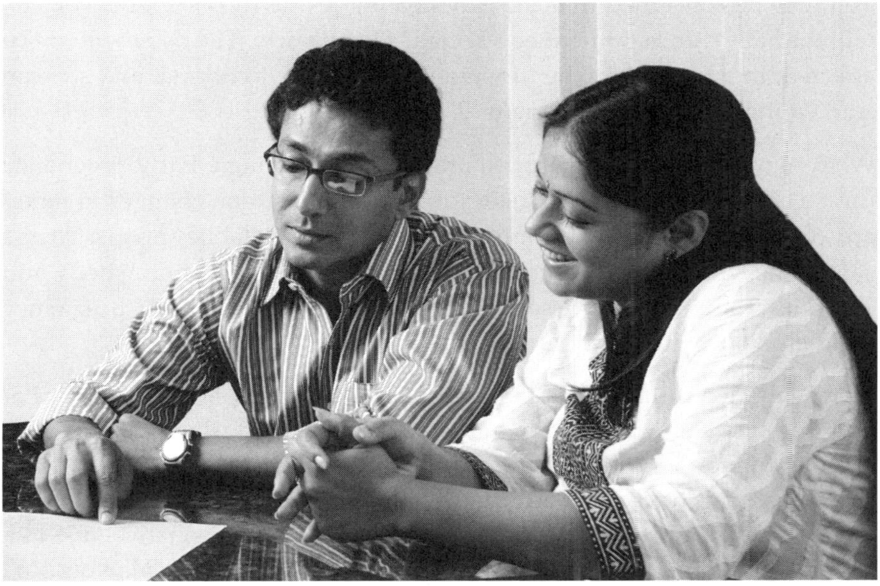

The father is important too

Children need their fathers as much as their mothers. A man's role as a father can begin long before the baby is born. A supportive husband can make his wife's pregnancy easier and healthier. There is no doubt that labour and delivery is easier and shorter for women whose husbands actively participate in the process.

A husband's role during labour and birth is to provide emotional support and to comfort his wife. Being part of the child's birth is a significant and incomparable experience.

The birth of your child is such an intense emotional experience that the significance doubles when the couple shares it.

Support in early pregnancy

> A husband who pitches in and let's his wife sleep a little longer, is worth his weight in gold!

Early in pregnancy your wife may feel tired, may need more sleep, urinate frequently and have sore breasts. Nausea and vomiting are quite common. Although it is known as 'morning sickness,' it can occur at any time of the day or night. Your support is important at this time. Try to spend as much time as you can with her. Take over some household chores so that she can sleep a little longer.

You may be concerned that she is not eating properly. If she does not eat, will the baby's development be affected? Don't worry. The baby will not be affected. In a few weeks, her appetite will be back to normal and she can start eating nutritious food again.

What may catch you by surprise are her mood swings! Early pregnancy can be an emotional roller-coaster for a woman. Sudden changes in mood are common. You may feel hurt and upset by her labile moods. At the same time, you may feel left out as she focusses on her changing body and emotions. Knowing that these changes are a natural part of early pregnancy will help you to support your wife and deal with her feelings.

These emotional upheavals may tempt you to spend less time with her and this may just worsen the situation. How do you deal with this? Speak to your friends who have been through a pregnancy. Just realizing that other husbands have also been through this will help ease the stress. If you have a cousin, a brother-in-law, an understanding older relative, just talk with them and get the emotional support you require. After all, you can't be expected to handle this all by yourself. Of course, this phase will pass once your wife learns to deal with the enormous surge of hormones in the first trimester.

Working together towards a healthy lifestyle will benefit you, your wife and your baby. You can both adapt your lifestyles to include a balanced diet and plenty of rest. Since she must stop any use of alcohol and tobacco, this is a good time for you to stop as well. Remember, if your wife inhales tobacco smoke from your smoking, this affects the baby.

Siddharth asked at Mala's booking appointment: We live by ourselves. Her parents are in Mumbai and mine are in Tanjavur. Should I send her to her parents' home? I am worried that I may not be able to take care of her. She is so tired and her vomiting is quite intense.

My answer: What Mala is facing is very normal. Since she is also working, it is doubly difficult. But does she really want to go to her parents' home? You can help her by sharing the household chores. If you can't cook, ask friends and relatives to pitch in with food. The vomiting will be under control with the tablets that will be prescribed. You both will get through these few weeks and then it will get much better! The sharing of all the changes that pregnancy brings about is a great bonding experience.

How can you help?

Just being there for her is an enormous mood elevator for the new mother-to-be. With words and deeds, let her know that you are delighted that she is pregnant. Help her out with housework because she may find it hard to do all the household chores due to the tiredness of early pregnancy.

Make sure that you go to all her antenatal check-ups with her. This will allow you to clear your doubts too. Knowing what is happening with her pregnancy will enable you to be a supportive and comforting husband.

The second trimester (14–28 weeks)

The second trimester is the good part of pregnancy. Your wife is energetic and will be able to carry on with all her work. She is still not very uncomfortable because of the size of the pregnancy. Her appetite is back to normal.

How can you help?

Make sure your wife gets a nutritious diet. At the same time, do not get carried away and force her to eat so much that she puts on unnecessary

Subhash asked: Is it okay for us to have sex? I am afraid that I might hurt her or the baby.

My answer: You are not alone in wondering this. Many couples ask if it is safe to have sex during pregnancy and if intercourse will harm the baby. In most pregnancies, sex is considered safe and healthy. In the first trimester, some women may find that tiredness and nausea turn their thoughts away from sex.

As she starts feeling better, she will be interested again. Your wife's comfort should be the most important guide during sex. As pregnancy advances, have intercourse in positions that do not put pressure on her abdomen, such as with her on top or lying side by side. If you have any concerns about having intercourse during pregnancy, talk to your doctor. If your wife is having bleeding in pregnancy, you might be asked to avoid sex for some time.

weight. If you insist on overfeeding her, the excess weight gain may leave you, at the end of the pregnancy, with more wife than you bargained for! Remember that the redundant weight put on during a pregnancy is difficult to get rid of and can be the beginning of lifelong obesity.

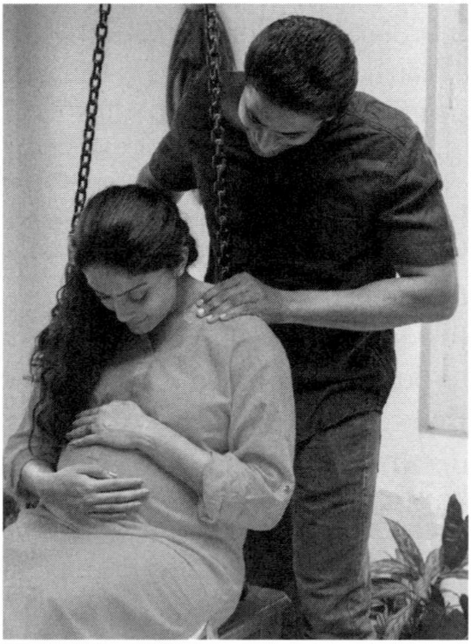

She may have leg aches and back pains. Help her exercise by taking time to walk with her. You can also help by massaging her shoulders, legs and low back.

Make sure that she takes her iron and vitamin supplement everyday.

Make sure to be there for the ultrasound scan

The second trimester is also the time when the targeted scan is done. By this time (20–22 weeks) your baby actually is recognizable on the scan as a tiny human being. With the help of the doctor, you will be able to identify the head, the spine, the arms and legs and you will see the little one kicking around. The most exciting part is watching the baby's heart beating away. This is an experience you should not miss out on! You will feel an intense bonding with your unborn child as you watch the scan.

After the third month (when your wife's energy levels are back to normal) and till the 8th month (when she should start getting prepared for labour), plan short weekend trips to nearby destinations. If you were thinking of a longer holiday, go ahead. Spend as much time together as possible. Once the baby is born, it can be quite a while before you can take a care-free holiday.

The third trimester (29 weeks to delivery)

The third trimester can be as stressful for you as it is for her. You might be worried about how she will handle labour. The reality of having a new baby is also sinking in.

How can you help?

Be prepared for labour by reading about it and by attending labour preparation classes with your wife. Have a checklist and make sure you are prepared when she goes into labour.

- Know the phone numbers of the hospital and the doctor and keep them handy
- Keep a packed suitcase to take to hospital (see **Chapter 17**, *Preparing to go to the hospital*)
- Make sure there is somebody who can take her to the hospital if she goes into labour when you are not around
- Do trial runs to see how long it takes to get to the hospital
- Make sure you always have fuel in the car!
- If you are going to use a call taxi, keep that number handy

Being in the labour room

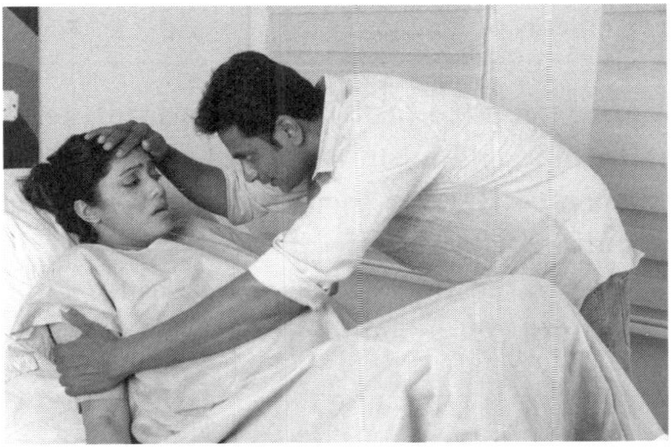

Talk to the obstetrician and request to be allowed into the labour room. Seeing your baby born before your eyes can be one of the most rewarding experiences of your life.

What if it is a caesarean?

The best way to minimize the chances of a caesarean section is to choose a doctor and hospital that has a reputation for low caesarean rates. However, you should be prepared for the eventuality of a caesarean. Nearly 20–25 per cent of pregnant women (and in some hospitals much more) may end up having a caesarean section. Make sure you have already discussed with your obstetrician what your wife will undergo if she needs a caesarean section. If your wife is undergoing a planned caesarean section for some reason, and blood is being reserved as is usually done, you can make arrangements for blood donors from your circle of friends or relatives.

As a husband, you may have eagerly waited to play a part in the birth of your baby. When you learn that your wife will be undergoing a caesarean section, you may at first feel a little cheated that you are not able to be in the labour room participating in the birth of the baby. Don't worry. You can provide emotional support for your wife after the baby is born, for there will be plenty of opportunities to participate in the bringing up of your baby.

Virendar asked: I really want to be in the labour room with my wife but my friends and family are discouraging me saying that I will not be able to handle seeing my wife in so much pain. They also tried to scare me that I will faint during the delivery. What do you think, doc?

My answer: The moral support that you can provide for your wife in labour is irreplaceable. I started practice in 1981 and we have had husbands in the labour room ever since. When the actual delivery actually happens, you only need to be near the head-end of the labour table, supporting her head and encouraging her to push. For me the most moving moment in the labour room is the quiet joy when the couple holds their baby and realizes that they have become parents. I strongly urge you to participate in the miracle of your baby's birth. When your wife can withstand the actual pain of labour, you will certainly be able to!

Being prepared for labour and delivery

Attending childbirth and labour preparation classes are quite helpful for husbands. It gives them a better understanding of the process. Understanding what your wife will be facing through labour and delivery gives you the ability to be able to better support and assist her through the travails of labour and delivery.

More than anything, a labour preparation class gives you the confidence to go through the childbirth experience. Many men are apprehensive that they may not be able to see their wife suffer. They are afraid they may not be able to handle the processes involved inside the labour room. If you are anxious and hesitant, attending the class will lay most of your fears to rest. You will feel more confident after seeing other men also participating in the classes.

Planning to be there for the delivery?

It is common for a woman to go to her mother's home for her delivery. What if you are in another city? How do you coordinate it so that you can get leave from your job and be with your wife for her delivery? This can be tricky.
It is difficult for your doctor to predict the exact date of delivery. Usually, if everything is going well, babies deliver between 37 and 40 weeks. If things are going as planned, you could schedule your leave to be with your wife in the last two weeks of pregnancy. Of course, babies are notorious for not sticking to the plans that we make! If you miss the delivery because your little one was in a hurry to come out, try to get to her side as soon as possible. You should not miss the first few days of your baby's life, a time when your wife also needs your support.

It is normal to be nervous!

Did you know that most husbands may be apprehensive about taking their wife through labour? You are not alone in that. This is a very normal and human reaction.

Your family may be worried that you might not be able to handle the sight of blood and other body fluids in the labour room. Do not worry. When your wife is in labour and when she is going to deliver, you will be so involved with encouraging her and giving her moral support that you will forget about everything else.

Remember that most of the times, you will be sitting or standing near your wife's head. You can turn your eyes away from anything else that is going on and only concentrate on talking your wife through her pains. Usually a chair or stool will be provided for you to be comfortably seated while you talk to your wife.

If a problem arises, you may be asked to leave the delivery room. In the best interest of the mother and baby, you should leave right away if asked.

Bond with your baby

Make sure you are allowed to hold the baby as soon as possible after the birth. This strengthens the bond between you and your newborn. It is important to cuddle your baby so that she can recognize your feel and touch.

After the baby's birth

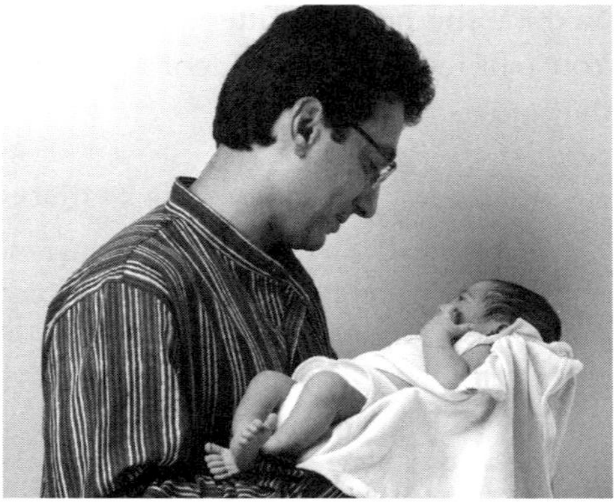
Never forget: all babies need their father as much as they need their mother.

The first six weeks after birth are considered the postpartum period. During this time, your wife's body again goes through dramatic changes as it recovers from the physical stress of pregnancy and birth. She will have some bleeding, for 4–6 weeks (see **Chapter 26**, *Taking care of yourself after birth*). If she has had an episiotomy, she may have pain and discomfort from the stitches. Her breasts may be sore. She may be anxious about breastfeeding and may worry whether the baby is getting enough milk.

If the baby was born by caesarean birth, the incision on the abdomen may be uncomfortable. It will take time for her to regain her usual strength.

How can you help?

If you do not have other family members to help out, the postpartum period can sometimes be overwhelming. New parents are often nervous about taking care of the newborn. It is important to maintain a sense of humour at this time to help both of you cope with the demands of your new baby.

Do not be afraid to take care of your baby. Bond with your newborn by changing diapers, bathing the baby and rocking him to sleep. Learn how to bathe the baby in the section on 'Giving baby a bath', **Chapter 42**, *Your new baby*. If you have older children at home, spend extra time with them to help them get used to being big brother or sister. By sharing the care of the baby with your wife, you will provide the support she needs and at the same time, gain confidence in your own parenting skills.

'Postpartum blues' is a term used when new mothers feel sad, afraid or anxious after childbirth. Most new mothers experience these feelings in a mild form. When these feelings are extreme and last longer, however, they signal a more serious condition called postpartum depression. **Postpartum depression** may require counselling and treatment.

Resuming intercourse after delivery

After a vaginal delivery or a caesarean section, it is usually safe to resume intercourse six weeks after birth. By that time, your wife would have had her postnatal check-up and her obstetrician would have made sure she has healed well. Your wife may be a little apprehensive about pain the first few times and it is important to make sure she is comfortable.

Remember that even if a woman is not having a period or is breastfeeding, she can become pregnant. Birth control should be used when you resume intercourse. Talk to your obstetrician about the safest and most suitable birth control option (see **Chapter 49**, *Methods of birth control*).

To-do list for dad

Pack a bag

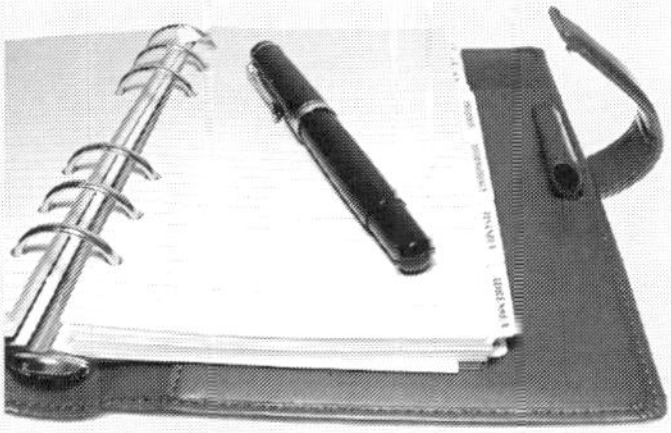

You may think you have all the time in the world to do this. Suddenly, your wife is in labour and you both have not completed putting together the hospital bag. Take time to discuss with your wife what she needs to take to the hospital (see the suggested list 'What to take to the hospital' in **Chapter 17**, *Preparing to go to the hospital*). Keep a suitcase handy in which you can pack all the essentials. As you buy things for the baby or for the delivery, keep placing them in the bag. Keep this bag in a convenient and prominent place so that you won't forget to take it when the time comes to go to the hospital.

Insurance and hospital payments

Do you have medical insurance? Find out if they will pay for pregnancy and pregnancy-related procedures. Check with the hospital whether they will accept payment by cash only, cheques or credit card.

Names for the baby

Shortlisting names for the baby can be fun. You have several months to decide but don't put it off for too long. Even when you think you have found the perfect name, you may change it as soon as you see your brand new baby. And please, choose names for both a boy and a girl! See the **For You** section in this book.

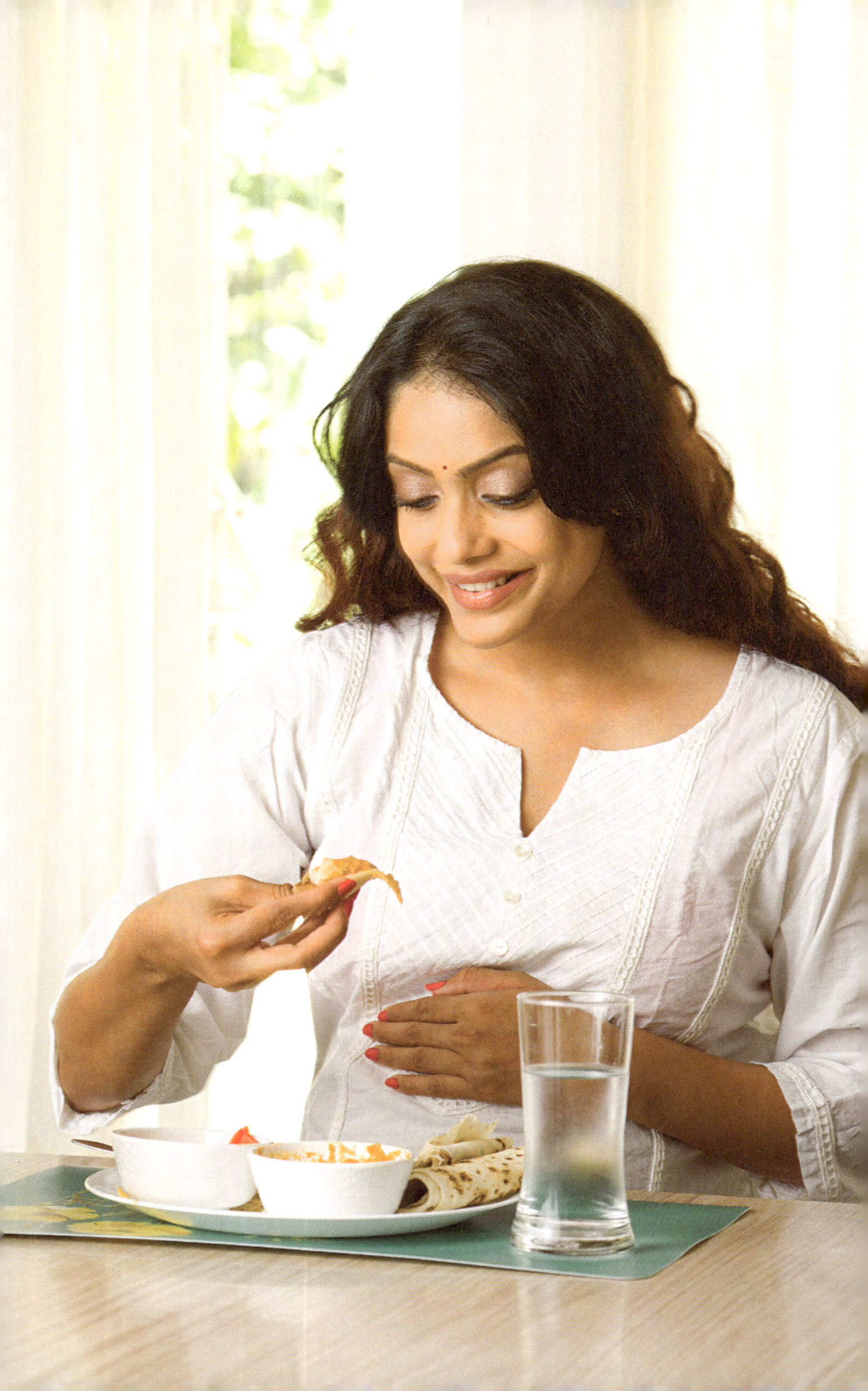

Taking care of yourself

CHAPTER 10

Eating healthy in pregnancy

Seetha is pregnant! She is excited and happy as she tells her family the wonderful news. There are smiles and an occasional tear of happiness as the news sinks in. The first reaction to the news is, 'Now you must take good care of yourself. You must eat for two, sleep well and be happy!' But does she really need to eat for two?

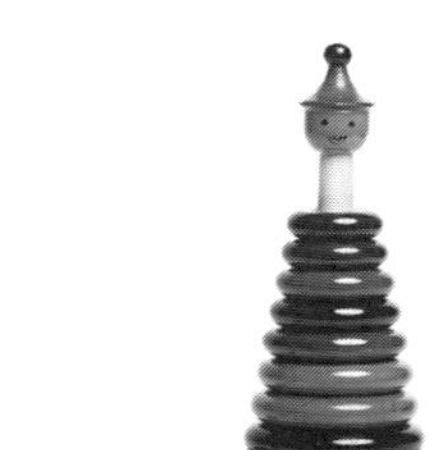

10

Eating healthy in pregnancy

There is no doubt that you definitely want the best for the little one growing inside you. You want to give your baby the optimal nutrition to ensure that her body and, equally importantly her brain, grow to their best possible potential. What you eat shapes the baby's future to a large extent.

Good nutrition also helps a woman's body prepare for motherhood. You need the right diet to help you deal with the increased demands of your body in pregnancy. The complex processes that occur during pregnancy require a rich supply of protein, vitamins and minerals not only for the baby but also for you. After you have delivered your little one, your body will need to gear up for feeding and providing proper nutrition for the baby. The foundation of good nutrition that you lay before and during your pregnancy will help enormously with this.

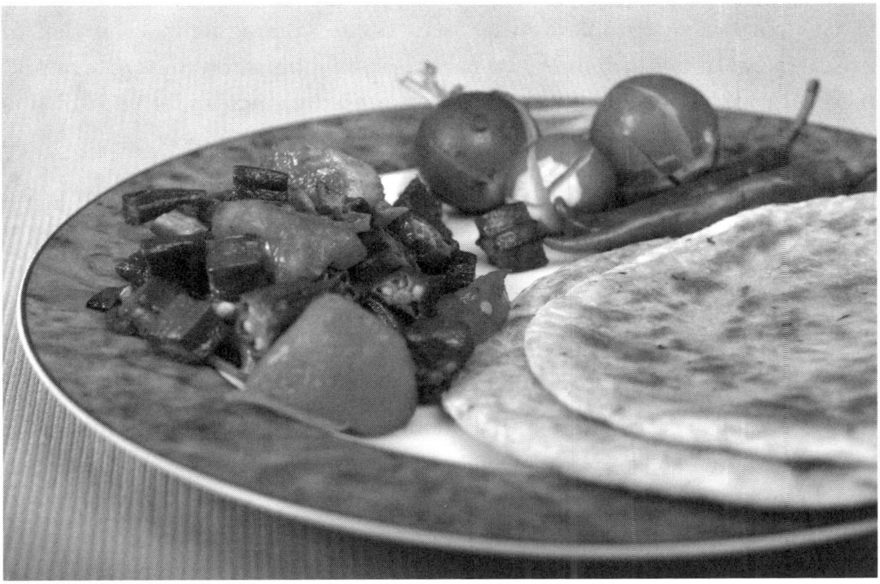

Getting an early start

When is the best time to start eating a healthy diet? The best results for your pregnancy would obviously be if you start paying attention to eating a healthy diet even before you become pregnant. This will ensure that both you and your baby start out with the right balance of nutrients required.

> Eating a balanced diet, rich in nutrients, during your pregnancy is one of the best things you can do for yourself and your baby.

Starting at the optimal weight

If you are underweight: It may be a good idea to start on a healthy diet plan to reach an optimal weight. Underweight women tend to have underweight babies. Add protein and healthy fats to your diet. Get a nutritionist to help you, if possible. Strength training with weights will also increase your muscle mass and will add healthy weight.

Proteins include all the dried beans (for example, rajma, kabuli channa), dairy products (milk, curds, paneer, cheese), eggs and lean meat. Healthy fats include safflower and sunflower oils, cold pressed oils (such as sesame, rice bran, coconut, mustard, and extra-virgin olive oil), butter and ghee, nuts and seeds (including walnuts, almonds, pistachio nuts, cashewnuts and peanuts).

If you are overweight: Being overweight (BMI $\geq$ 25 kg/m^2) puts you at risk for certain problems that may occur in pregnancy. The risk of miscarriage, difficult delivery or caesarean section, preterm delivery and medical problems (diabetes, high blood pressure) increase if your BMI is $\geq$ 30 kg/m^2 at the start of your pregnancy.

Being overweight also means that the baby may be overweight at birth. This not only adds complications at the time of delivery (forceps delivery or caesarean section), it also has an impact on the baby's future health. Overweight babies grow up to be overweight adults and tend to have an increased risk of diabetes, high blood pressure and heart disease.

The most important dietary change would be to decrease your carbohydrate intake. Did you know that Indians eat way too many carbohydrates? If you notice, the average Indian plate will have more rice or chapatis than vegetables and proteins. Reducing your carbohydrates and increasing your intake of vegetables, dals and dairy products will help shed the extra pounds. Healthy fats are fine when combined with protein (omelettes made with butter or olive oil); they only make you gain weight when they are combined with carbohydrates (rice with ghee).

Adding a healthy exercise regimen to your daily routine will also help you attain your weight goal.

The importance of folic acid

If you are planning a pregnancy, it would be a good idea to start taking a daily supplement of **folic acid**. This vitamin prevents certain spinal defects called neural tube defects, that can lead to disability in the baby. A healthy level of folic acid in your body, *before* you get pregnant, can prevent this.

> Folic acid supplements should contain at least 0.4 mg (400 mcg) of folic acid. Many brands contain up to 5 mg per tablet. Vitamin B-12 is also combined with folic acid in some supplements and is recommended. If a woman has had a previous child with a neural tube defect, she should be on a supplement that contains at least 4 mg of folic acid.

Folic acid is found naturally in green leafy vegetables, citrus fruits or dried lentils. In addition, your doctor will prescribe a folic acid supplement. It is recommended to start this at least 1–3 months before you get pregnant and to continue it for the first three months of the pregnancy.

If you had not started folic acid before you got pregnant, your doctor will prescribe folic acid at your first visit.

A commonly asked question is: 'How do I start the folic acid when I don't know when I will become pregnant?'

Folic acid is also known as the engagement vitamin! We recommend that once you get engaged and are planning a pregnancy, you should start taking folic acid. If you are using some form of birth control method, you should start folic acid 1–3 months before you discontinue birth control. The idea is to have a good level of folic acid in your blood stream when you conceive so that the baby will not have a problem as its organs are forming. If you have not been on folic acid before you became pregnant, you should start it as soon as the pregnancy is confirmed

Do I need to eat for two?

This is a time that is exciting and yet a bit scary. Having a baby means so much more than just carrying around some extra weight for the next nine months. That new life growing inside you will depend on you for

everything he needs, to be healthy and strong, before and after he is born.

The extra 300 calories per day: how can you get them?

2 cups of cow's milk	200 calories
2 medium chapatis with small cup of vegetables	300 calories
100 gm of cooked rice	325 calories
3 idlis with ½ cup of sambar	300 calories
2 small vegetable sandwiches	300 calories
Egg (whole)	75 calories
White of egg	15 calories

Do you really need to eat for two? Not really. The growing baby doesn't 'eat' food! He only absorbs the essential nutrients he requires from the blood circulating through the placenta. In the last six months of a normal pregnancy, you require 300 calories more per day. These 300 calories are really not much in terms of food quantity (see box). There is no need to overeat to achieve this.

Do remember that if you started out overweight, you should check with your doctor on how much weight you need to gain during pregnancy. The extra calories that are recommended are for women who have started out with a weight that is appropriate for their height.

Even women who have been very careful about eating right, even before they became pregnant, tend to get a little lax with their food habits in their pregnancy. 'I'm pregnant, I can eat dessert every day, can't I?' they ask. Their family says, 'Don't deny a pregnant girl, let her eat what she wants.' Unfortunately you may consume more calories than you need. Of course, it is okay to have an ice-cream or a dessert once in a while, but even when you are pregnant, you have to pay attention to whether you are eating healthy.

I don't want to gain too much weight during pregnancy!

Many women today are conscious about their weight. They dread getting out of shape during pregnancy. It is difficult to expend too much energy

A healthy weight gain for the entire pregnancy would be between 8-10 kilos for someone with a BMI less than 25 kg/m^2 at the start of the pregnancy.

If you are overweight (BMI between 25 and 29 kg/m^2) it is better to restrict the weight gain to 8 kilos.

If your BMI is 30 kg/m^2 or more, your weight gain should not be more than 6 kilos.

If you are underweight to begin with (BMI less than 23 kg/m^2), it might be advisable to put on 10–12 kilos.

while being pregnant. Therefore, there's no need to increase your intake drastically. If your weight is appropriate for your height, a healthy weight gain is between 8–10 kilos for the entire pregnancy. After the first three months, a healthy weight gain is usually between 1–1.5 kilos per month.

It is not all baby

During her monthly check-up, Shantha was found to have put on 4 kilos in one month. Her husband was happy because he had visions of a cute, chubby baby. He believed if the mother put on a lot of weight, the baby would be 'healthy'. He had to be gently reminded that the weight gain could not be all baby. In fact, if she continued to put on too much weight, at the end of the pregnancy he would have more wife than he had bargained for!

Where does the weight gain come from?

Average sized Indian baby	2.5–3.5 kilos
Uterus, placenta and amniotic fluid	1.5 kilos
Blood and retained water	2.5 kilos
Body stores (mostly fat)	4.0–4.5 kilos

The extra fat stores are difficult to get rid off after a pregnancy. If there has been too much weight gain due to fat accumulation, then a strict diet regimen needs to be followed after the delivery.

Remember, the seeds of future obesity are found in excessive weight gain during pregnancy.

The first three months

The first three months of pregnancy are tough. The levels of estrogen are rising rapidly in your blood stream and this makes you want to throw up all the time. The sight and smell of food can be difficult to handle and may make you retch.

Getting through those first three months

Eat low fat foods that are rich in carbohydrates such as idlis or chapatis. Bland, dry foods, for example, salt biscuits, crackers and dry toast will keep your nausea under control. Avoid strong smelling, oily, spicy foods. If you can tolerate milk, have a bowl of cereal with cold milk.

A mid-morning and mid-afternoon snack keeps the acidity down and can decrease nausea. It can be a fruit juice, salt or sweet biscuits or fresh

Sahana asked: I am 2 months pregnant. I have severe nausea and hate the sight of food. I can't stand the smell of milk. My husband and mother-in-law are forcing me to eat saying that the baby will be affected if I don't drink milk and eat well. This only makes me vomit more. What should I do?

My answer: You definitely are not harming your baby by eating less than usual! In the first three months, pregnant women may not like the smell and taste of many foods and at the same time, may develop strange cravings. You may find it easier to eat small meals at frequent intervals rather than three big meals a day. This also may help avoid nausea. It is enough to avoid getting dehydrated and feeling run-down. Avoid long periods of starvation because this will increase acidity and therefore you will be even more nauseous. Don't worry, your appetite will usually come back after the third month of pregnancy. You can resume drinking milk after that.

fruits. Dried fruits like raisins, dates and apricots are also good. Identify healthy snacks that you can eat during the day. This is a good way to get the nutrients and extra calories you need.

If you are vomiting a lot, you may tend to get dehydrated. This will make you feel exhausted and can also lead to constipation. Try and consume at least two litres of fluid every day. You may not even like the taste of water, so you can drink other fluids: diluted buttermilk, tender coconut water, thin soups and juices like sweet lime (musambi) or lemon.

Your obstetrician will prescribe medication to control moderate to severe nausea and vomiting. This will definitely help you get through the first few weeks of pregnancy.

The good news

Did you know that having nausea and vomiting is a good sign that your pregnancy is growing well? Studies have shown that nausea and vomiting are a good indication that the estrogen levels are high, that it is a healthy pregnancy, and the chances of miscarriage are low.

A balanced diet

A healthy diet in pregnancy should include proteins, carbohydrates, fats, vitamins, and minerals. To ensure that your diet provides you with the right nutrients, learn which foods are good sources of each.

Dairy products

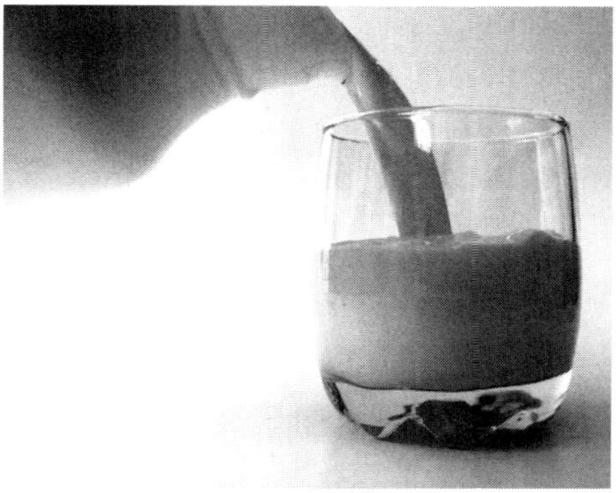

Pregnant women should try to drink two glasses of milk and eat two cups of curds (yogurt) a day. Dairy products are an excellent source of protein and calcium. If you are trying to control your weight, then low-fat milk and curds will give you the protein and calcium you require, without the fat. Cheese and paneer are also good sources of milk protein.

If you cannot drink milk by itself, you can try to camouflage the taste by adding coffee or tea. If no flavouring helps, then you can try to have 4 cups of curds daily instead of the recommended 2 cups of milk and 2 cups of curds.

What about women who have never liked or tolerated milk all their lives? How can they manage to meet their calcium needs? If you are unable to have any dairy products, then you should make sure that you get 500 mg of calcium twice daily (1000 mg per day) as a supplement in tablet form.

Sadly ice-cream and milkshakes cannot be your milk substitutes! Though they are dairy products, they contain too many calories (from sugar and fat) for them to be healthy substitutes for milk.

The caffeine confusion

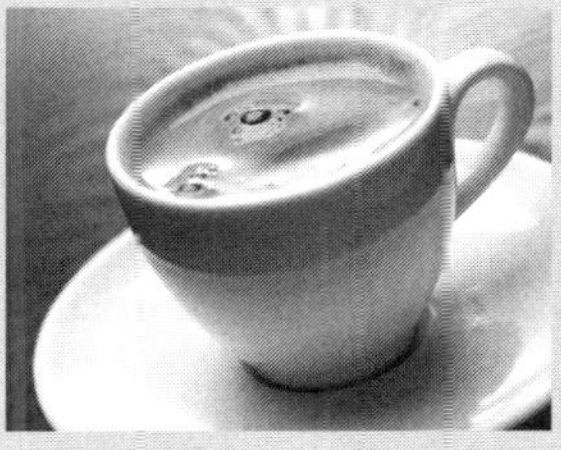

If you are a coffee or tea drinker, you are sure to get the most confusing and conflicting views from friends and family on whether caffeine affects the baby! Here's the good news: 2 average cups of coffee or tea in a day are perfectly safe to have. In early pregnancy coffee or tea may aggravate acidity but you can start drinking them when the nausea subsides.

Are you one of those who need a caffeine jolt to start the day but pregnancy has made milk intolerable? No problem. You can have black coffee or tea without milk, if you want.

Protein

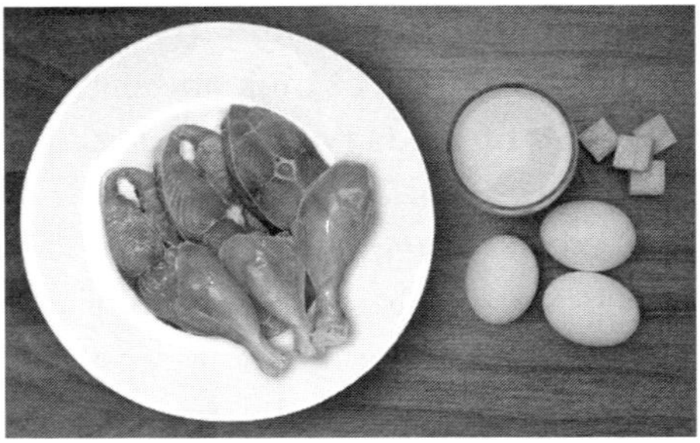

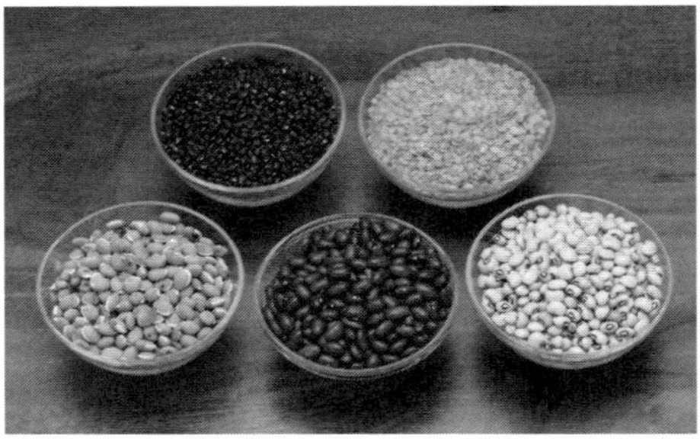

Proteins are the building blocks for the baby. Make sure your diet includes dairy products, grains, nuts, pulses, meat, fish or poultry.

What about vegetarians?

Vegetarians can have perfectly healthy babies. You can get proteins from milk, curds, paneer, whole pulses (e.g., channa, rajma) and nuts. Almonds are a great source of protein and also provide omega-3 fatty acids. If you are willing to experiment, tofu is also a good source of protein and does adapt itself to Indian dishes.

Protein supplements

There is absolutely no reason to waste money on 'protein powders'. The recommended serving size by the manufacturers is generally 10 g (containing 8 g of protein and providing 36 calories). A single serving therefore costs approximately a whopping Rs 40! The protein in these powders is usually provided by soy and milk protein. Compare this to the cost of 1 cup of yogurt (11.9 g protein and 144 calories), the white only of 1 large hard-boiled egg (6 g of protein, 30 calories) or ½ cup cooked rajma beans (7.6 g protein, 112 calories). Eat healthy and eat smart!

Carbohydrates

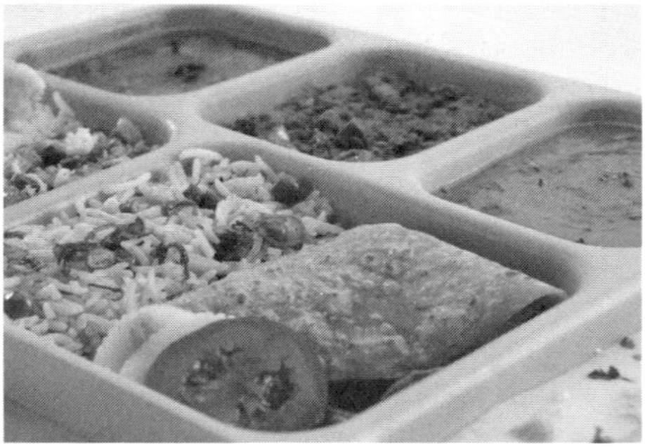

Carbohydrates provide you with energy. When taken in larger quantities, you will only get empty calories. You need not increase the quantity of rice you normally take. Substitute chapatis for rice at one meal, if you are gaining too much weight.

Madhu's husband asked: You are saying Madhu is putting on too much weight in pregnancy. She only eats 4 idlis for breakfast, rice for lunch and then 3–4 dosas, idlis or chapatis for dinner. She feels weak if she eats anything less. My mother and I have to make sure she eats well because she is such a poor eater. Won't eating less affect the baby?

My answer: I think there is a basic problem here in your perception of how much Madhu needs to eat! 'Only' 3–4 idlis? She really needs only 2–3 idlis, with the dal in sambar providing the protein. She can have two small katoris of cooked rice in the afternoon with a large cup of vegetables, sambar or dal and curds. Non-vegetarians can have meat or fish. The night meal must be eaten early (preferably before 8 pm) and should consist of two chapatis with a vegetable. Fresh salads including cucumber and tomatoes can round off a meal.

Feeling 'weak' is a misconception. Blood sugars in pregnancy can fluctuate rapidly and when Madhu's blood sugars drop she may feel a little light-headed. To avoid this, make sure that she eats small quantities at short intervals. The mid-morning snack can consist of a fruit. The evening snack can be a cup of sprouts or a small bowl of channa. Unless Madhu is involved in strenuous physical labour (and nowadays who is?), she will not be able to use up the calories that she is ingesting. Madhu should incorporate a brisk walk in her daily routine to burn off the extra calories.

Gaining excess weight in pregnancy puts the mother and baby at risk.

Vegetables and fruits

Vegetables provide vitamins, minerals and roughage. Try to include 3–4 servings per day. A salad with fresh, raw vegetables is highly recommended.

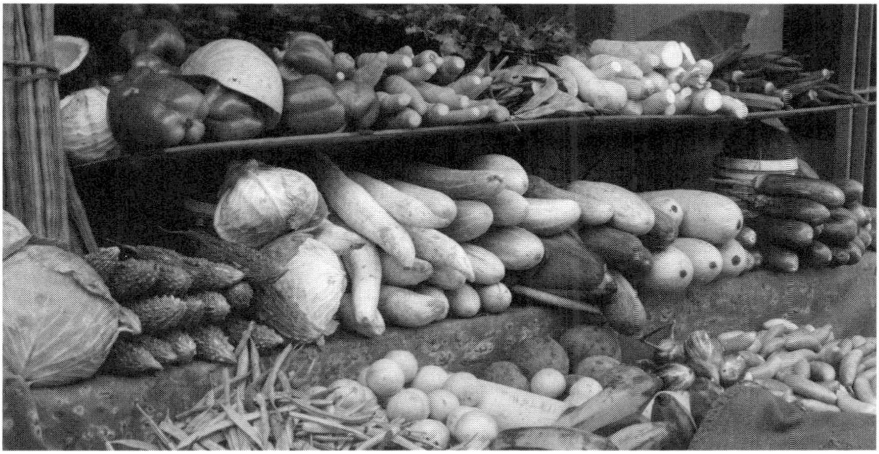

Vegetables, especially salads will provide the fibre and roughage that will prevent constipation. About 2–3 servings of fruit should be included daily.

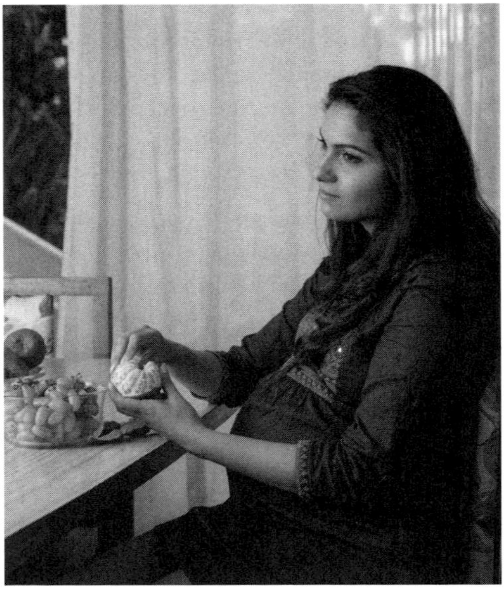

In Indian culture there is an old wives' tale that fruits like papaya, pineapple and mango, and seeds like sesame create 'heat' in the body and hence lead to miscarriage. This has no basis in fact. If it were so easy to abort a pregnancy by eating one of these, women would find it easy to get rid of an unwanted pregnancy!

How much iron and folic acid should you take daily?

Did your sister send you iron capsules from the U.S? Does your father-in-law want to buy you the most expensive capsules? Remember that the important thing is not the cost but how much iron and folic acid are present in the capsule. An iron and folic acid supplement should contain a minimum of 60 mg of elemental iron and 0.4 mg of folic acid. The best absorbable forms of iron are ferrous fumarate and ferrous sulphate. Look for all this information on the label. Most multivitamin supplement that contain iron and folic acid also contain B-complex.

The iron and folic acid supplement is best taken on an empty stomach. You can take it 2 hours after lunch or dinner. It is also better absorbed if you take it along with a glass of orange or lemon juice. On the other hand, calcium should be taken with a meal.

Do not take iron and calcium supplement at the same time. The absorption of both will be decreased. A good option would be to take the iron 2 hours after lunch and calcium along with dinner.

Many women have a problem with taking iron supplements. Iron can cause nausea and also constipation/diarrhoea. The best thing to do is to take the iron regularly for 15 days in spite of the discomfort. The body usually adapts within 10–15 days and and the problems resolve. If the constipation persists, your doctor can give you a stool softener to relieve the discomfort.

Pramila asked: My sister-in-law has sent me fish oil capsules from abroad. She says the DHA in it will make my baby smart. Is this true?

My answer: Sadly, that's not true. DHA or omega-3 is found in cold-water fish like salmon, tuna, and herring. These fish are not even available to Indians but we have done well without them, haven't we? DHA is also found in nuts like walnuts and almonds. DHA is a necessary structural component of the brain, nervous system, and eye. However, there is no scientific evidence to show that taking DHA supplements improves brain or language development in early childhood.

Vitamins and minerals

Many women of childbearing age have low iron stores. It is important to be on a combination supplement of iron, B-complex and folic acid. Calcium requirements double during pregnancy. A mother's body adapts to absorb more calcium from the foods eaten and so keep up your intake of dairy products. In India, women may have low levels of calcium. In that case, a supplement of calcium, 500 mg twice daily, may be recommended.

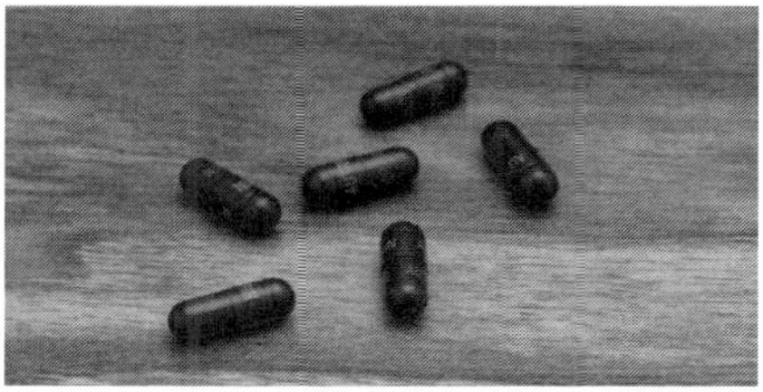

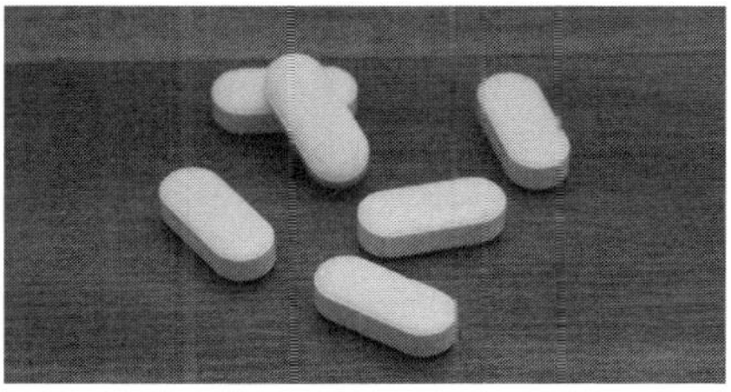

Pregnant women need extra iron and folic acid, and these are usually prescribed in the form of tablets or capsules. A prenatal supplement that contains these two nutrients plus B-complex vitamins is recommended.

Women who have had a child with a neural tube defect are more likely to have another child with this problem. These women need much higher doses of folic acid—4 mgs daily. It should be taken for 1–3 months before pregnancy and during the first 3 months of pregnancy. Women who need 4 mgs should take folic acid as a separate supplement, not as part of a multivitamin.

Healthy eating also means avoiding things that may be harmful. This includes alcohol (beer, wine, or mixed drinks) that may cause birth defects and other problems for the baby. Smoking cigarettes is especially harmful to a pregnant woman and her baby.

Nutrient	How does it help?	Best sources
Iron	Helps in producing red blood cells which carry oxygen to your baby	Green leafy vegetables, dates, iron supplements
Calcium	Helps build strong bones and teeth	Milk, curds, paneer, cheese, calcium supplements
Vitamin A	Healthy skin and good eyesight	Carrots, dark-green leafy vegetables
Vitamin C	Helps in absorption of iron; promotes healthy gums, prevents colds	Citrus fruits, tomatoes, amla
Vitamin B6	Helps body utilize protein, fat, carbohydrates and helps in formation of red blood cells	Whole grains, bananas
Vitamin B-12	Important in the formation of red blood cells, maintains nervous system	Found only in animal foods—vegetarians need to take a supplement
Folic acid	Prevents spinal abnormalities in the foetus. Needed to produce blood and protein	Green leafy vegetables, dark yellow fruits and vegetables, legumes and nuts
Vitamin D	Low levels may result in preeclampsia/diabetes in mothers and may cause low calcium levels in the newborn	Eggs, oily fish, meat. Vitamin D supplements are not routinely given

I have the urge to eat the strangest things!

It is commonly known that women have a craving for some foods that they may not even like when they are not pregnant. Most women feel like eating sour or spicy food, especially in the early months of pregnancy. Occasionally, some may take a violent dislike to what used to be their favourite food.

A strange phenomenon called **pica** occurs sometimes in pregnancy, where women feel strong urges to eat non-food items such as clay, ice, mud or chalk. Pica can be harmful to your pregnancy. It can affect your intake of nutrients and can lead to constipation and anaemia. Luckily, pica lasts for only short periods of time.

Old wives' tales

- Saffron makes your baby fair skinned. **Not true!** No food that you eat can have any effect on the colour of your baby's skin. That is determined by genetics.
- Mangoes, pineapples and papayas can cause a miscarriage. **Not true!**
- Sesame seed can cause a miscarriage. **Not true!**
- 'Eat sweets for a baby boy and sour things if you want a baby girl'. Sadly, giving birth to a baby boy is considered the pinnacle of a woman's purpose in life! Towards that end, many myths have sprung up including the one that eating sweets will ensure the birth of a baby boy. Remember that the sex of the baby is already determined on the day the sperm fertilizes the egg. What you eat or don't eat is not going to change that.

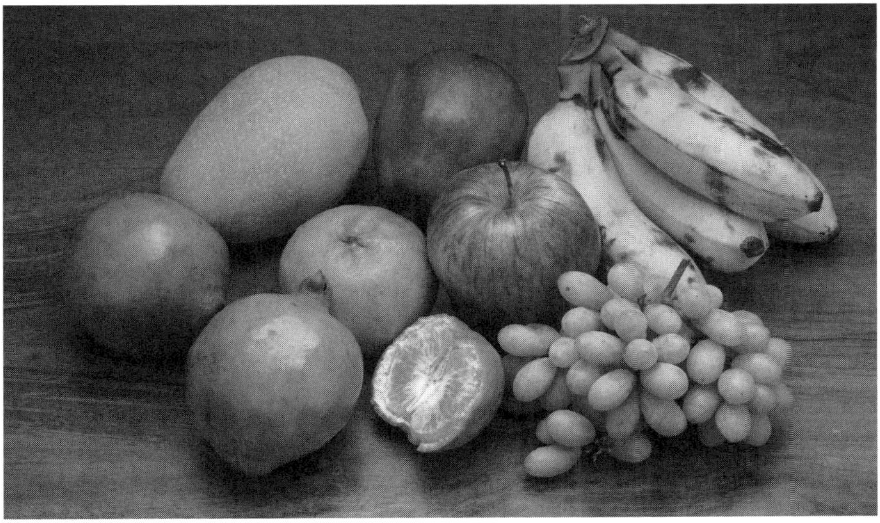

CHAPTER 11

Exercising in pregnancy

Santoshini is pregnant for the second time. She was active throughout her first pregnancy, keeping up a regular exercise programme. Her friends were amazed at how fit she was through her pregnancy and how quickly she lost the pregnancy weight after delivery.

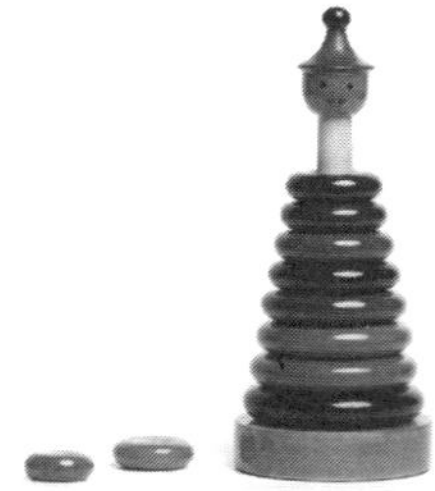

11

Exercising in pregnancy

Pregnancy is a time you should be full of energy and should keep yourself active. The first three months of pregnancy, however, can leave you feeling exhausted. This is due to the surge of hormones in your body. The hormone, progesterone, leaves you feeling sleepy and tired. Luckily, most women will start to regain their energy after the third month. The nausea and vomiting will also be under control by that time.

It does not matter if you take it easy and don't exercise in the first trimester. Stay as active as you possibly can. After that, you should set up some exercise schedule. Starting with walking, you can incorporate many other exercises into the regimen.

It is an erroneous belief that exercise can harm a pregnancy. Childbirth is among the most physically stressful challenges a woman ever faces. Being active and exercising at least 30 minutes, at least 4–5 days in the week can benefit a pregnant woman's health. Regular activity helps keep you fit during pregnancy, strengthens muscles needed for labour and delivery and may improve your ability to cope with the pain of labour.

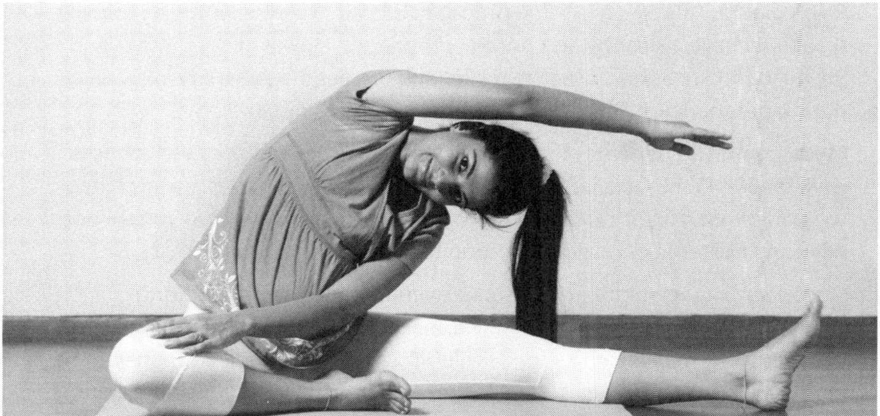

Exercise improves posture, helps reduce backaches, constipation and bloating. Regular exercise actually makes you feel less tired and improves sleep.

There is no doubt about it: exercising throughout pregnancy has great benefits. The level of exercise you do depends on how fit you were before your pregnancy. Discuss with your obstetrician what adjustments you need to make to your normal exercise routine. Even if you did not have a regular exercise routine earlier, you can keep yourself fit with a sensible fitness regimen. Walking is an excellent form of exercise and should be part of your fitness programme.

If at the monthly check-up, your doctor says that your weight gain is not adequate, it is still okay to continue exercising. You just have to make sure that you increase your healthy calorie intake. Exercising will not make you lose weight. On the contrary, it will help you maintain your muscle mass and keep you fit.

Why exercise?

It is common knowledge that exercise has immense benefits at any stage of life. In pregnancy, exercise can:

- **Make you feel better** by boosting your energy levels. As the pregnancy progresses, your sense of balance will be challenged because of your changing posture. Exercise improves your balance
- **Relieve backaches and improve your posture** by strengthening and toning muscles in your back, buttocks and thighs. As your body under-

Rupa asked: This being my first pregnancy, I want to do everything to make sure that I have a healthy and normal pregnancy. However my mother and my husband are asking me to rest a lot and are dead against my exercising during pregnancy. Is there any reason why I should not exercise?

My answer: The benefits of regular exercise are tremendous. Even a brisk walk for 30–45 minutes per day will ensure that your muscles are stretched regularly. Your doctor can examine you and can assure you that you do not have any obstetric or health condition that would limit your activity.

Of course doctors might advise some women not to exercise during pregnancy because they have had vaginal bleeding recently in their pregnancy, or may be at risk for developing preterm labour. Women who had high blood pressure even before pregnancy or those who develop it during pregnancy should avoid strenuous exercise.

goes changes, you will develop aches and pains caused by the growing uterus. There is additional strain on the muscles of your back, abdomen and legs. Exercise will help relieve these pains

- **Reduce constipation** by improving intestinal movement
- **Help you sleep better** by releasing muscle tension and relieving stress
- **Prepare you and your body for birth** by strengthening your muscles and gently stretching your pelvic muscles
- **Help you return to your pre-pregnancy shape faster** because you will not gain unnecessary weight

What is the best exercise plan?

Brisk walking

Nothing beats the benefits of brisk walking. You should build up your stamina till you are walking at least 30–45 minutes a day, at least five times a week. If you are just starting, begin with a moderately brisk pace for a kilometre, five days a week. Add five minutes every few days till you are walking for the optimal time. As the pregnancy progresses, especially in the last few weeks, you might find yourself tiring easily and getting breathless. Pace yourself and modify your regimen but do not give up completely. Remember—walk slowly for the first five minutes as a warm-up. Similarly, slow down in the last five minutes to cool down.

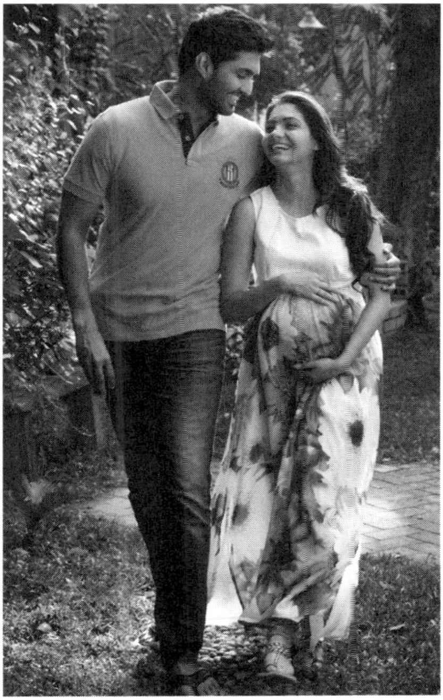

Antenatal exercises

A combination of cardio (aerobic), strength and flexibility exercises is the best for you. Find out if there are any antenatal exercise classes near you and enrol in one of them.

In your enthusiasm to exercise, do not overdo things as soon as you start. With the proper guidance, start with a gentle regimen and then work up to a more strenuous routine. Begin with as little as 15 minutes of exercise a day and add 10 minutes each week until you can stay active for at least

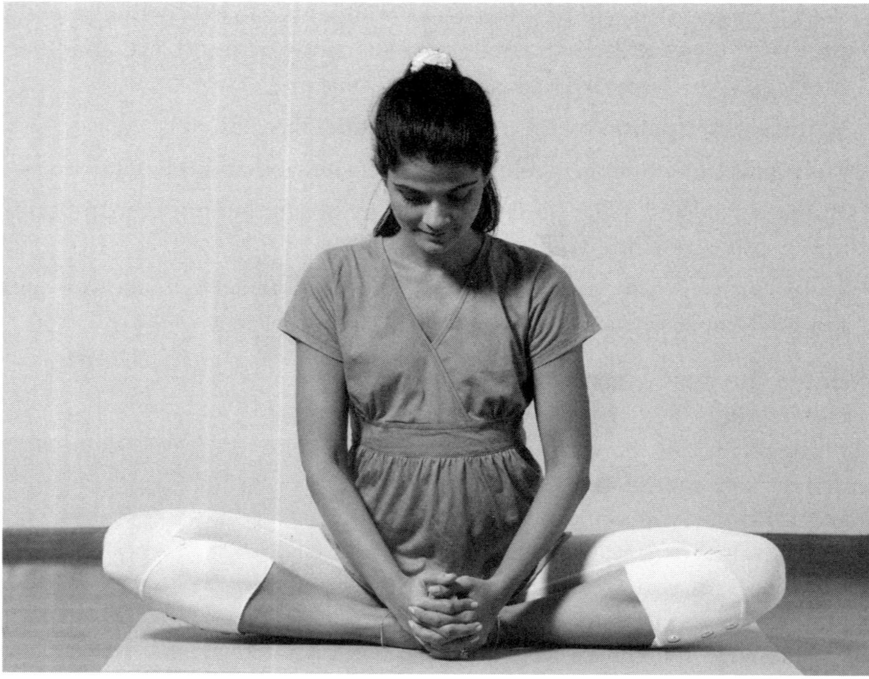

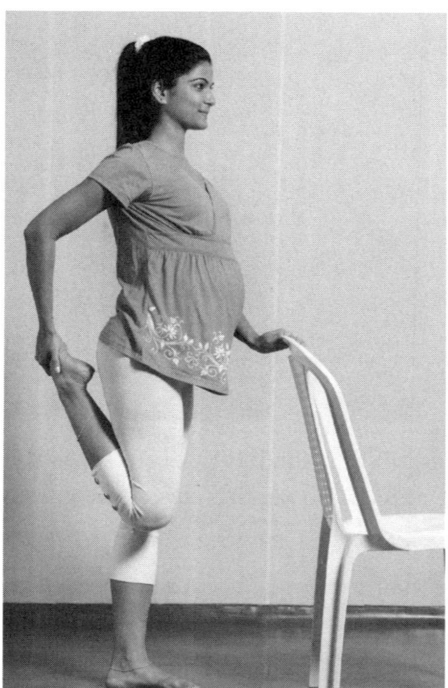

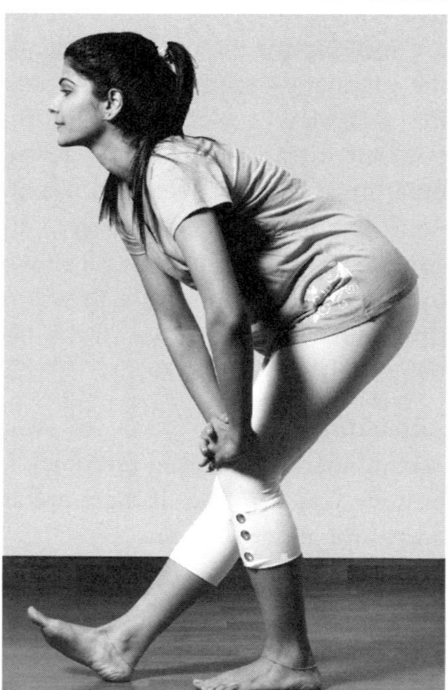

30 minutes a day. Regular exercise (at least 4–5 times a week) is better than bouts of exercise followed by long periods of inactivity.

Exercise during pregnancy is most practical during the first 7 months. It is normal to find exercise difficult during the last few weeks. Walking should be continued throughout pregnancy. Always begin each exercise session with a warm-up period for 5–10 minutes. Light activity, such as slow walking, prepares the muscles. It is also important to cool down for 5–10 minutes. During the warm-up and the cooling-down, stretching the muscles avoids stiffness and soreness.

Drink water often before, during, and after exercise to prevent dehydration.

When you exercise, extra care must be taken not to hurt the back. In pregnancy, the normal curve of the small of the back is exaggerated because of the growing size of the uterus. There is a tendency to get low back pain. Avoid positions and exercises that increase the curve in your back. Make sure that a person who is trained to teach pregnancy exercises supervizes your exercise regimen.

Kanchana asked: I am 4 months pregnant. I want to join a prenatal exercise class. What should I be aware of so that I don't overdo it?

My answer: Pregnancy causes many changes in the body and some of these changes will affect your ability to exercise. Hormones produced during pregnancy cause the ligaments that support joints, particularly the ones in the lower back, to become relaxed, making the joints more at risk for sprains. Make sure you avoid jerky, bouncy, or high-impact exercise. This will decrease the risk of injury.

The extra weight in the front of the body shifts the centre of gravity and places stress on joints and muscles, especially those in the pelvis and lower back. This can make you less stable, and more likely to lose balance and fall, especially in later pregnancy. The right exercises will help with balance and stability.

What should working women do?

Even if you are a working woman, you can squeeze at least 30 minutes out of your day for a brisk walk. Do you have stairs at your work place? During lunch break, walk up and down the stairs for 15 minutes. Take the stairs at home or the office instead of the lift. Recruit your husband or a friend to be your walking buddy. It is easier to motivate yourself when someone walks along with you.

If your working hours allow it, join an antenatal exercise class because exercising with other pregnant women will really elevate your mood and make you feel more enthusiastic about exercising.

I am sure you want the best for your baby. We know that excessive weight gain in pregnancy has an adverse effect on the health of the child. If a mother starts her pregnancy already overweight and then proceeds to put on more weight in pregnancy, this may even result in the child having health problems once it becomes an adult.

Stretches and yoga

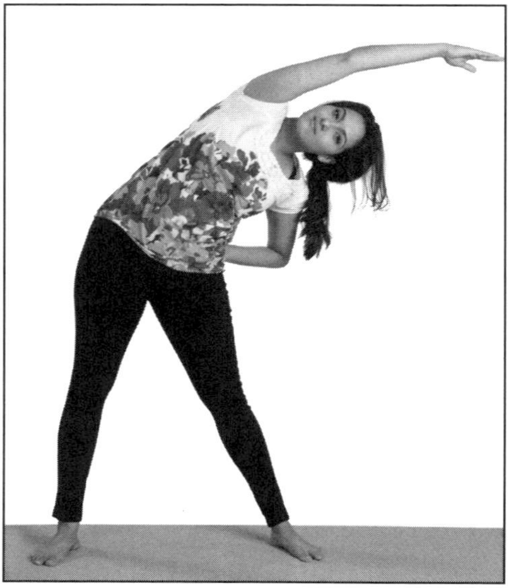

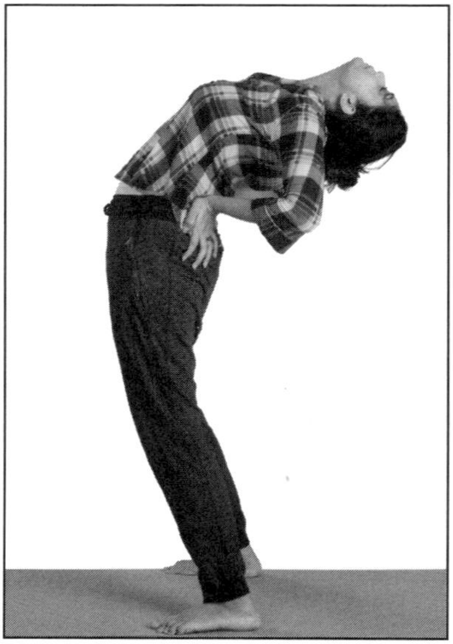

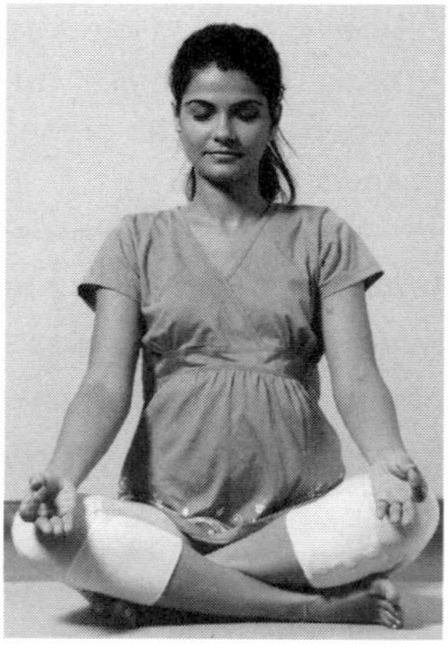

During pregnancy, it is important to gently stretch the major muscle groups and ligaments of the body. Yoga is one option to stretch different muscle groups. **Pranayama** (rhythmic deep breathing) improves oxygenation to all parts of the body and also to the uterus.

If you have any concerns about exercising, discuss them with your obstetrician.

Swimming

If you are a regular swimmer, there is no reason to give up swimming in pregnancy. In fact, as the pregnancy grows and you feel heavier and heavier, swimming is a great exercise because floating in water lightens the weight you are carrying. Be careful when stepping into the pool because the change in your centre of gravity may make it easier for you to slip. You will also need to get appropriate swimwear to cover your expanding waistline.

When should exercise be avoided?

Your obstetrician may ask you to limit your exercise if you have:

- Pregnancy-induced high blood pressure
- Early contractions
- Vaginal bleeding
- Premature rupture of membranes (leaking of the amniotic fluid)

Tips for healthy exercising in pregnancy

- Warm-up and cool down
- Wear loose fitting, comfortable clothes
- Wear non-skid shoes that support your arches
- Use a well-fitting bra or a sports bra
- Watch your centre of gravity and always keep your balance
- Bouncy or jerky exercises are best avoided
- Don't get dehydrated—drink plenty of water before, during and after exercising
- Listen to your body when something hurts or doesn't feel right
- Your heart rate should stay below 130 beats per minute
- You know you have reached the target of exercise when you are mildly breathless but still able to carry on a conversation. This is known as the aerobic zone

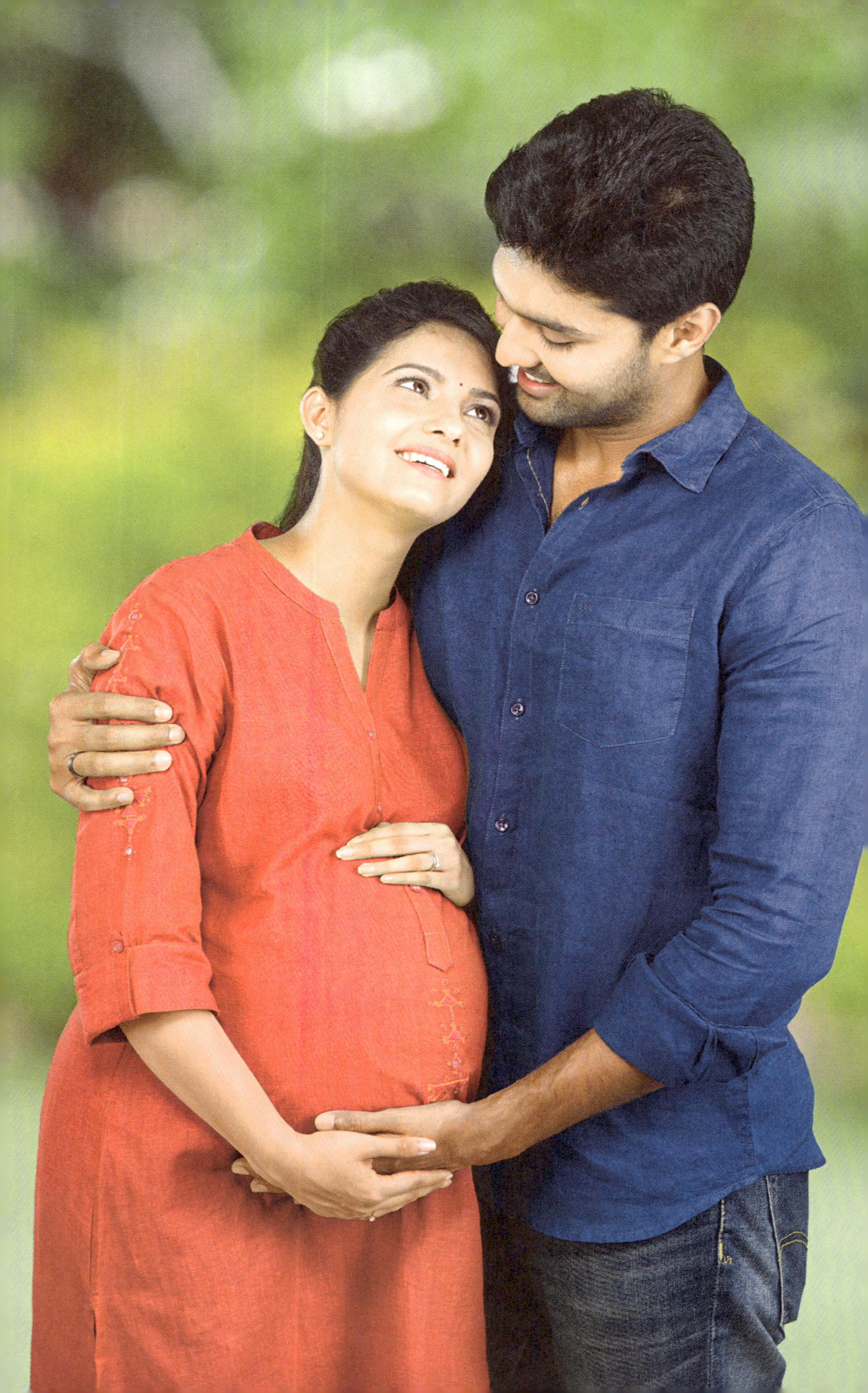

How is the baby doing?

CHAPTER 12

Could my baby have a problem?

The fear that haunts every parent-to-be is: Will my baby be healthy and normal? At every check-up, you look for reassurance that the baby is normal and growing according to schedule. Waiting for each test result is stressful because you worry that it may reveal a defect in the baby.

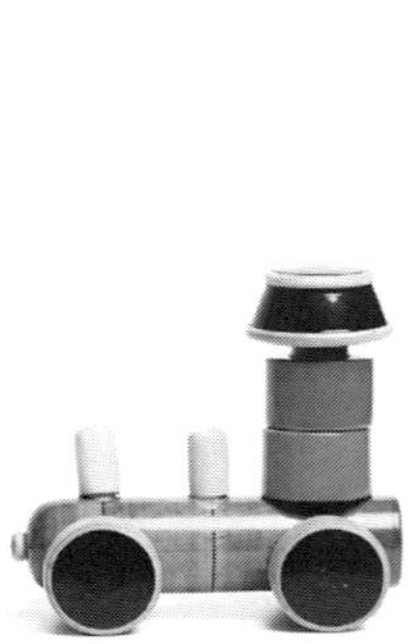

12

Could my baby have a problem?

The good news: out of every 100 babies born, only four will have a birth defect and of these, only two will have a serious or major one. Most birth defects are small and insignificant, like an extra finger, or a tiny heart defect that will disappear soon after birth without causing any problem for the baby.

What is a birth defect?

A birth defect (also called a **congenital abnormality, anomaly** or **malformation**) is a problem in the baby that may impact on its physical or intellectual development. A birth defect can be detected before birth, at birth or any time after birth. In about 70 per cent of babies the cause for a congenital abnormality is not known. In other cases, birth defects are inherited through genes or chromosomes. Occasionally, the defect can be caused by the mother being exposed to an infection or a harmful drug in early pregnancy.

Birth defects are caused by a mishap in the way the baby develops. A birth defect may affect the structure of a body part (for example, a cleft lip) or its function (for example, learning disabilities or autistic spectrum disorders). The baby's organs develop in the first three months of pregnancy and this is when most birth defects occur. Birth defects are most often mild, but some can be severe enough to jeopardize the baby's life. Some babies with birth defects may need surgical or medical treatment after birth.

Some congenital anomalies can be identified before birth with special screening tests. Other defects may be recognized only at birth or later in a person's life.

Types of birth defects

More than 3,000 different birth defects are known. They can be divided into several types, such as structural, genetic and those caused by exposure to an infectious disease or a harmful chemical agent.

Structural defects

With a structural birth defect, some part of the baby's body is not formed properly. Such a defect can be internal such as a heart defect, or external such as a clubfoot or an extra finger. There is no single cause for structural defects.

Heart defects are the most common type of birth defect. Some of the problems are mild. Others are complex and may require surgery. Neural tube defects are another common structural birth defect.

Genetic defects

Genetic defects can be caused by errors in one or more genes passed on by the parents (inherited defects), by a missing, damaged or extra chromosome (chromosomal disorders) or by a combination of factors (multifactorial defects).

Chromosomal disorders

Chromosomal disorders are most often the result of an error that occurs at the time of fertilization. The risk of having a child with a chromosomal disorder increases with age. The most common chromosomal disorder is Down syndrome. In this condition, there are three chromosomes 21, instead of two.

What causes birth defects?

If you consider the fact that just two cells (the egg and the sperm) combine to form a complex being made of billions of cells and with intricate functions, it is astounding that only 2–3 per cent end up with a major abnormality!

> Two cells—the egg and the sperm—get fertilized and develop into a complex organism composed of billions of cells with intricate organs that can see, hear and taste, among other things, and perform complicated tasks. It is not surprising that sometimes the process can go awry and some part of the body may be deformed or there is a chromosomal abnormality. What is amazing is that this so uncommon!

Birth defects are caused by an error in the way complex organs such as the heart, kidney, bone, muscles, brain or skin develop. A birth defect may affect how the body looks, functions or both. Rarely, the birth defect can be so complex that the baby may not survive.

Multifactorial causes

The coming together of many small factors when the baby is being formed causes some conditions like cleft lip and cleft palate. They are said to have a multifactorial cause.

Defective gene

Defective genes can result in conditions such as β-thalassaemia, Duchenne's muscular dystrophy and cystic fibrosis.

Exposure to infections

Some birth defects can occur when the mother develops an infection such as Rubella (German measles) during pregnancy, especially in the first three months. The latest viral infection that has been implicated in causing birth defects is the Zika virus that can result in the baby having a very small brain (microcephaly) and intellectual disability.

Diabetes before pregnancy

If you are a diabetic and are contemplating pregnancy, it is absolutely essential to have your sugar levels under strict control. Women who have high sugar levels when they conceive have a greater chance of either miscarrying or having a baby with birth defects.

Mamta asked: There is going to be a solar eclipse next week. My mother-in-law insists that I must stay inside a darkened room the whole day and refuses to let me go to work that day. Can the solar eclipse really harm my baby and cause it to have a defect?

My answer: Long before people understood that the solar eclipse is simply the shadow of the moon passing between the earth and the sun, they dreamt up superstitious explanations. In the 21st century, should we still fall prey to these superstitions? Certainly not. The answer to your question is simple: neither the solar nor the lunar eclipse has any effect on the baby inside your womb and will not cause birth defects.

Medications

Some medications taken during the first three months of the pregnancy (the most susceptible time of the baby's development) may result in birth defects. For example, drugs taken for epilepsy may have to be changed to the one that has the least harmful effects.

Alcohol

Alcohol is an absolute no-no once you find out that you are pregnant. Did you have a glass or two of wine before you confirmed your pregnancy? That will not affect your baby. However, knowing that alcohol can cause the *foetal alcohol syndrome* leading to intellectual disability, it is very important that you do not consume any alcohol after you have confirmed that you are pregnant.

What are the commonly detected birth defects?

Ultrasound scanning is the commonest modality used to detect birth defects during your pregnancy (see **Chapter 13**, *Ultrasound in pregnancy*). Additional screening tests are performed to try and detect chromosomal abnormalities in the baby. These are called screening tests (see **Chapter 14**, *Screening tests in pregnancy*). Some of the most common birth defects found through prenatal testing include:

- **Neural tube defect:** There is incomplete closure of the foetal spine that can result in *spina bifida*, or the bony skull does not form (*anencephaly*)
- **Abdominal wall defects:** One type of defect occurs when the muscle and skin that cover the wall of the abdomen are missing and the bowel protrudes through a defect in the abdominal wall (*gastroschisis*). Another type is when the tissue around the umbilical cord is weak and allows organs to protrude into this area (*omphalocoele*)
- **Heart defect:** The chambers or blood vessels of the heart are not properly developed
- **Kidney defects**
- **Down syndrome:** An extra chromosome 21 causes the child to be intellectually disabled, with abnormal features of the face and medical problems such as heart defects
- **Trisomy 18:** There is an extra chromosome 18, which causes severe problems with growth and development

Are you at risk of having a baby with a birth defect?

Though many babies with birth defects are born to couples with no risk factors, the risk of birth defects increases in the following situations:

- Family or personal history of birth defects
- Previous child with a birth defect
- Diabetes before pregnancy
- Woman aged 35 years or older at the time of delivery
- Infection with Rubella, toxoplasmosis, cytomegalovirus or Zika virus in pregnancy
- Certain medicines used around the time of conception

Couples with these risk factors should have counselling and testing. Some genetic disorders occur more often in certain communities, and testing may be offered to detect them. However, most birth defects occur when there is no history of problems. There are many genetic disorders that cannot be detected by testing.

Some women, or their husbands, may be carriers for a genetic disorder e.g., thalassaemia or cystic fibrosis. Carrier testing can be done before, during and after pregnancy to see if a woman is at risk for these genetic disorders. If the test results show that both parents are carriers, genetic counselling is needed to identify the risk of having a baby with the disorder. Diagnostic testing of the baby can show if the defect is present.

If a woman is at risk for a specific disorder such as haemophilia, the cells of the foetus can be tested by a special prenatal procedure, to see if the baby will have this condition.

Preventing birth defects

Most birth defects cannot be prevented. You do not have control over the way the baby is formed. However, being careful about medications you take during the first three months of the pregnancy (the most susceptible time of the baby's development) can reduce the risk of a birth defect. If you are thinking about getting pregnant and are on regular medications for a health condition, visit your doctor first.

A pre-pregnancy visit is especially important for women who have medical problems, such as diabetes or epilepsy. Find out what changes in medication need to be made to bring your condition under control before you try to get pregnant. If diabetes is not well controlled at the time of conception, the baby has an increased risk of having birth defects (see **Chapter 1**, *Preparing yourself for pregnancy: pre-pregnancy counselling*).

Tell anyone who prescribes drugs for you that you are pregnant. That includes any doctors you see for non-pregnancy problems.

Folic acid

Taking folic acid supplements can help prevent neural tube defects like spina bifida and anencephaly. To do this, folic acid must be taken before you get pregnant and in early pregnancy. The time when the developing neural tube needs the folic acid often occurs before a woman knows she is pregnant.

Genetic counselling

Shreyasee has a baby with thalassaemia major. Seeing her child having to undergo repeated transfusions, she wants to know if she can have a normal baby in her next pregnancy.

Shreyasee needs to be seen by a genetic counsellor. There is more and more knowledge being uncovered about the genetics of common diseases and how these diseases run in families. A genetic counsellor can also help them learn what testing, surveillance or prevention strategies are available.

Do you need to see a genetic counsellor?
If you have a genetic condition, have a family history of an inherited disease, or have other risk factors for a genetic condition or birth defect, you may benefit from consulting a genetic counsellor. If your family history indicates the possibility of an inherited disease, your obstetrician may refer you to a genetic counsellor.

How does genetic counselling help?
The genetic counsellor takes a detailed family history. This allows her to draw up a family tree or pedigree chart that helps clarify the way the genetic disorder is being passed from generation to generation. This diagram also helps to determine your baby's risk for inheriting that particular disease.
If you do have an increased risk, the counsellor will make sure that you understand the basic genetic concepts that affect how the disease runs in families, educate you about the disease itself, and explain the level of risk for you and your family.

Let us take the case of Shreyasee and her husband. To assess their risk for having another baby with thalassaemia, the genetic counsellor discussed their family history. Shreyasee came from a community where there was a lot of intermarrying among close relatives. This increased the chance of both being carriers of the disease. (A carrier is a person who has both a normal and a defective gene. The carrier is therefore normal in all ways but can pass on the disease to the baby). The genetic counsellor tested Shreyasee and her husband to find out if they were carriers of thalassaemia. After DNA testing, both were found to be carriers of thalassaemia. The counsellor told them that they had a 25% chance of having an unaffected (normal) baby, a 25% chance of having an affected baby and a 50% chance of a baby who will be a carrier. With their next pregnancy, Shreyasee underwent a chorionic villus sampling. This showed that the baby was a carrier but did not suffer from the disease. This meant that the baby had inherited a defective gene from one parent but also a normal gene from the other parent. The baby was born healthy and has continued to stay healthy.

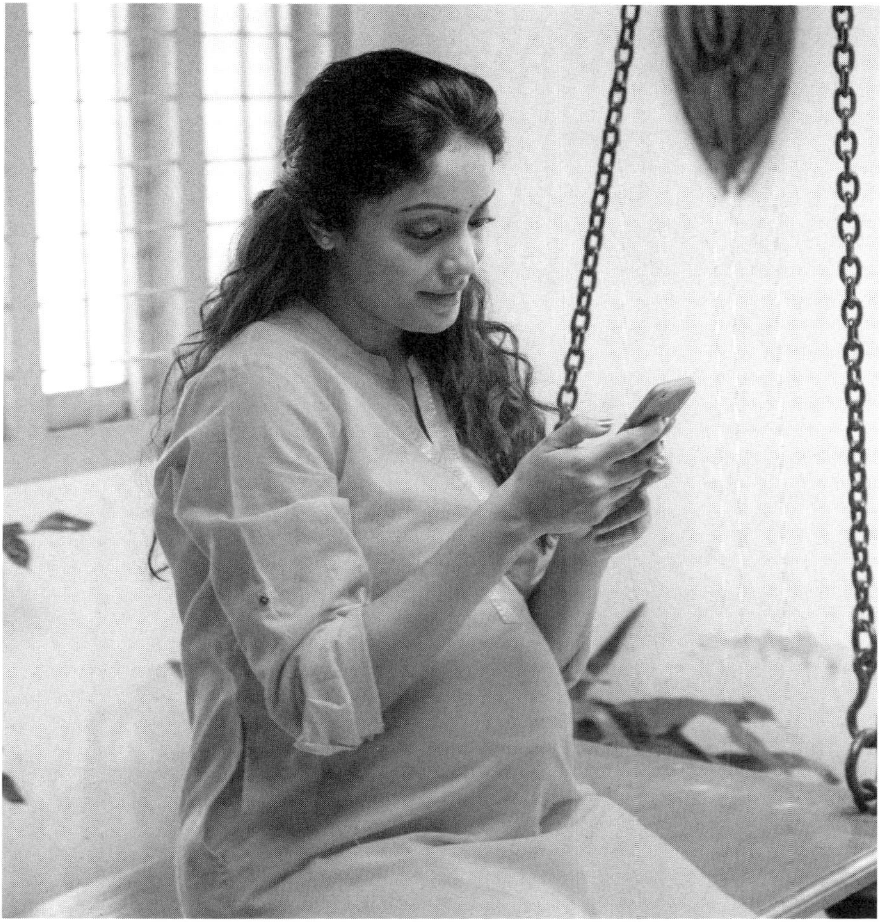

Old wives' tales

Birth defects are **NOT** caused by:

- Eclipses
- Sewing during pregnancy
- Being frightened by any incident
- Riding in autorickshaws
- Using a cellphone
- Eating certain foods
- Using a microwave
- Working on the computer
- Flying on a plane

CHAPTER 13

Ultrasound scans in pregnancy

Sumithra is excited. She is three months pregnant and has been scheduled for an ultrasound examination. She and her husband will actually be able to see the baby! However, little niggling doubts gnaw at her: Will the baby be normal? Will the doctor be able to tell her that the baby is growing normally? What if she has twins?

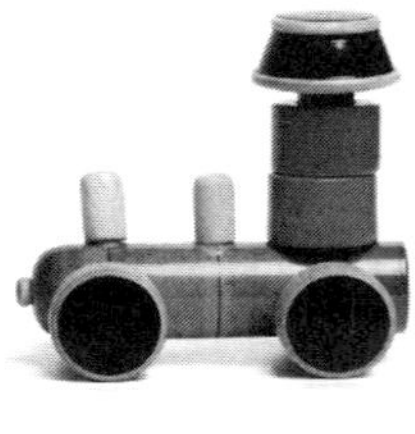

13

Ultrasound scans in pregnancy

In the 70s, ultrasound scanning was introduced to image the baby growing inside the uterus. Prior to the introduction of ultrasound scans, the obstetrician could only depend on hearing the baby's heart beat to predict if the baby was doing well or not. Ultrasound scans literally threw a new light on the growing baby. We are now able to get a peek into the hitherto hidden world of the unborn one.

We use ultrasound to determine the age of your little one. Apart from measuring his growth, we can determine whether his organs are functioning well. We can see him moving, blinking his eyes, breathing, swallowing, waving his fingers, sucking his thumb and even urinating inside! The excitement of seeing his heart beating is something you will remember for a long time.

Ultrasound scan is a safe, non-invasive, accurate and cost-effective investigation in a pregnancy. It has increasingly become an indispensable

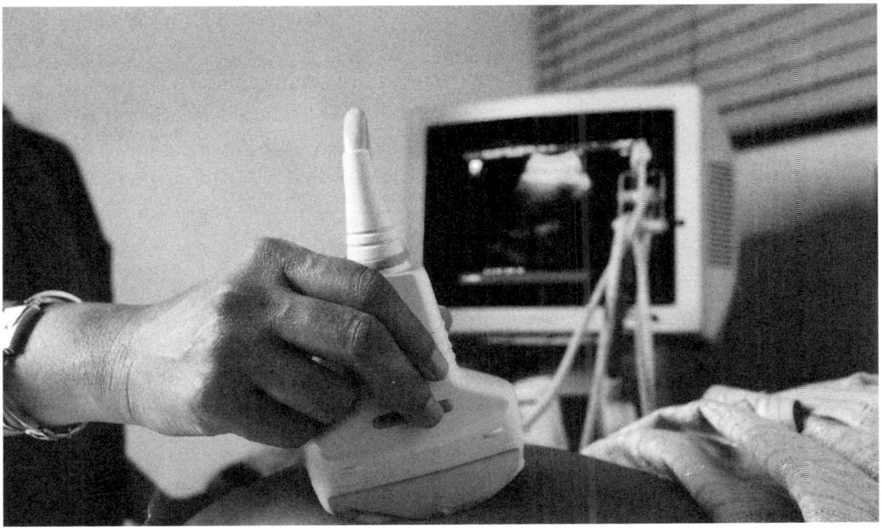

obstetric tool and plays an important and vital part in the care of every pregnant woman.

How does ultrasound scanning work?

The term **ultrasound** is used for sound waves with frequencies that make them inaudible to humans. These very high frequency sound waves are generally used for scanning the uterus and the baby. These sound waves are generated from a **transducer** that is placed in contact with the mother's abdomen (transabdominal scan) or inserted into the vagina (transvaginal scan). Ultrasound beams scan the baby in thin slices and are bounced back on to the same transducer.

The information obtained is recomposed back into a **picture** or **image** on the monitor. Using these images, measurements of the different parts of the baby can be made accurately. Abnormalities in the baby can be assessed. The movement of the baby's heart can be seen. Other movements and functions of the baby can also be monitored.

Kajal asked: Why have I been asked to come for my scan with a full bladder? I have also been told that I might require an internal scan. What does that mean and will it be painful?

My answer: When we do an **abdominal** ultrasound scan before 12 weeks (3 months), a full bladder is required for the procedure. The urine-filled bladder acts as a window for the sound waves and allows the baby to be seen clearly.

You will be asked to empty your bladder for an internal scan. From 5 weeks to 12 weeks, an internal or **transvaginal** scanning may be more accurate in visualizing the baby. This is done by using a probe that is inserted into the vagina. The procedure may be a little uncomfortable and it helps if you relax your pelvic muscles. Do remember that this will not hurt you or harm the baby.

Can ultrasound scanning harm the baby?

Since ultrasound scanning only uses sound waves, it does not harm the growing baby in any way. This method has been used for many decades, and on many millions of babies, and to date no harmful effects have been documented.

How often will I have a scan?

There is no hard and fast rule as to the number of scans a woman should have during her pregnancy. Normally, in the absence of any complication either for you or your baby, you will have two to three scans during the course of your pregnancy.

Time of scan (in weeks)	Reason for scan
6–8 weeks (for specific indications)	• Confirmation of pregnancy • Confirmation of the baby's age (most accurate) • Checking for heartbeat • Number of babies • Find out cause for bleeding • Rule out ectopic or molar pregnancy
11–14 weeks (highly recommended)	• Confirmation of the baby's age (very accurate) • Nuchal translucency • As part of combined first trimester screening for Down syndrome • Identification of certain birth defects
20–22 weeks (mandatory)	• Confirmation of the baby's age (+/- 1 week) • Presence of anatomical defects or other birth defects • As part of second trimester screening for Down syndrome • Location of the placenta • Baby's growth • Assessment of twin or triplet pregnancy
28 weeks onwards (for specific indications)	• Baby's growth • Baby's weight • Amount of amniotic fluid in the uterus • Baby's body movements, breathing movements, and heart rate to assess the baby's health • Baby's position • Placental position

Early pregnancy scan

An early scan may be done at around 6 weeks to **confirm pregnancy**, when there is a specific indication. A scan between 6 and 8 weeks can help **exclude ectopic** or **molar pregnancies** (see **Chapter 29**, *Bleeding in pregnancy*), measure the **crown-rump length** for dating, **confirm the presence of a heart beat**, and **confirm the number of foetuses**. The **age of the foetus** can be most accurately assessed between 6–10 weeks of pregnancy.

First trimester scan

A scan between **11–14 weeks** of pregnancy is useful to check nuchal translucency and can be combined with blood tests to rule out Down syndrome. Advances in ultrasound technology now also allow doctors to identify many birth defects at this stage. The age of the foetus can be determined with great accuracy at this stage.

Second trimester scan

An ultrasound scan at **20–22 weeks (targeted scan or anomaly scan)** is important to rule out **foetal abnormalities**. The **growth** is monitored using a growth chart. The **age of the foetus** can be determined with an accuracy of ≥ 1 week. Placental position is also determined. Further scans may be necessary if abnormalities are suspected.

Placental position

In the first and second trimester scans the placenta can be easily seen and we can determine where it is attached. Do not be alarmed if the placenta is reported as 'low lying' or 'covering the cervix'. As the pregnancy progresses, the placenta will also move away from the lower part of the uterus. A scan done at 36 weeks will confirm this. A low lying placenta in the first and second trimester does not require any restriction of activity or avoidance of intercourse.

In rare cases, the placenta may not move away from the cervix and may cause bleeding (see **Chapter 31**, *Bleeding in pregnancy*)

Third trimester scan

Your obstetrician may ask for an ultrasound scan in the third trimester for the following reasons:

- To **assess the baby's growth** and also to **evaluate baby's size** and **weight.** The most common reason for having more scans in the later part of pregnancy is **foetal growth restriction**, a condition where the baby is smaller than it should be and is not growing at a normal rate inside the womb
- If you have diabetes or hypertension in pregnancy, you most definitely will require a scan in the third trimester
- **To follow up on possible abnormalities** seen at an earlier scan
- To assess **the baby's position** (is the baby head-down or are the buttocks entering the birth canal?)

- To assess **placental position**
- To **measure amniotic fluid volume** because that gives important information about the condition of your baby
- To **determine the health of your baby** by observing foetal body movements, foetal breathing movements and foetal body tone (see **Chapter 16**, *Is the baby tolerating pregnancy well?*)

Common reasons for having an ultrasound scan in pregnancy

Ultrasound has become an integral part of modern obstetric care. It helps in answering many questions that arise regarding your pregnancy.

Am I pregnant?

The gestational sac can be recognized as early as four-and-a-half weeks of gestation and the yolk sac at about 5 weeks. The embryo may be observed and measured by about five-and-a-half weeks, and definitely by 6 weeks of pregnancy.

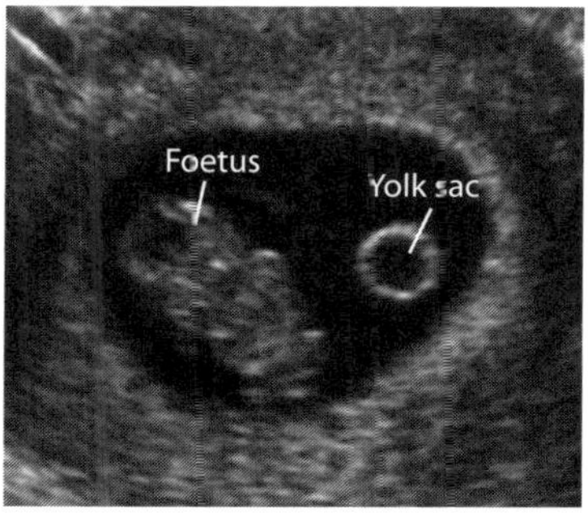

One of the important uses of ultrasound in early pregnancy is to confirm that the pregnancy is growing inside the cavity of the uterus and not in the tube (ectopic pregnancy, see **Chapter 31**, *Bleeding in pregnancy*).

Amrtha asked: My last period was on March 1st. I had a positive pregnancy test on April 7th. I rushed to my local obstetrician and she did a scan. She says there is a sac but no heartbeat is seen. Is something wrong? Should I worry?

My answer: It seems like you have been in a bit of a hurry! If you had just waited another week there would have been no confusion. At 5 weeks your baby is so tiny, it may not be seen on a scan. An abdominal scan may just show the amniotic sac. A vaginal scan may reveal the presence of the yolk sac. A confirmatory scan is best done after 6 weeks so that the baby can be seen and measured. The heartbeat can also be identified at or after 6 weeks.

Occasionally, the foetus may not be seen even at 6 weeks. This may happen if you have conceived later than is usual in a normal cycle, or you have irregular cycles. In that case, you have missed a period for 6 weeks but are not really 6 weeks pregnant. The doctor will ask you to come a week later and then the foetus and its heartbeat will be clearly seen. The doctor will adjust your due date based on that scan.

How many weeks pregnant am I?

Foetal body measurements give us the gestational age of the foetus. A scan done between 6–12 weeks of gestation will give us an accurate age of the foetus. In women who have irregular periods or who do not remember the first day of the last period, such measurements must be made as early as possible in pregnancy to arrive at a correct **dating** of the pregnancy.

In early pregnancy

In early pregnancy, assignment of foetal age by measuring the foetal crown-rump-length (see box) is based on the fact that a normal foetus will grow at the rate of 1 mm per day after the 6th week of gestation. For example, a CRL of 10 mm would correspond to a gestational age of 7 weeks and 3 days (6 weeks plus 10 days = 7 weeks and 3 days).

Foetal age assignment in early pregnancy

Crown-rump length (CRL) is a measurement of the foetus from the tip of the head to the buttocks. This measurement can be made between 7 to 13 weeks and gives an accurate gestational age. When the due date has been set by an accurately measured CRL, it should not be changed by a subsequent scan.

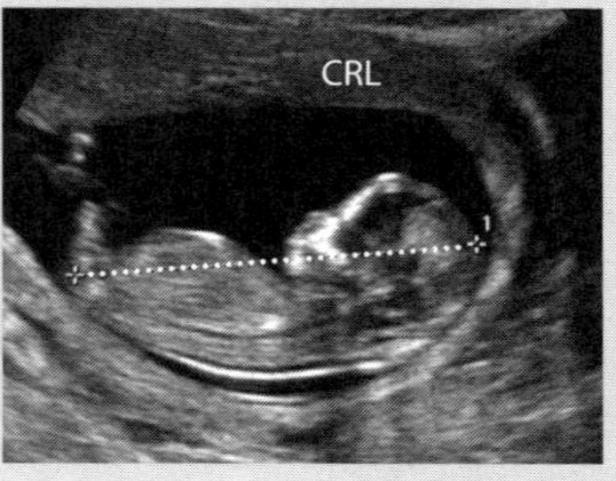

In the second half of pregnancy

In the second half of pregnancy, measuring certain foetal parameters will allow assessment of the size and growth of the foetus. The measurements help in determining if the baby is growing normally or not. The commonly measured parameters are: biparietal diameter, head circumference, femur length and abdominal circumference (see box). Other measurements are required in special cases when a problem is suspected.

Am I having a miscarriage?

When there is **vaginal bleeding in early pregnancy**, ultrasound examination is important for confirming the viability of the foetus. In a normally growing pregnancy, the heartbeat can definitely be identified by 6 weeks of pregnancy. If the heartbeat is identified, the chance that the baby will go to term is almost

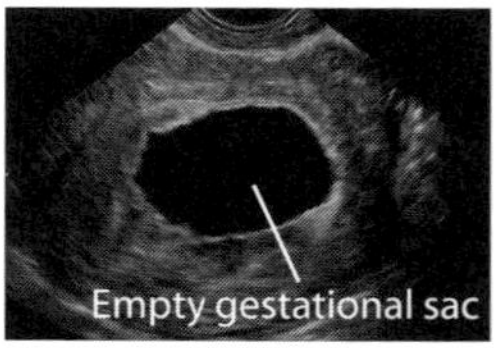

Empty gestational sac—blighted ovum

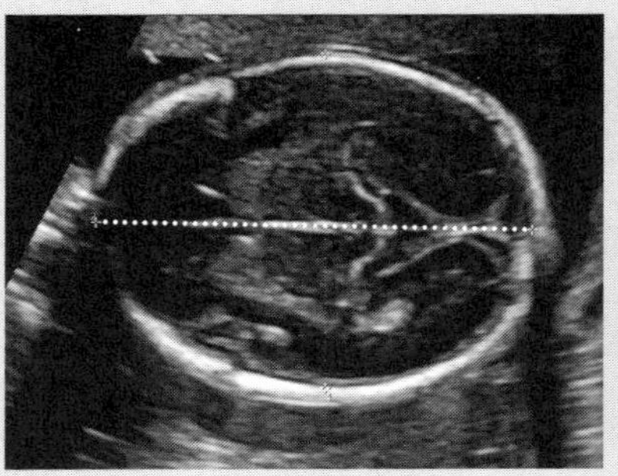

Biparietal diameter (BPD) is the diameter between the 2 sides of the head.

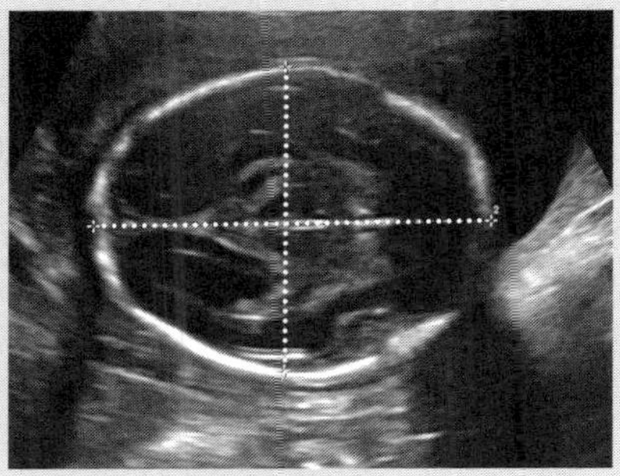

Head circumference (HC) is the circumference of the skull and is measured along with the BPD.

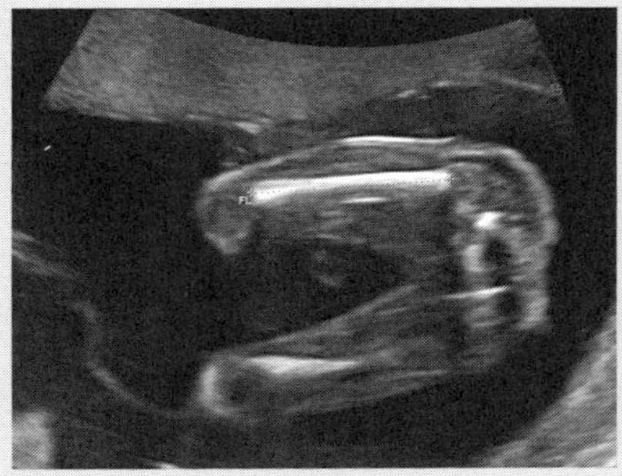

Femur length (FL) measures the thigh bone.

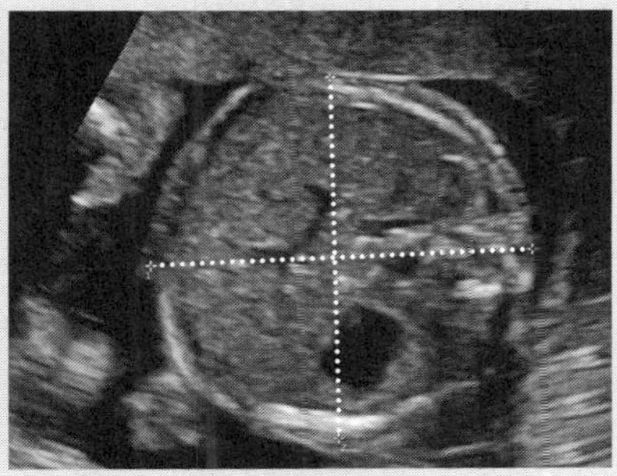

Abdominal circumference (AC) is the single most important measurement to assess foetal growth and weight.

95 per cent. In case the pregnancy is not growing well, the gestational sac may be irregular and the foetus may not be identified. This is called a **blighted ovum**. If the foetus is seen but there is no heartbeat, a diagnosis of **missed miscarriage** will be made (see **Chapter 30**, *Miscarriage*).

Since some women do not have regular periods, the findings after a single scan may be interpreted with caution. You may be asked to repeat the ultrasound scan in 7–10 days to confirm a missed miscarriage.

Occasionally, the pregnancy may not be growing inside the uterus but may actually have formed inside the tube. This is called an **ectopic pregnancy** (see **Chapter 31**, *Bleeding in pregnancy*). In the presence of first trimester bleeding, an ultrasound scan, along with a blood test for pregnancy, can help in the early diagnosis of an ectopic pregnancy.

Is my baby normal?

This is the first question that pops into a parent's mind when the doctor suggests an ultrasound scan in the fifth month! Don't forget that the vast majority of parents will have scans that will be reassuring.

Many physical abnormalities in the baby can be reliably diagnosed by a properly done ultrasound scan. A few abnormalities can be seen even at 11–14 weeks but the best time to look for most anatomical defects is between 20–22 weeks of pregnancy.

Ultrasound cannot diagnose all malformations

Ultrasound cannot diagnose all malformations and problems of an unborn baby. A 'normal scan' report is not a guarantee that the baby will be completely normal. Some abnormalities are difficult to find or to be absolutely certain about. Even with the most advanced ultrasound technology, nearly 25 per cent of foetal defects may be missed. However, most life-threatening anatomical defects, can be seen or identified at 20–22 weeks.

Increased abdominal fat in a woman can make it hard for the sound waves to penetrate and may make it difficult to diagnose abnormalities. When the amniotic fluid around the baby is decreased for some reason, it makes it difficult to see all organs in detail. It is easier to see the baby clearly in a thin patient with plenty of amniotic fluid.

Some conditions, like hydrocephalus (where the baby is born with fluid collected in the brain), may not be obvious at the time of a 5th month scan and may develop late in pregnancy.

Manisha asked: During my 5th month scan, the doctor said the baby was lying in the wrong position and not moving well. She asked me to walk around for a while. After half an hour, she made me lie down again and finished the scan. Why did she do that?

My answer: Just like adults, babies too have their cycles of sleeping and waking. If the baby is sleeping in a position when certain organs such as the heart, face and spine cannot be seen properly, the doctor may ask you to walk around. This will wake up the baby and make it turn around to a position that makes it easier for the organs to be seen. Sometimes a repeat examination has to be scheduled the following day, in the hope that the baby has moved and made it easier to visualize certain parts. Eat before you go for a scan because a well fed baby is an active baby!

Am I having more than one baby?

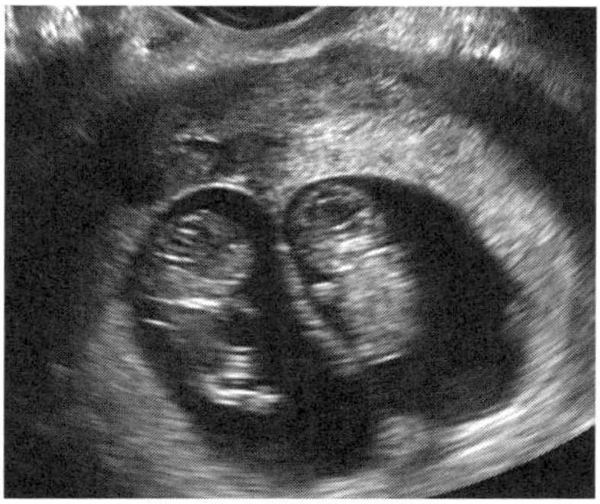

Twins at 8 weeks

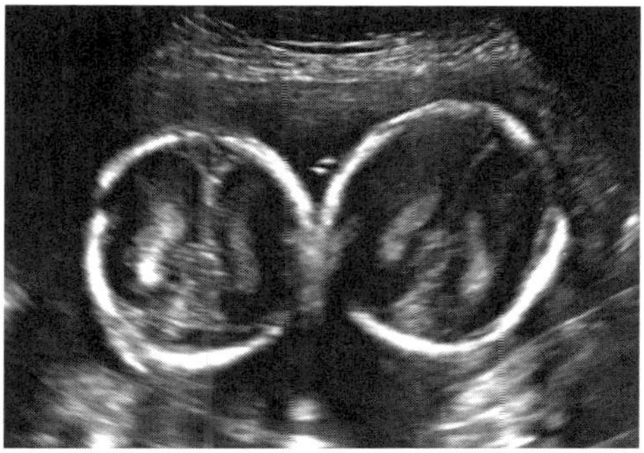

Twin heads seen side-by-side at 20 weeks

Ultrasound scanning is invaluable in the diagnosis of twins or triplets and is used to monitor the growth of the babies. Most twins will do well in pregnancy. Some twins do tend to have their own specific set of problems that can be picked up by ultrasound (see **Chapter 36**, *Twins: double trouble?*).

Screening and diagnostic procedures

Ultrasound scanning is an important part of screening for chromosomal abnormalities such as Down syndrome (see **Chapter 14**, *Screening tests in pregnancy*).

Ultrasound can also assist in other diagnostic procedures in prenatal diagnosis such as amniocentesis, chorionic villus sampling and foetal blood sampling (see **Chapter 15**, *Diagnostic tests in pregnancy*).

Assessment of amniotic fluid

The amniotic fluid around the foetus is a good indicator of the health of the baby. Ultrasound helps in assessing and measuring the amount of amniotic fluid. Too little fluid (oligohydramnios) and too much fluid (polyhydramnios) may both be indicators of foetal problems (see **Chapter 16**, *Is the baby tolerating pregnancy well?*). Measuring the amniotic fluid volume is extremely useful in foetal growth restriction.

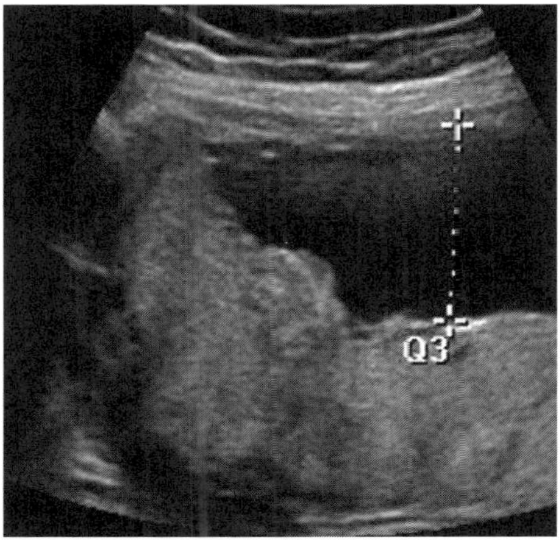

Measuring amniotic fluid volume

Other uses for ultrasound in pregnancy

In situations where your obstetrician is not sure which part of the baby is coming down into the birth canal, ultrasound is used to confirm the position of the baby. It is also used to assess foetal health by evaluating movements, tone and breathing movements of the baby. In some cases, where foetal movements have stopped and the heart beat is not heard, ultrasound is used for confirmation of intrauterine death. Ultrasound scanning also helps in diagnosing the presence of fibroids and ovarian cysts in pregnancy.

Special ultrasound scans

Doppler ultrasound: This imaging technique is used to measure the flow of blood in the blood vessels of the placenta and the foetal blood vessels (see **Chapter 16**, *Is the baby tolerating pregnancy well?*). Commonly, the uterine arteries of the mother, and the umbilical and middle cerebral arteries of the baby are imaged.

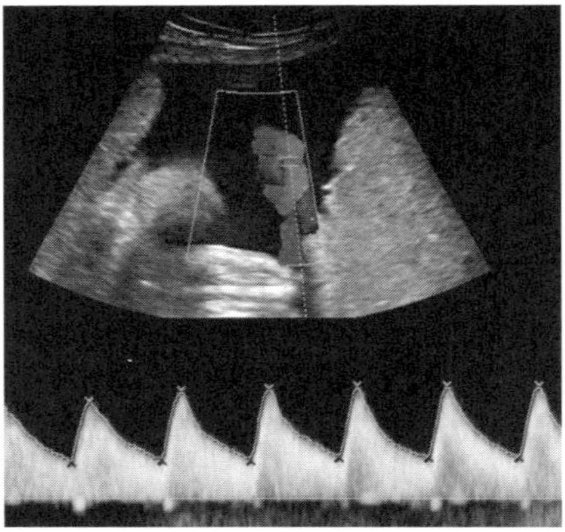

Doppler waveform for baby's umbilical artery

3-D ultrasound: This technology uses specially designed probes and software to generate 3-D images of the developing foetus. It helps in clearly defining certain foetal abnormalities, for example, cleft lip.

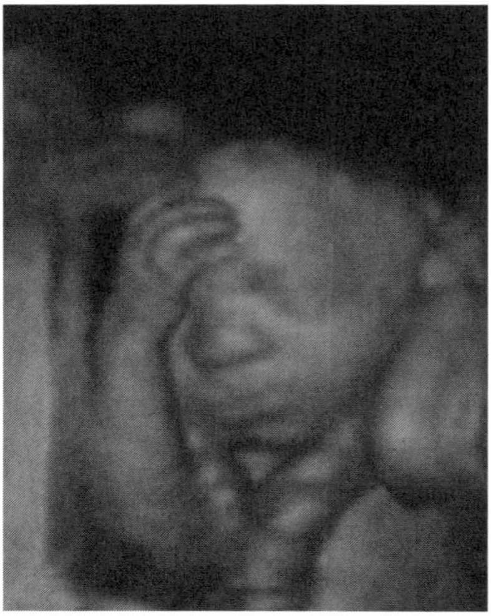

3D image of baby's face

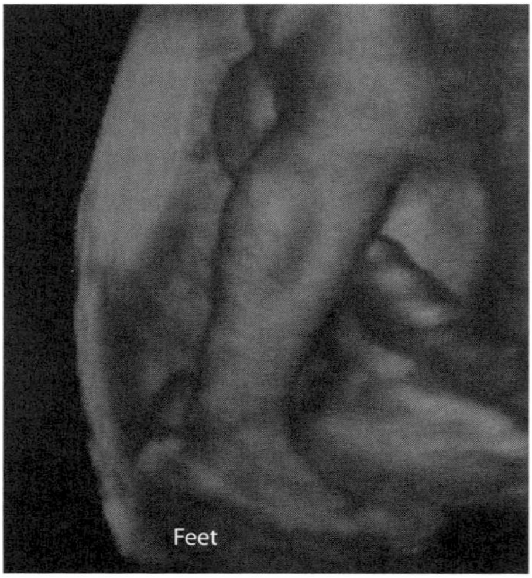

3D image of baby's legs and feet

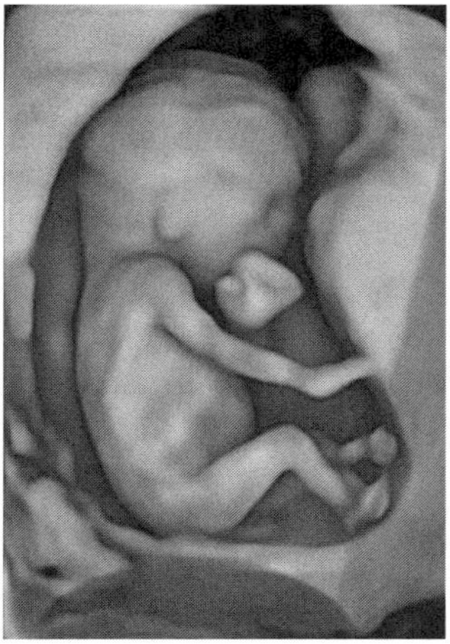

3D image of 3 month old baby inside the womb

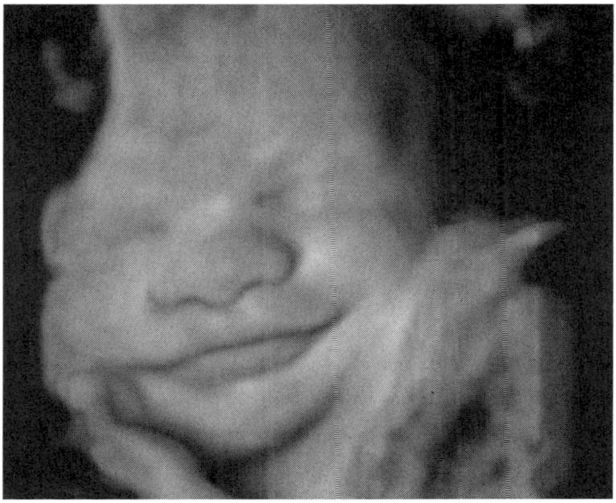

3 D image of smiling baby

4-D or dynamic 3-D ultrasound: This uses specially designed scanners to combine 3-D images with imaging of the movements of the baby.

Foetal echocardiography: This technology is extremely useful to assess the baby's heart structure and function. This is used to help assess suspected congenital heart defects.

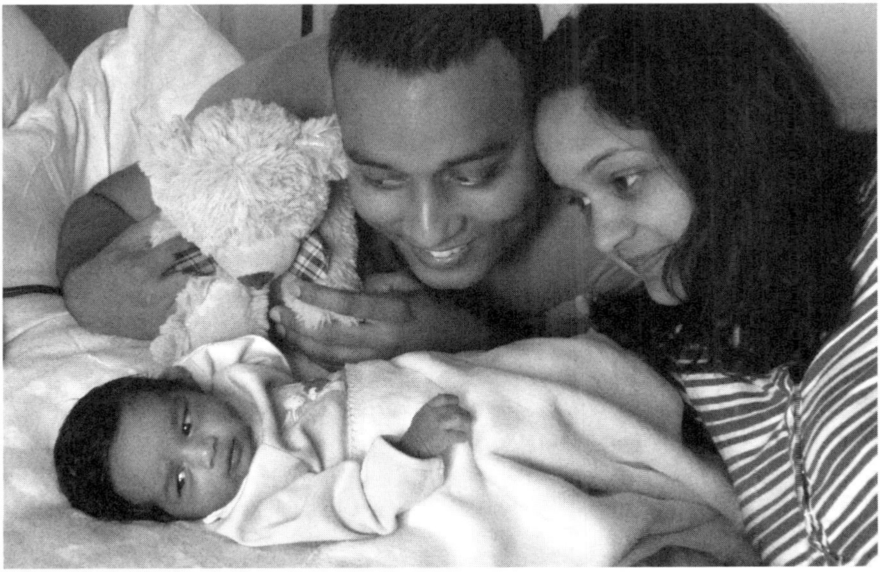

CHAPTER 14

Screening tests during pregnancy

Sheri is pregnant for the first time. She heard from her cousin about a friend who had a baby with Down syndrome. Like all mothers-to-be, Sheri is concerned.

Will her baby be perfect in every way? Is there any way she can find out if her baby has a genetic defect? What tests should she undergo in pregnancy to ensure that the baby is normal?

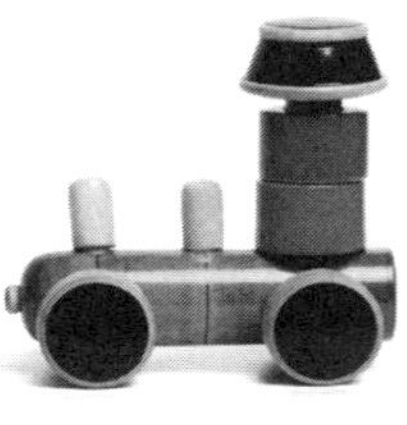

14

Screening tests during pregnancy

There is no doubt that a pregnant couple worries about the baby constantly. They want the baby to be born without a birth defect or any intellectual disability. **Down syndrome** is the commonest chromosomal defect that results in intellectual disabilities in humans. In Down syndrome an extra chromosome 21 causes the child to be intellectually and developmentally disabled, with abnormal features of the face and medical problems such as heart defects. That is why it is important to screen for Down syndrome in pregnancy.

Though the risk of Down syndrome increases with increasing age of the mother, even younger mothers can have a baby with Down syndrome. It is therefore important for all women to undergo this test.

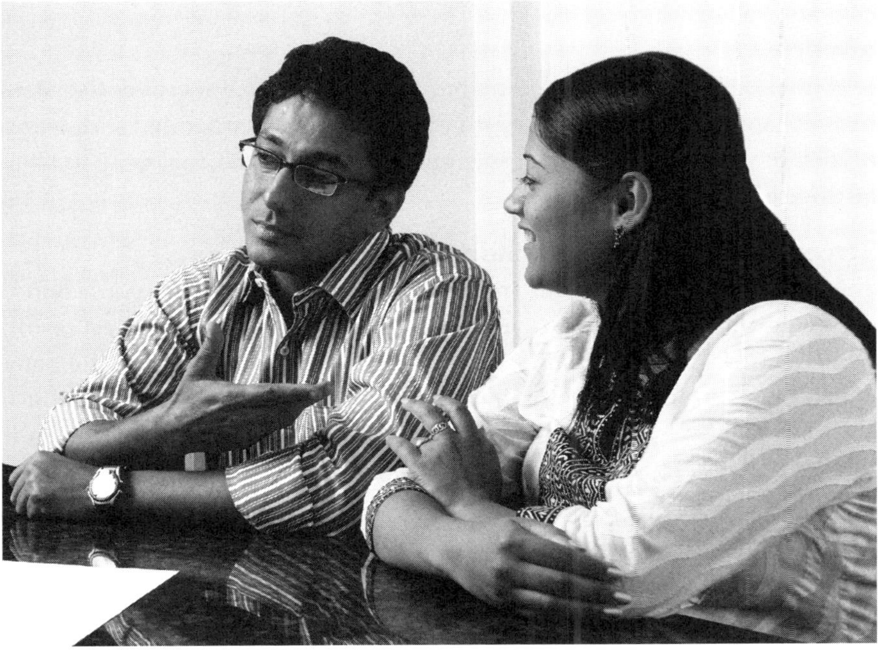

What are genetic disorders?

These can be of two types:

Chromosomal abnormalities

Chromosomes carry all our genetic material. We should all have 23 pairs of chromosomes (a total of 46). When your baby was conceived, 23 from your partner's sperm and 23 from your egg came together to form a new life. Occasionally, mistakes can happen during this process and when they do, the pregnancy may often end in miscarriage. Sometimes though, the pregnancy continues with a baby that has either too many or too few chromosomes, or sometimes with pieces of chromosomes mixed up or missing.

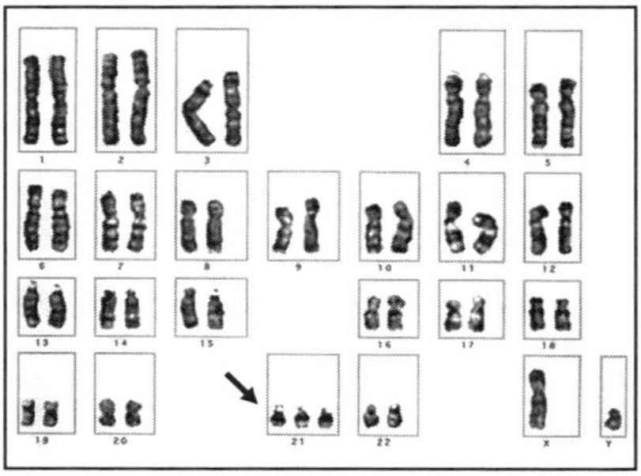

Chromosomal analysis showing trisomy 21 (Down syndrome). The arrow indicates the three chromosomes 21

Down syndrome is the commonest chromosomal abnormality that is screened for. Babies with Down syndrome have three of chromosome number 21 instead of two. The next two most common chromosomal abnormalities are trisomy 18 and trisomy 13.

Inherited disorders

Inherited disorders are caused by mutations in genes. Inherited disorders include **sickle cell disease, cystic fibrosis, β-thalassaemia**, and many others. In most cases, both parents must carry the abnormal gene to have an affected child.

Screening test for Down syndrome

A screening test is done for all pregnant women and will assess your chance of having a baby with Down syndrome. An abnormal screening test result, while alarming, only signals a possible problem. In most cases, the baby is healthy even if there is an abnormal screening test result (*false positive result*). In a very small number of women, a birth defect can occur even if the test result does not reveal a problem (*false negative result*).

If a screening test reveals a high chance of having an affected baby, further tests may be used to diagnose or confirm the problem. Diagnostic tests are usually invasive tests. In other words, tissue or cells are collected from the baby's own placenta or amniotic fluid and a confirmed diagnosis is obtained (see **Chapter 15**, *Diagnostic tests in pregnancy*). These tests are more accurate in detecting chromosome abnormalities like Down syndrome.

Screening for Down syndrome uses

- Ultrasound scans
- Maternal serum screening (blood tests)
- Cell-free DNA testing or non-invasive prenatal testing (NIPT)

Ultrasound scanning

Ultrasound scan at 11–14 weeks

An ultrasound scan done at this time is important as a screening test because it checks the ***nuchal translucency***. This is the measurement of the thickness of the skin at the back of the baby's neck. This is an important indicator of chromosomal abnormalities and possible heart defects.

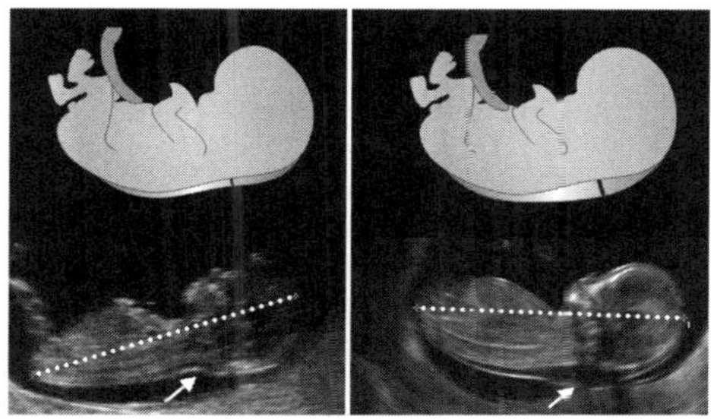

The foetus on the left has a normal nuchal translucency measurement (black line) The foetus on the right has an increased nuchal translucency measurement (black line)

Absent nasal bone

Another ultrasound marker for Down syndrome is the **absence of the nasal bone** at 11–14 weeks. This means that the bone that forms the bridge of your baby's nose is not seen. Just because the nasal bone is not seen does not mean that your baby definitely has Down syndrome. Babies with normal chromosomes can also appear to be missing a nasal bone on an early ultrasound scan. If the blood screening test for Down syndrome is reported as low-risk, your doctor will ask for a repeat scan at 16 weeks. The nasal bone sometimes appears late and will certainly be seen at 16 weeks.

Understanding the results of screening tests

A positive screening test result means that your baby is at a higher risk of having the disorder compared with the general population. It **does not mean** that your baby definitely has the disorder. A further diagnostic test will be required to confirm or rule out the disorder.

A negative result means that your baby is at a lower risk of having the disorder compared with the general population. It does not rule out the possibility that your baby has the disorder.

Ultrasound scan at 20-22 weeks

Certain 'soft markers' are considered indicative of chromosomal abnormalities. Soft markers are slight deviations from the normal anatomy seen on an ultrasound that may or may not indicate a chromosomal problem.

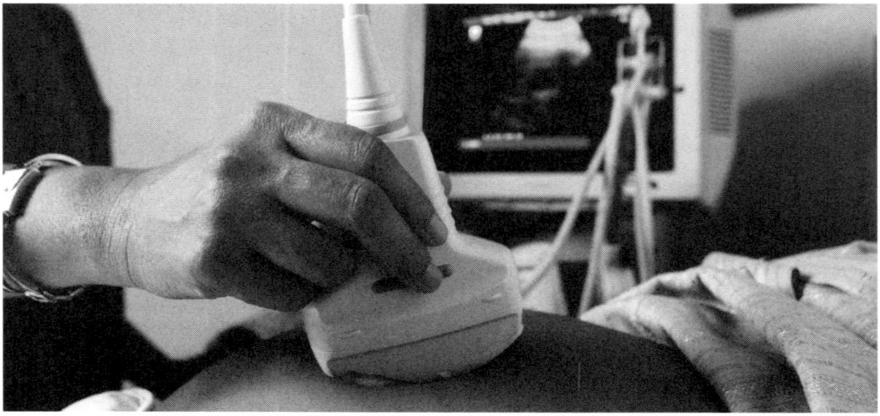

Maternal serum screening

Maternal serum screening tests are done to find out if there is a higher-than-normal risk of having a baby with Down syndrome, trisomy 18, trisomy 13, or neural tube defects. Down screening can be done in the first trimester or the second trimester.

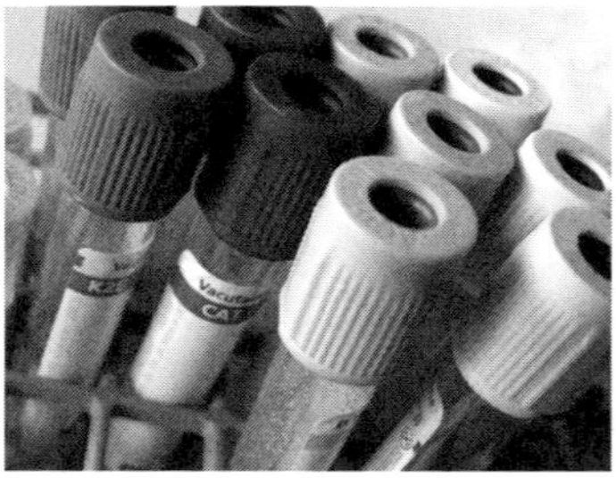

First trimester combined screening at 11–14 weeks.

An ultrasound scan for nuchal translucency (NT) is combined with blood tests **on the same day**. This test is done between 11–14 weeks of pregnancy.

The blood tests measure the level of two substances in the mother's blood:

1. Pregnancy-associated plasma protein-A **(PAPP-A)**
2. Human chorionic gonadotropin **(hCG)**

The factors that are combined to calculate the risk of Down syndrome are:

- Your age
- Nuchal translucency
- Presence or absence of the nasal bone
- The levels of PAPP-A and hCG.

In the first trimester, the combined test will identify 85 per cent of pregnancies with Down syndrome.

Increased NT with normal blood tests
When the nuchal translucency is increased but the blood tests are normal, the baby still has a small chance of a defect of the heart, abdominal wall, or skeleton. In this case, a more detailed ultrasound exam around 20–22 weeks of pregnancy is essential to detect any abnormality.

Quadruple screening test at 15–22 weeks
If you missed having the first trimester screening for Down syndrome, a quadruple test can be done between 15 and 22 weeks. Blood levels of the following 4 serum markers are tested:

1. Estriol
2. Human chorionic gonadotropin
3. Alpha-foetoprotein (AFP)
4. Inhibin-A

The blood levels of these markers are put through computerized testing which calculates your chance of having a baby with Down syndrome, trisomy 18 or neural tube defects.

In the second trimester, the quadruple screen will detect 80 per cent of pregnancies with Down syndrome.

Triple screening test
In some centres, the inhibin-A test is not performed and only three blood tests are done (the triple screening test). The triple screening test has now been replaced by the quadruple test in most centres.

The triple screening test will identify 70 per cent of pregnancies that have Down syndrome.

Interpreting results of Down screening

The test result will tell you whether you are

- At **high-risk** (the chances are higher than the general population that you may have a baby with Down syndrome) or,
- At **low-risk** (chances are lower than the general population of having a baby with Down syndrome)

The report will mention what the expected risk is at your age and also the risk predicted after the test.

For example a typical report will read:

Risk of Down syndrome at 27 (maternal age): 1: 1111

Risk of Down syndrome based on test: 1: 4000

This means you are **low-risk** for having a baby with Down syndrome.

If the risk of Down syndrome is more than 1:250 (e.g.1: 100 or 1 in 70), you are **high-risk** and will be advised to have further tests.

Cell-free DNA testing or non-invasive prenatal testing (NIPT)

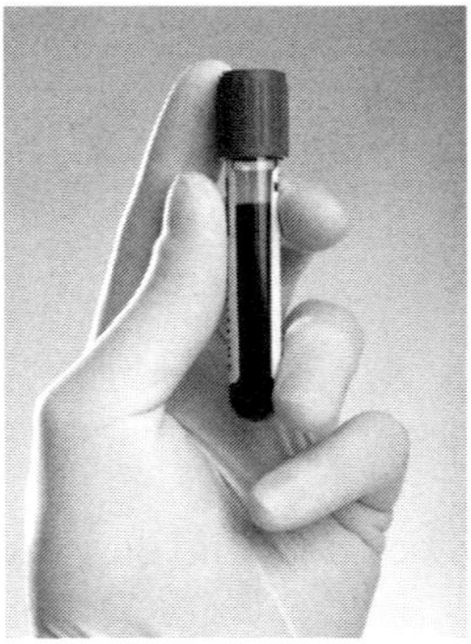

When you are pregnant, a small amount of DNA from your baby is released into your blood stream. This is called **cell-free DNA** and since 2011, it has become possible to analyze this genetic material. The cell-free DNA in a sample of the mother's blood can be screened only for Down syndrome, trisomy 13, trisomy 18, and problems with the number of sex chromosomes.

This test can be done starting at 10 weeks of pregnancy. It takes about 1 week to get the results. If the cell-free DNA test result is positive, it should be confirmed by a diagnostic test with amniocentesis or chorionic villus sampling.

Is cell-free DNA testing for everyone?

Due to the fact that this test is very expensive (Rs 30,000 and above), and has not proved to be better than the conventional screening tests already discussed, this test is **not recommended for everyone**. For a woman at low risk of having a baby with a chromosome disorder, conventional screening remains the most appropriate choice.

The current recommendation is that this test should only be offered to women who have an increased risk of having a baby with a chromosome disorder. This includes women:

- 35 years or older
- Who have had a previous baby with a trisomy
- Who have a family history of trisomy
- With abnormal ultrasound findings indicating increased risk (for example, increased nuchal translucency)
- With an abnormal first trimester or triple screening test who do not want to undergo amniocentesis or chorionic villus sampling

Cell-free DNA testing is not recommended for a woman carrying twins or triplets.

Carrier screening for genetic disorders

Some birth defects are inherited, just as a baby can inherit the shape of the nose or the colour of the skin from one of the parents. A carrier is a person who has no manifestation of a particular disorder but carries the defective gene and can pass the gene on to his or her children. Carrier screening is done to see if the husband, wife or both carry a defective gene for certain inherited disorders. A carrier screening test can be done if there is a strong history of a particular genetic disorder in a family e.g., ***thalassaemia, cystic fibrosis, sickle cell anaemia, fragile X syndrome, Duchenne muscular dystrophy, haemophilia*** and ***Huntington's disease.***

Going directly to a diagnostic test

Are you at an increased risk of having a baby with a chromosomal abnormality? If you are, then an amniocentesis or chorionic villus sampling may be offered directly instead of a screening test (see **Chapter 15**, *Diagnostic tests in pregnancy*).

You are at high risk for having a birth defect if you have:

- A family or personal history of birth defects
- A previous child with a birth defect or genetic condition
- Infection with Rubella, toxoplasmosis, or cytomegalovirus in pregnancy

Is it safe to marry a close relative?

In India, tradition and cultural norms sometimes dictate that women are married to a close family member i.e., a cousin or an uncle. Sometimes this is carried out generation after generation. When close relatives marry, it increases their chance of having a child that has inherited a genetic disease.

This is how it happens: the mother may have a defective gene, but it may not reveal the disease in her because she also has a corresponding normal gene. Similarly, the father may be normal appearing but, may also be carrying the defective gene. When the baby gets the mother's defective gene as well as the father's defective gene, the baby will have the genetic disorder. It is therefore safer to avoid marrying close relatives.

CHAPTER 15

Prenatal diagnostic tests

Sathya has just confirmed her pregnancy. Instead of being happy, she is consumed with worry. Sathya's brother has Down syndrome. Will her baby also have Down syndrome?

Santhoshi is 37 years old. This is her second pregnancy. Her first child suffered from cystic fibrosis, which is a lung condition that can prove fatal. She wants to know if this baby is normal.

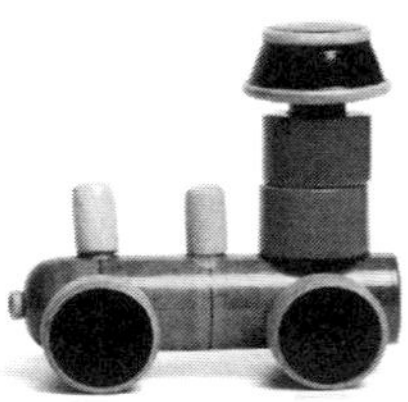

15

Prenatal diagnostic tests

During your regular antenatal check-ups, several tests may be offered to screen for and rule out abnormalities in the baby. The commonest test done is an ultrasound scan (see **Chapter 13**, *Ultrasound scans in pregnancy*). In addition to this, there are a number of special screening tests (see **Chapter 14**, *Screening tests in pregnancy*)

If either the ultrasound scan or the screening is suggestive of an abnormality, diagnostic tests are offered to confirm or rule out the chromosomal or genetic defect.

Diagnostic tests

These tests serve two purposes. If the doctor suspects a problem in the baby, or if you or your husband has a family history of a genetic problem, these tests can reassure you that the baby is normal. On the other hand, the tests may also reveal a problem that may require some serious thought on whether to continue with the pregnancy or not.

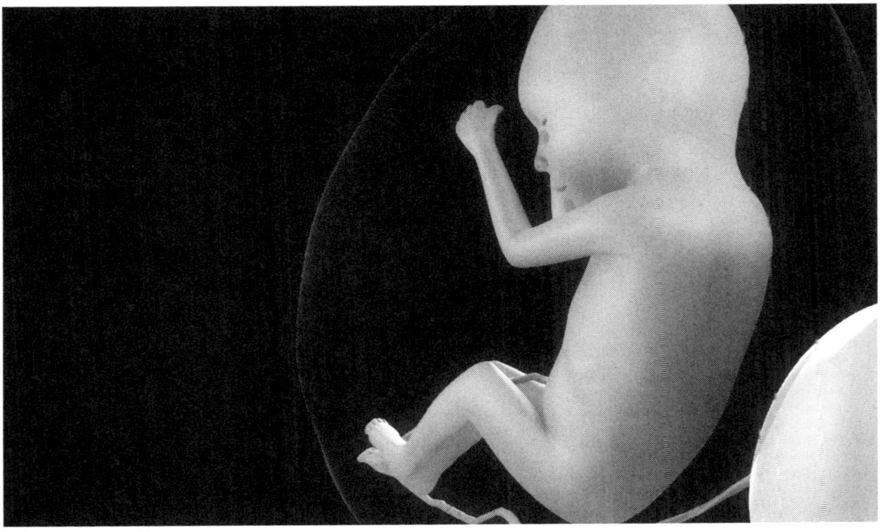

It is important to understand why these tests are done. You must discuss with your obstetrician the implications of an abnormal result and the choices that you will have. Most birth defects occur even when there is no history of problems. There are many genetic disorders that cannot be detected by testing.

A woman or her husband or both may be carriers for a genetic disorder e.g., thalassaemia or cystic fibrosis. Carrier testing can be done before, during and after pregnancy to see if a woman is at risk for these genetic disorders. If the test results show that both parents are carriers, genetic counselling is needed to identify the risk of having a baby with the disorder. Diagnostic testing of the baby can show if the defect is present.

It is important that you and your husband have counselling about the implications and suitability of these tests before you go ahead with the testing.

Commonly offered diagnostic tests	Performed at gestational age (in weeks)
Amniocentesis	Between 15 and 20 weeks
Chorionic villus sampling (CVS)	Between 10 and 13 weeks
Foetal blood sampling (FBS)	After 18 weeks

Amniocentesis

Amniocentesis is the procedure where amniotic fluid is withdrawn from the amniotic sac surrounding the baby. Amniocentesis is the most common diagnostic test offered when a chromosomal or genetic disorder needs to be ruled out.

The baby is constantly shedding cells into the amniotic fluid from its skin and other organs. These cells are extracted from the amniotic fluid and analyzed.

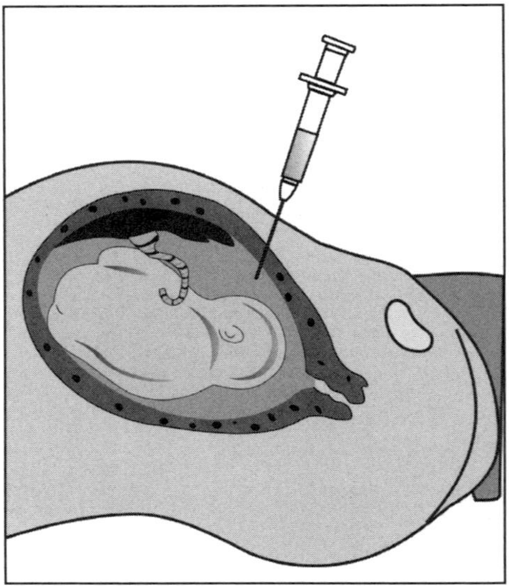

Amniocentesis

When is amniocentesis advised?

Amniocentesis is offered as an option if a screening test has come back positive, if you are 35 years or older or if an ultrasound scan reveals an abnormality which may be caused by a chromosomal aberration or an infection.

Analysis of amniotic fluid

- The cells from the amniotic fluid can be cultured and tested for chromosomal abnormalities. This is known as **karyotyping**
- The amniotic fluid can be tested for the presence of certain intrauterine infections such as Rubella, cytomegalovirus or toxoplasmosis. These infections can cause major problems in the baby. These tests are done when the mother is suspected of having had the infection and there is a chance that it may have crossed over to the baby

How is an amniocentesis done?

Amniocentesis is usually done between 15 and 20 weeks. At this time, there is enough amniotic fluid around the baby so that withdrawing a small amount will not harm the baby. Using ultrasound guidance, a needle is inserted into the amniotic sac through the abdominal wall. About 20 ml of amniotic fluid is withdrawn.

The amniotic fluid is processed to separate the cells from the fluid and then these cells are cultured. **Chromosomal analysis** is then carried out. It may take up to three weeks for the results to come back. A special technique called **fluoroscopic in-situ hybridization (FISH)** can be used to confirm specific chromosomal abnormalities like Down syndrome. The results of this test can be obtained in 48 hours.

Pallavi asked: My quadruple test came back as high-risk for Down syndrome and now I have been asked to undergo an amniocentesis. Will the procedure harm my baby?

My answer: Amniocentesis carries a very small risk of causing a miscarriage. This risk is less than 1 in 100. Rarely, leakage of amniotic fluid and slight bleeding can occur after amniocentesis. In most cases, both stop on their own. The benefit of knowing whether your baby is normal or not far outweighs this slight risk.

Chorionic villus sampling (CVS)

CVS is used when an early diagnosis is required because it can be done between 10 and 13 weeks of pregnancy. Chorionic villi are fingerlike outgrowths on the developing placenta. These are genetically identical to the baby. Getting a sample of the chorionic villi helps in identifying specific abnormalities in the baby.

When is CVS advised?

A CVS sample can be used to rule out or confirm a chromosomal abnormality like Down syndrome. Blood diseases such as sickle-cell disease or thalassaemia can also be diagnosed with CVS. Inborn errors of metabolism are caused by an enzyme deficiency, and direct enzyme analysis of the chorionic tissue can give a diagnosis. Inherited genetic disorders such as cystic fibrosis, haemophilia, Huntington's chorea and muscular dystrophy, can be detected with the use of CVS.

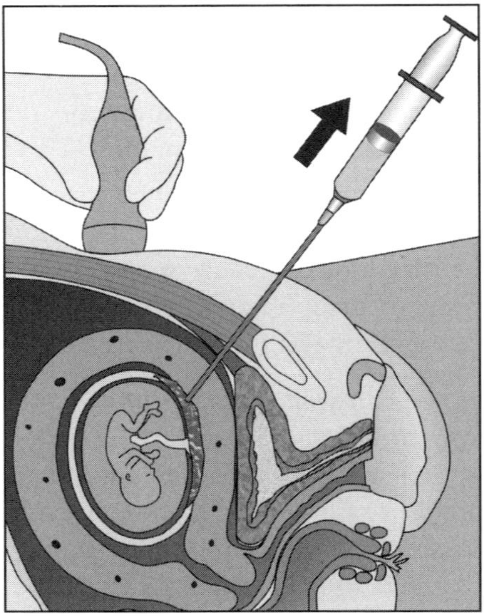

Transabdominal chorionic villus sampling

How is a CVS done?

CVS is performed under ultrasound guidance. The sample is obtained from the edge of the placenta using a needle. The tissue is then sent for analysis.

The sample obtained is sent to a lab, where it is grown in a culture. This usually takes about seven days. The sample is then studied under a microscope to check for chromosomal defects. DNA analysis can also be done for inborn errors of metabolism or for other genetic abnormalities.

Risks of CVS

The risk of miscarriage following CVS is very low and is just 1 per cent higher than the spontaneous miscarriage rate. The advantage of a CVS is that it is done early in pregnancy and you do not have to wait too long to find out if the baby has an abnormality.

Foetal blood sampling (FBS)

Foetal blood sampling is a procedure where a sample of blood is obtained from the umbilical cord of the baby. This allows us to perform blood tests for the baby. The blood can also be used for chromosomal analysis.

When is FBS advised?

Foetal blood sampling can be used for chromosomal analysis but is usually reserved for situations where the blood sample needs to be tested for specific blood-related problems.

When a foetal infection is suspected with Rubella, toxoplasmosis, or cytomegalovirus, FBS can help detect the presence of infection. In cases of Rh incompatibility (see **Chapter 37**, *Rh factor: how it can affect pregnancy*), assessing the baby's haemoglobin level is one of the methods to determine the severity of foetal anaemia and whether a blood transfusion is required for the baby while it is still inside the uterus.

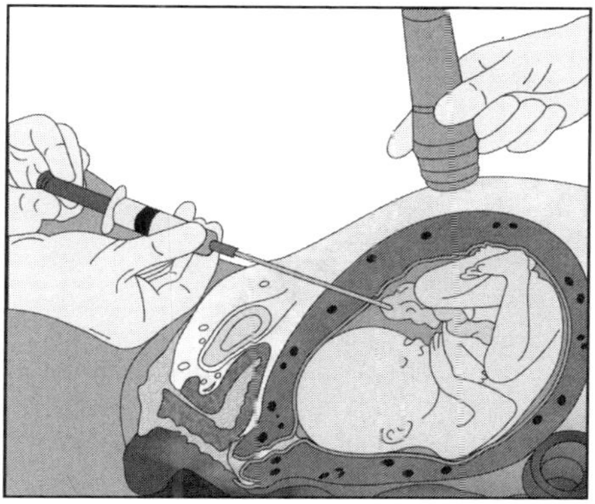

Foetal blood sampling

How is an FBS done?
This test may be done at 18 weeks of pregnancy or later. Under ultrasound guidance, a needle is passed through the mother's abdomen and uterus, and into a blood vessel in the baby's umbilical cord. A small quantity of blood can then be drawn for testing.

Risks of FBS
The risk of miscarriage is about 1–2 per 100.

Follow up of diagnostic tests

When a problem is detected following a diagnostic test, your obstetrician or a genetic counsellor will discuss the problem with you. Depending on the severity of the problem, a decision will need to be made about carrying on with the pregnancy. If the problem detected is so severe that the baby will not survive, you might be counselled about terminating the pregnancy. If the defect is compatible with life, you might be asked to meet a specialist who can give you more information about the implications of the defect. Sometimes, surgery or treatment is possible. You can then make an informed decision about the pregnancy. Testing can help prepare you so you can plan for any special care that the newborn may require.

CHAPTER 16

Tests of foetal well-being

Sushma has developed high blood pressure in the 8th month. An ultrasound scan shows that the baby is not growing as well as he should be. The obstetrician told her that the baby has foetal growth restriction. She has been asked to undergo tests to make sure that the baby is healthy. These tests of foetal well-being are important in determining how long the baby can stay in the womb and when the decision has to be made to deliver the baby without further delay.

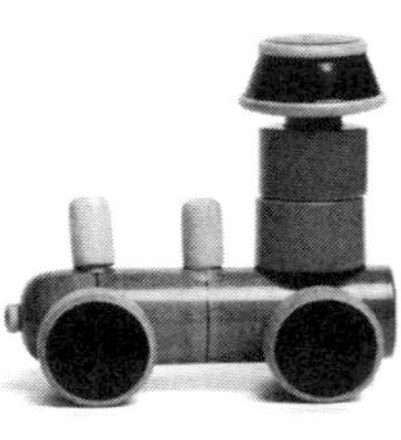

16

Tests of foetal well-being: is the baby tolerating pregnancy well?

In a high-risk (complicated) pregnancy, tests of foetal well-being check whether your little one is tolerating the pregnancy well. These tests are essential in determining if the baby should be allowed to stay in the womb, or is better off being delivered.

The placenta and its role in the unborn baby's health

The placenta is an amazing organ. It is a fully functioning organ but is present only for the duration of the pregnancy. It connects the baby to the mother and is the pipeline through which the baby gets nutrition and, most importantly, oxygen from the mother.

As the pregnancy nears 40 weeks, the placenta functions less and less. As the pregnancy goes past 40 weeks, the placenta becomes less capable of providing nutrition and oxygen to the baby.

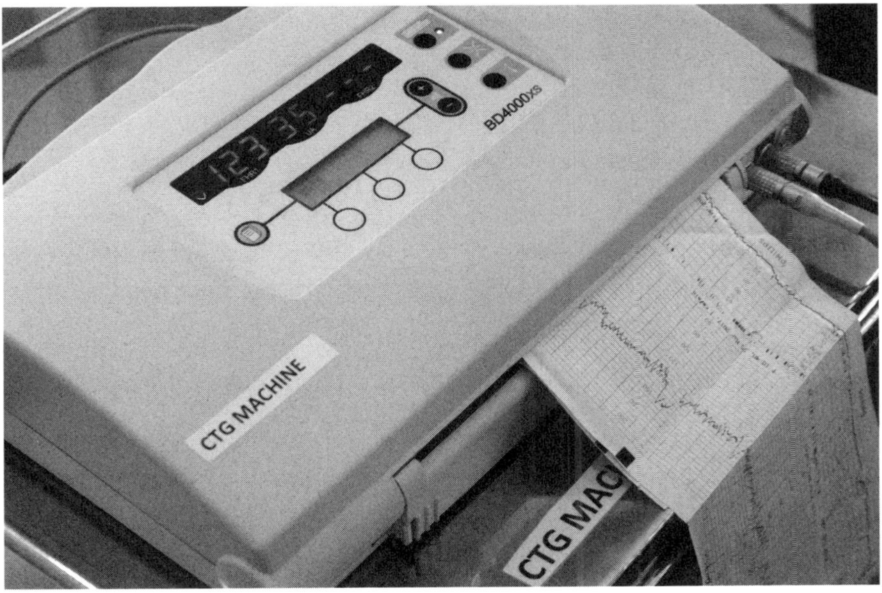

In certain conditions, the placenta loses its function much earlier in pregnancy. This **placental insufficiency** (or **placental dysfunction**) can have a harmful effect on the baby. The baby starts showing signs of undernutrition and decreased oxygenation.

> **How does the baby react to poor placental function?**
>
> When you have run up a flight of stairs and are breathless, what do you do? You stop moving. That is exactly what the baby does. The first thing that the baby does to conserve oxygen is to stop moving. If the oxygen supply does not improve, the baby starts protecting its brain by shunting most of the blood to the brain. In the process other organs, like the kidney, receive less blood and suffer. Tests of foetal well-being basically test the baby's reaction to decreased oxygen supply.

Conditions that affect placental function

Sometimes a pregnancy can develop complications (see **Section 5**, *When things go wrong*). Some common conditions where the placental function is affected are:

- Postdates
- Diabetes that requires insulin in pregnancy
- High blood pressure in pregnancy
- Antiphospholipid antibody (APLA) syndrome

Tests of foetal well-being

In a high-risk, (complicated) pregnancy, tests of foetal well-being allow us to choose the right time to deliver the baby. They basically identify when the baby is being affected by lack of oxygen.

Some complications occur when the baby is still premature. This requires an important decision to be made. If the baby is allowed to stay in the womb then the lack of oxygen may harm her. On the other hand, if she is delivered too prematurely, she will have problems after delivery.

The tests are in addition to the routine antenatal check-ups that you undergo:

- Daily kick count
- Nonstress test
- Amniotic fluid assessment
- Biophysical profile
- Doppler studies for blood flow

Tests of foetal well-being are extremely important in determining whether it is more dangerous for the baby to stay in the womb or safer to be delivered right away. These tests are more effective in reassuring us that the baby is healthy than in telling us that the baby is in trouble. What does that mean? *A sick baby can never give a good result,* so if the test shows that the baby is healthy, she definitely is.

When are these tests advised?

- The mother has had an unexplained stillbirth in a previous pregnancy
- The pregnancy has gone beyond the due date
- High blood pressure in pregnancy
- Diabetes requiring insulin in pregnancy

Sometimes the tests are done if the baby has developed problems:

- Movements have decreased
- The growth is affected (foetal growth restriction)
- The fluid around the baby is too little
- One twin is not growing as well as the other one

Usually these tests are done from **32–34 weeks of pregnancy**. In some women these tests may be initiated earlier.

Daily kick count

Rationale

Why is it important to see if your baby is moving well? The rationale behind the daily kick count is that when the placenta stops functioning well, there is decreased oxygen reaching the baby. To conserve oxygen, the baby stops moving around.

Counting movements

If every thing is going well with the baby, you can start counting the kicks from 36 weeks onwards. If you have a complication, you might be asked to count kicks from 32–34 weeks.

There are many ways to count the baby's kicks but this is the method I recommend:

- From the time you wake up in the morning till 12 noon: you should be able to count at least 10 movements.
- From 12 noon to 6 in the evening: you should be able to count at least another 10 movements.

You might feel 10 kicks in a very short period or it may take longer if the baby is sleeping. Once you have counted 10 movements, you can stop counting for that half of the day. If you feel the movements are less than normal, lie on your side for an hour. If you feel at least three movements in that hour, then your baby is healthy.

If you find that the daily kick count is less than it should be, you should go immediately to the hospital.

> **Alka asked:** I am a working woman. How do I monitor the baby's kicks?
>
> **My answer:** In that case I recommend that you track the kicks for an hour at a time: for example between 10 and 11 am, 2 and 3 pm and 5 and 6 pm. If you feel at least 3 kicks in each observed hour, the baby is fine.

What happens if the daily kick count is low?

- A CTG will be done to record the foetal heart rate and perform an NST (see below)
- An ultrasound will be done to show you the baby's movements, to record the amniotic fluid volume and maybe do a BPP (see below)

Non-stress test (NST)

An NST is one of the commonest tests done to ascertain the baby's health.

Rationale

In a healthy, well oxygenated baby, the heart rate will increase in response to the baby's movement.

How is the NST done?

During an NST, you will be monitored with a foetal monitor strap on your abdomen to detect and record the foetal heart rate (***cardiotocograph*** *or* ***electronic foetal monitoring***, (see **Chapter 23**, *Monitoring the baby's well-being during labour*). This may last 20 to 40 minutes. You will be asked to press a button when you feel the baby kick or move, so your doctor can see how the baby's heartbeat changes while moving.

During the test, a healthy baby shows a specific pattern called a **reactive pattern**. The heartbeat graph will show a nice arcing upwards of the heart rate when the baby moves. If this does not happen, it is called a **non-reactive test.** This can even happen if the baby is sleeping. The doctor will attempt to wake the baby up by shaking it or by applying a vibratory sound stimulus to the abdomen. Sometimes you will be asked to eat or drink something and the test will be repeated after an hour.

If the NST continues to stay non-reactive, the NST may be repeated after 4 hours or additional testing may be carried out.

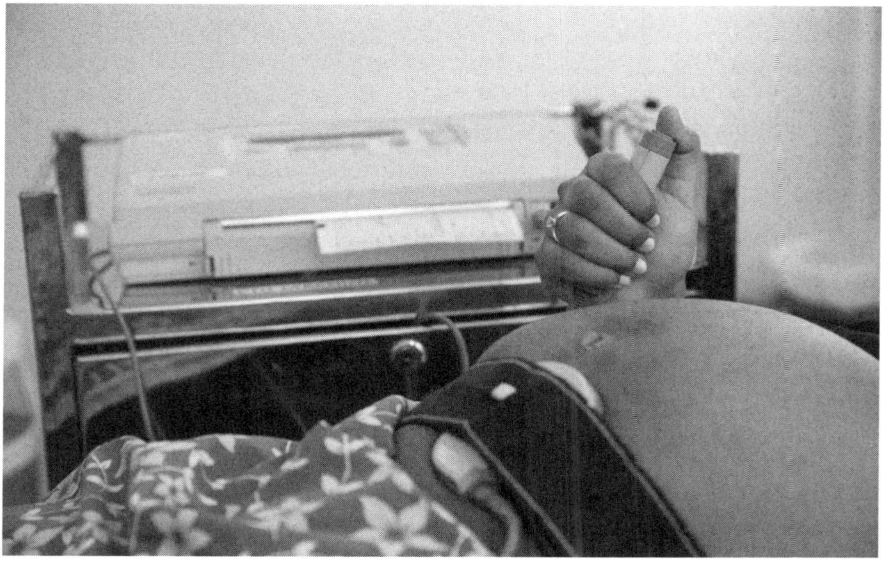

Cardiotocograph being done. The mother presses the button when the baby moves

Amniotic fluid volume

Amniotic fluid volume (AFV) is evaluated by ultrasound and is an important indication of foetal well-being.

Rationale

The amount of amniotic fluid around the baby reflects the function of the baby's kidneys. When the oxygen supply to the baby decreases, the blood is shunted to the brain as a protective step. This diverts the blood away from the kidneys, resulting in decreased production of urine. The amniotic fluid volume will start dropping. Decreasing amniotic fluid is an indicator of decreased placental function.

How is amniotic fluid volume measured?

The amniotic fluid volume is measured using ultrasound. It is reported as **amniotic fluid index** (AFI) or **single deep pocket** (SDP). The fluid is considered low if the AFI is less than 5 cm or SDP is less than 2 cm. It is an indication that the baby should be delivered as soon as possible.

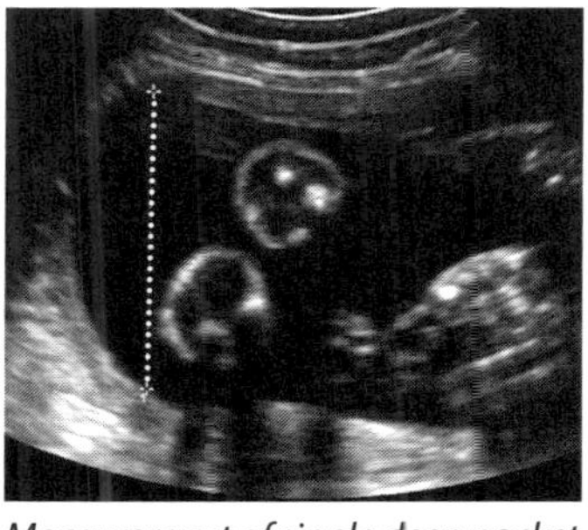

Measurement of single deep pocket

If the amniotic fluid is low even though the baby is otherwise normal, and you have no complications of pregnancy, there are two situations to be considered:

1. Amniotic fluid volume can sometimes drop in hot summer months if you do not drink enough water. Drinking an extra 1500–2000 mL of fluid per day increases amniotic fluid.
2. Some anti-inflammatory painkillers, particularly nimuselide, can drastically affect the baby's kidney function. The baby's urine production decreases and this affects the amniotic fluid volume. When being prescribed anti-inflammatory drugs, always let your doctor know that you are pregnant.

Biophysical profile (BPP)

Rationale

As the oxygen supply to the baby's brain decreases, there will be a progressive effect not just on the heart rate but also other functions, like movements of the arms and legs, breathing movements, and muscle tone.

How is the BPP done?

Using ultrasound, the baby is observed and a score is assigned to four specific parameters:

- Foetal breathing movement
- Foetal body movement
- Foetal tone
- Amniotic fluid volume

A score is also assigned to the 5th parameter, an NST that is tested with a foetal monitor.

The final score will help the doctor decide if it is to safe to leave the baby in the womb or the baby has to be delivered right away.

Modified biophysical profile

Most doctors will do a modified BPP that consists of:

- Measuring the amniotic fluid volume
- Performing an NST

It has been found that these two tests are excellent predictors of foetal health and it takes less time to do these two tests as compared to a complete BPP.

Doppler flow studies

Doppler flow studies are a specialized form of ultrasound scan (see **Chapter 13**, *Ultrasound scans in pregnancy*). The blood flow through the umbilical artery to the baby is measured. The blood flow to the baby's brain is also measured.

Rationale

As the placenta loses the ability to function, the blood supply to the baby decreases. This is shown by decreased blood flow in the umbilical artery. As the oxygen supply to the baby decreases, the blood flow to the baby's brain increases. This is a mechanism to prevent damage to the brain.

When are Doppler studies done?

Doppler blood flow studies are particularly useful when there is foetal growth restriction. The obstetrician depends on this information to decide when to deliver the baby.

How often are these tests done?

If you have a high-risk pregnancy (for example, your pregnancy has gone beyond the due date or your baby has growth restriction), you may have these tests done every week or twice a week, depending on your medical problem and the baby's condition.

What if the tests are non-reassuring?

If the tests suggest that the baby is not tolerating pregnancy well and is showing the effects of low oxygen levels, your obstetrician may decide to deliver the baby. The decision is easier after 36–37 weeks because the baby will not face the additional problem of prematurity. If there are good facilities for intensive care for the newborn, the baby can be delivered after 32–34 weeks. The decision to deliver before 32 weeks depends on the condition of the mother. For example, if the mother has severe high blood pressure that may cause harm to the her, the decision will be taken to deliver the baby early.

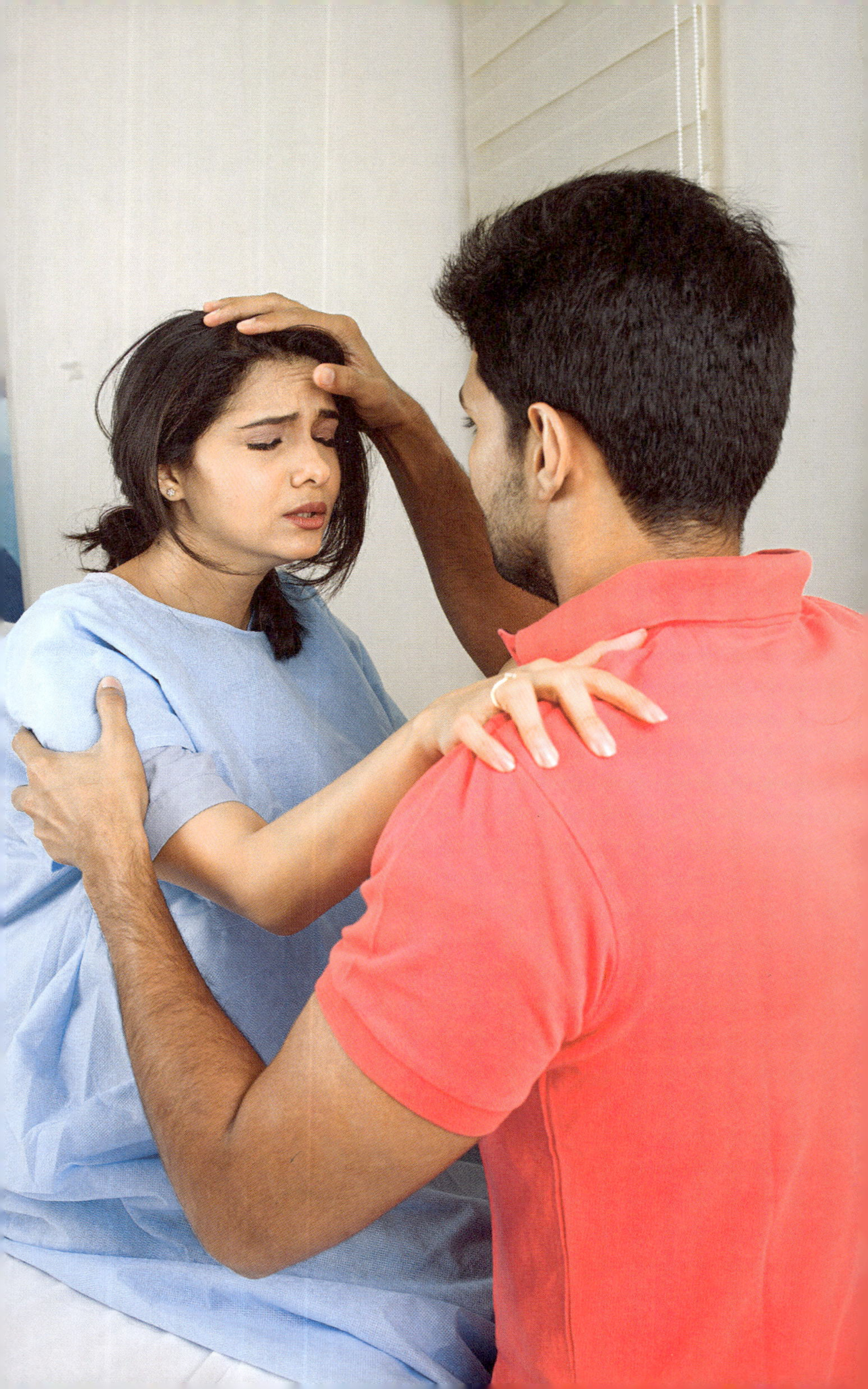

Labour and delivery

CHAPTER 17

Preparing to go to the hospital

Smriti and her husband worry constantly about being prepared for getting to the hospital on time when labour starts. There are certain steps that they can take to make sure that she is ready for going to the hospital. Being prepared will decrease the stress and anxiety that are so common in the last weeks of pregnancy.

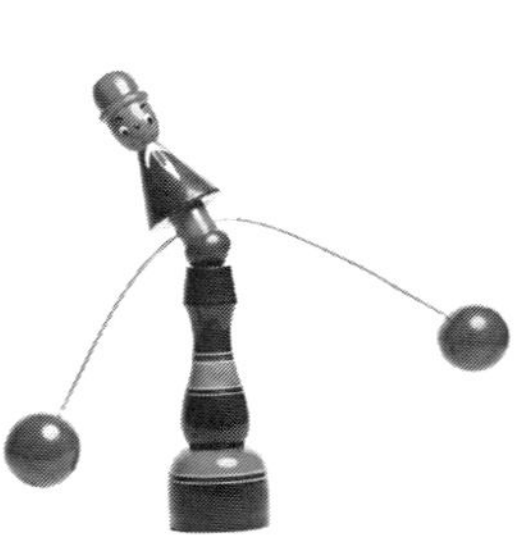

17

Preparing to go to the hospital

These are the last few weeks of your pregnancy and the countdown has begun! The anticipation is overwhelming. You want to be prepared for when the first contraction hits, you want the admission process to go smoothly, you want to be able to handle labour well and of course, you want an easy, smooth delivery.

As you plan for the birth of your baby, you can take steps to go through your hospitalization without a hitch. It is best to discuss these questions about the labour process with your obstetrician before the time comes. Some of these questions probably have already occurred to you.

When should I call the doctor?

It helps to know the signs of labour (see **Chapter 19**, *Labour and delivery*). Your doctor will probably bring this up closer to your delivery date. If you have not had this conversation, it is never too early after 34 weeks to bring it up! Several hospitals offer labour preparation classes that you and your partner can attend. You will find them very useful in understanding the labour process and particularly, when to head out to the hospital.

If your water bag breaks (rupture of membranes) or if your pains are coming regularly, call your doctor and check when you should leave for the hospital. Learn how to differentiate between true and false labour in **Chapter 19**, *Labour and delivery*. If you see a little spotting or bleeding mixed with a mucus discharge, you have passed what is known as the 'mucus plug'. This may happen up to 48 hours before labour starts. You do not have to rush to the hospital but you can call your doctor and inform her.

How can I contact the doctor or hospital after clinic hours?

Make sure you have the phone numbers of your obstetrician and and all the numbers of the hospital.

Should I go directly to the hospital or call first?

If you think you are in labour and the pains are coming at regular intervals, you can go directly to the hospital. Check with your obstetrician, and the hospital that you are delivering at. Knowing their protocols ahead of time will save you worry when you go into labour.

Most hospitals offer an orientation tour of their facilities. A few weeks before your due date, walk through the process of admission. Ask particularly to be taken to the labour room so that it does not look completely unfamiliar to you when you actually go into labour.

Are there any special steps I should follow when I am in labour?

- Put on a clean sanitary pad if your water has started leaking
- Start timing your contractions
- Make sure you take the suitcase or bag that you have packed for the hospital
- Do not eat or drink anything if you suspect you are in labour. Once you have been examined and it has been determined that you are in labour, your obstetrician may allow you to drink liquids. Tender coconut water is a great choice since it is not only refreshing but packed with electrolytes!

Brinda asked: My aunt says that once my pains start, I should have a good meal since I won't be able to eat again for a few hours. Is that right?

My answer: Not at all. Once labour starts, digestion in the stomach comes to a halt. The food that you have eaten will stay in your stomach. Carbohydrates (like rice) tend to just sit in the stomach in labour. As the cervix dilates, you may tend to vomit and if you have eaten a full meal, this can be uncomfortable for you. More importantly, if you have to have a caesarean, having a full stomach can be a problem in case anaesthesia has to be given.

Packing the hospital bag!

Remember that your due date is just an estimate—do not wait till the last minute to pack your bag in case your little one decides to surprise you! The hospital bag with essentials can be packed as early as 34 weeks. Whenever you think of an essential item, make sure that you put it into the hospital bag. Several hospitals make some of these items a part of the package, so be sure to check ahead of time what they will provide.

For-mom-to-be

Consider packing the following things for yourself in the hospital bag:

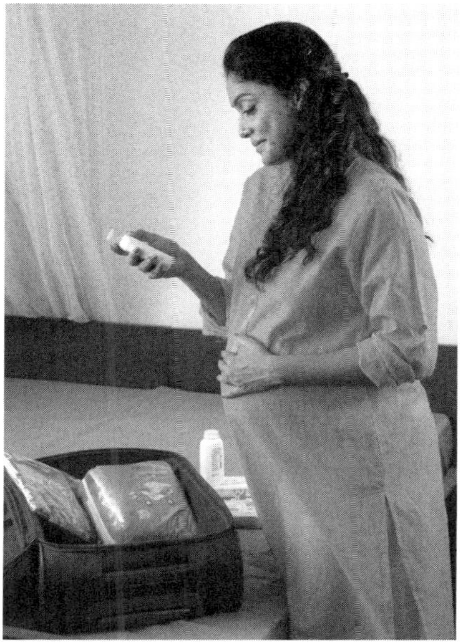

- Three sets of nightclothes. You can use something with openings in front (front openings are helpful for breastfeeding and for examinations by the doctor)
- Three nursing bras—they have a flap in front that allow you to feed the baby without having to remove the whole bra. They are now available in any store selling women's clothing or newborn needs
- Several pairs of panties, in case of blood stains (disposable paper panties are available in the market)
- Large sanitary pads (you will not be able to use tampons for 6 weeks after your delivery). Remember that the pads you buy have to be soft so as to not abrade the perineum in case of a vaginal delivery—maternity towels or the old-fashioned, thicker sanitary napkins are the ones that are best used at this time. Reusable cloth napkins have made a resurgence now and are available in larger sizes too
- Lanolin cream to apply on the nipples after breastfeeding
- Feeding pillows that allow the baby to be placed comfortably for nursing (see **Chapter 27**, *Breast feeding*)
- Loose-fitting clothes (you won't have your pre-pregnancy figure back yet) and comfortable slippers (your feet may still be a little swollen) to wear when you are leaving the hospital for home
- Hand sanitizer for your visitors to use it if they insist on handling the baby
- Mosquito repellent (essential in India!)
- Bathroom slippers
- Soap, shampoo and conditioner
- Cosmetics (don't forget toothbrush and toothpaste!)
- Comb/hair brush/nail clipper

- Glasses (contact lenses will be removed during labour and in case of a caesarean section)
- Books or magazines to distract you while you are in the early stages of labour
- Music and ear phones if you want to zone out during early labour
- Pad and pencil (good for writing down questions to ask doctors when they make rounds)
- Your mobile phone charger
- Any prenatal reports, insurance information, and papers related to your stay at the hospital

Do not take large sums of money or valuables with you to the hospital.

Pack a small bag for the labour room

For you

Though you will be in a hospital gown for delivery, you can wear comfortable clothes once you are done with the delivery and out of the labour room. The nurses will help you change after the delivery.

- A comfortable gown that opens in front
- Panties and sanitary napkins
- You can even carry your favourite music into the labour room to keep your mind off the pain!

For baby

- One dress (a simple tie-on jabla will do)
- A diaper (some hospitals prefer disposables)
- A cloth cap to cover baby's head and ears
- A soft baby sheet to wrap the baby in (soft, old sarees, appropriately cut to size will also do)

For baby

- Tie-on jablas, simple cotton dresses
- Baby sheets or soft, old sarees (appropriately cut to size) to snugly wrap the baby in
- A receiving blanket (to carry her home safely)
- Baby soap, baby shampoo, baby lotion
- Diaper pins and rubber or nylon pants, if you are using nappies—cloth diapers that come with water-proof covers are also a popular option

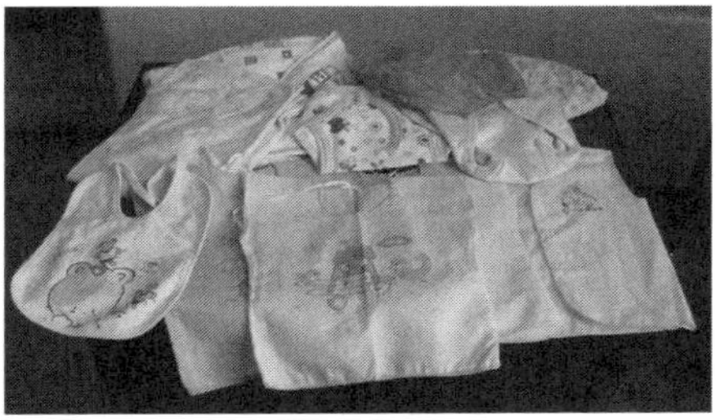 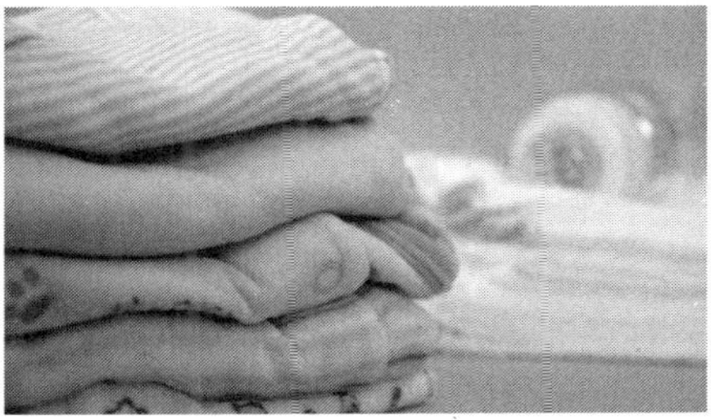

- Disposable diapers
- Cotton roll/wet wipes (buy the non-scented, alcohol-free wipes for baby)
- Waterproof sheets to place under the baby
- Soft blanket (always tuck firmly around the baby)
- Baby towels
- Small soft cloth hand towels
- Mosquito net for the cradle (small mattresses fitted with mosquito nets that you can also use at home are available in the market)

Where will the baby sleep?

While you are in the hospital, the baby may be kept in a crib in your room. When you get home, where are you planning to have the baby sleep?

Choice 1: Baby sleeping in your bed

Advantages of having the baby sleeping in your bed

- You don't need to buy a crib
- You can feed the baby without getting up from the bed

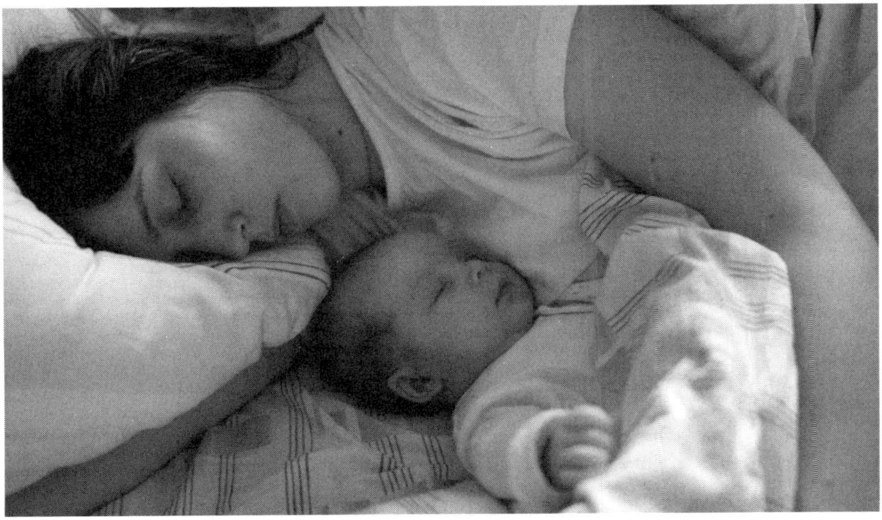

Disadvantages of having the baby sleeping in your bed

- It is difficult for you to sleep with the baby lying next to you
- The bed can get soiled frequently. Make sure that you have leak-proof rubber sheets or plastic bedding to place under the baby
- You will always worry that you might roll over the baby in your sleep or that the baby will roll off the bed. If you have no choice or if you really want the baby next to you, keep a pillow on either side of the baby after she falls asleep. This will prevent you from moving too close to the baby in your sleep and will also prevent the baby from rolling off the bed
- You and your husband will find it difficult to resume physical relations if you have the baby in the bed with you

Choice 2: Baby bed, crib or cradle

Your family may already have a cradle that has been used for many babies in the family. There are also a variety of cribs and baby beds available in the market. Choose the one that suits your space and your budget. Before you spend too much money, remember that a baby grows really fast and will outgrow the cradle in a few short months. Get something that will accommodate your baby as she grows for a few years.

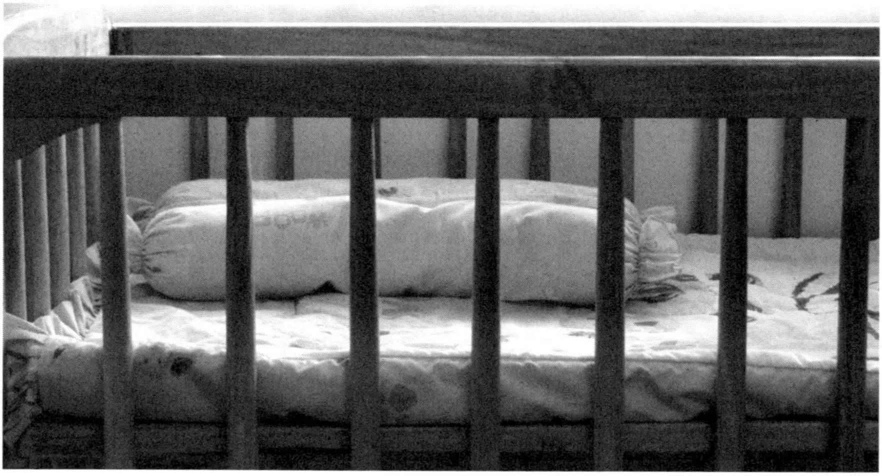

What you should look for in a crib

Your baby will spend much time in the crib unattended, so you must make certain it is a safe crib.

Most commercially available cribs come with the following features:

- Adjustable heights so that you can lower the height of the mattress base as the baby grows. When the baby reaches the stage of sitting up and standing, a low mattress height will prevent him from climbing and falling out of the crib

- Slats that are not more than 6–7 cms apart to prevent the baby from getting stuck between the bars (applicable for cradles also)

There are cribs available that are covered all around. These covered cribs protect the baby against mosquitoes and flies. The mattress should be firm and should fit the bottom of the crib well. It is better to place a waterproof (rubber or plastic) sheet between the baby sheet and the mattress.

Make sure to load the phone numbers of friends and family on to your phone because you will want to call them after the delivery. You can also create a group on WhatsApp for all those you want to inform. If you do that, a single birth announcement will be all that you need to send out.

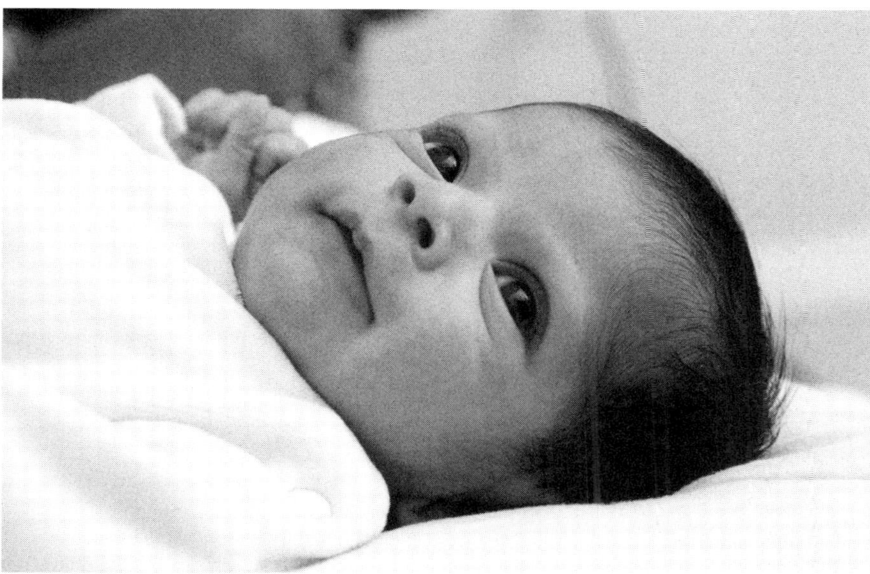

CHAPTER 18

Planning for labour

Sahana is ready and packed for the hospital. She knows that she may not have time to think about all the details once she is in labour. She has informed her office. She has also made arrangements at home for the new baby. She is smart to be ready ahead of time.

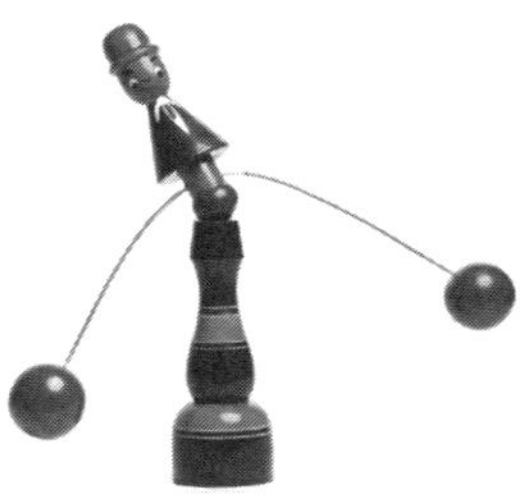

18

Planning for labour

Before it is time to go to the hospital, there are many things to think about. You may not have time to think about them once you are in labour, so it is best to consider them ahead of time.

Distance: how far do you live from the hospital?

If you stay close to the hospital where you are going to deliver, it will be easy enough to get to the hospital on time. The problem arises if you stay far from the hospital. It is important that you make arrangements to get to the hospital and know these arrangements ahead of time.

How long will it take to get to the hospital?

Make sure you know how long it will take you to reach the hospital during the peak traffic hours so that you can give yourself extra time. Have your husband do a practice run at different times of the day, so you know the best route to reach the hospital. In this day of frenzied traffic, one-way traffic, and traffic jams, it is prudent to figure out all these things. You do not want to be taking this ride for the first time when you are in pain. Your husband will be in full panic mode thinking that it is taking too long to get to the hospital!

> Even if you are getting delayed, remember that it usually takes a few hours to deliver (especially for a first-time mom-to-be), so there is no need to panic.

Transportation

When you go into labour, any mode of transportation is safe to take to reach the hospital (you probably shouldn't be on a two-wheeler though!).

Is there someone who can take you to hospital at any time, or do you have to call and find someone? If you have somebody who has offered to drive you to the hospital in their car at the time of labour, warn them beforehand as you near your due date.

If you are planning to take a taxi, speak to a taxi service and make arrangements so that they can send a car as soon as you call. Some local auto drivers also help out labouring women, so it's a good idea to come to an arrangement with one of them.

Time of day

Depending on where you live, it may take longer during rush hours than at night.

Do you need to get admitted ahead of time?

Check with your obstetrician if you need to be admitted before your due date. If you have a complication of pregnancy, admission may be advised before labour starts.

Occasionally, your obstetrician may suspect that you may end up having a fast labour and if you live far away, she may ask you to get admitted a few days before your due date.

Arrangements at home

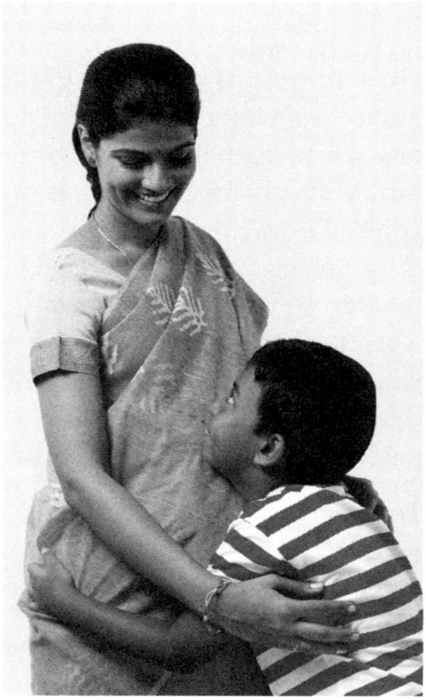

Do you have other children to take care of at home, and do you have to make special arrangements for them? In these days of the nuclear family, where both the husband and wife are working, and live by themselves, you need to get yourself organized before you go into labour. You may need to inform the person who will be coming and helping with your home arrangements, well in advance. Is your mother or your sister planning to stay with you? Have her come at least 2 weeks prior to your due date.

Who will be there to help you when you get home?

In India, a new mother is usually lucky enough to have her mother or mother-in-law around to help with the baby. New fathers are also very enthusiastic and eager to help with the baby. Make sure that your husband is in the hospital with you during and after the delivery so that he can get used to the baby's feeding, sleeping and diaper changing routines.

Remember that your sleep patterns will be altered because of your baby's demands. It will help to have somebody around who will let you sleep for a few hours between the baby's feeds.

Arrangements at work

Maternity leave

Working women should be aware of the rules regarding maternity leave in their workplace. As of March 2017, the Maternity Benefit (Amendment) Act raised maternity leave from the current 12 weeks to 26 weeks. The prenatal leave is also extended from six to eight weeks.

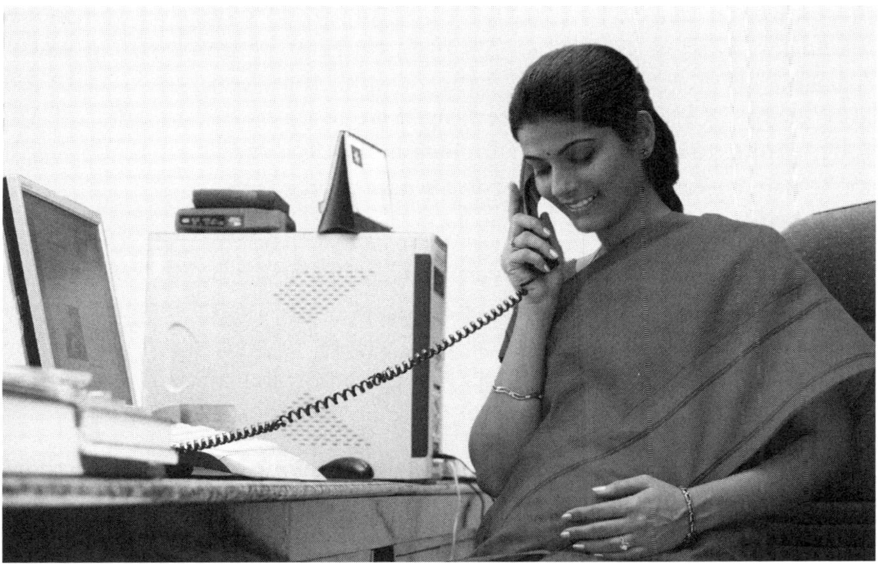

Amba asked: I have a month to go for my due date. My mother-in-law says I should quit going to the office. I am reasonably comfortable and I will quite frankly go bonkers sitting at home. How long can I continue to work?

My answer: You can work as long as you are comfortable. It might be a smart idea to work for as long as possible so that you can avail the maximum leave after the baby is born. This will allow you to bond with your baby for a longer period of time after delivery. If you plan to go to work till you go into labour, make sure you have a colleague who will take you to the hospital in the event that you get pains while at work.

If you are feeling exhausted in the last weeks of pregnancy, by all means take time off from work 1–2 months before your due date.

Talk to your office to see if there is a sabbatical policy that allows extending the duration of leave if required. Discuss whether you can get an option to work from home after delivery. Women working in large corporations (employing 50 or more women) will also find the new rule mandating crèches in offices a boon!

Readying your home for a new baby

The pregnancy has passed faster than you expected. It is almost time to bring the baby home. Are you sure that your home is organized and ready for the baby?

Once the baby arrives, you may have not much time to organize the house. Take a few days to plan what you need to do to keep everything ready. Will you be moving to your mother's home for a few weeks after the baby is born? Do you have everything there to take care of the baby? Are you planning to be in your own home after the delivery? Have you thought about where everything for the baby is going to be kept?

A place to sleep

A little time spent in planning everything will relieve you of a lot of stress and anxiety. You will need to prepare your room for the baby. You may purchase a crib to ensure that the baby sleeps in your room during the initial stages. The baby needs a crib that is comfortable and a firm mattress to sleep in (see **Chapter 17**, *Preparing to go to the hospital*).

Once the baby is a bit older you may consider moving him to another room or share a room with your first child, if you have one.

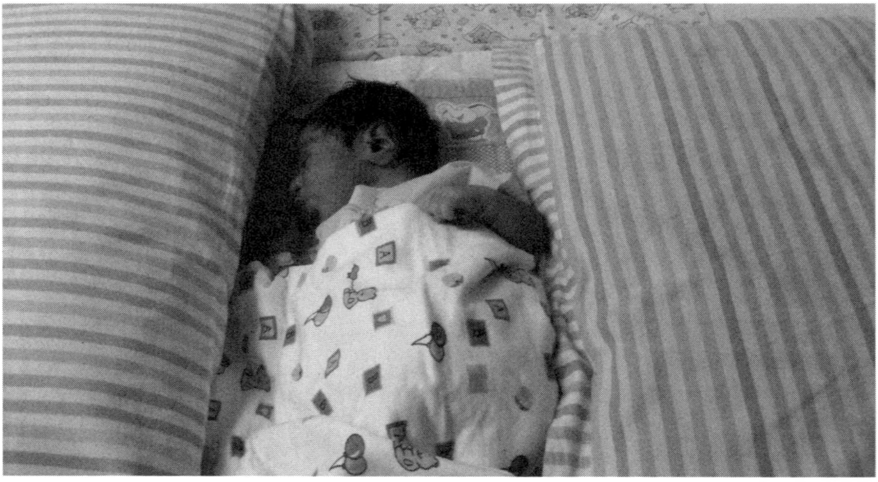

A place to change diapers

You may need to decide where you will be changing the baby's diapers (see more on changing diapers in **Chapter 46**, *Your new baby*). If it is going to be on your bed, make sure that you have enough rubber or plastic sheets so that your bed does not get soiled. If you are going to use a table, then it has to be at a convenient height. The table has to be solid and wide enough for you to change the diaper comfortably. A soft blanket (covered with a plastic sheet) may be placed on top to make it comfortable for the baby too.

Where will the baby's supplies go?

Get one part of your cupboard cleaned out so that you can keep the baby's supplies there. There must be enough place to hold the baby's clothes, diapers, blankets, powder, soap, shampoo and creams.

Getting your house ready

Once the baby is home, you will be so busy getting adjusted to the baby's schedule, that you may not have any time for regular household chores. Make sure that you have everything organized in your home so that you do not have to waste any time on routine chores. It will be better to find the right place for all items and to get into the habit of placing things in the place meant for them. This way the house may need little attention apart from regular cleaning.

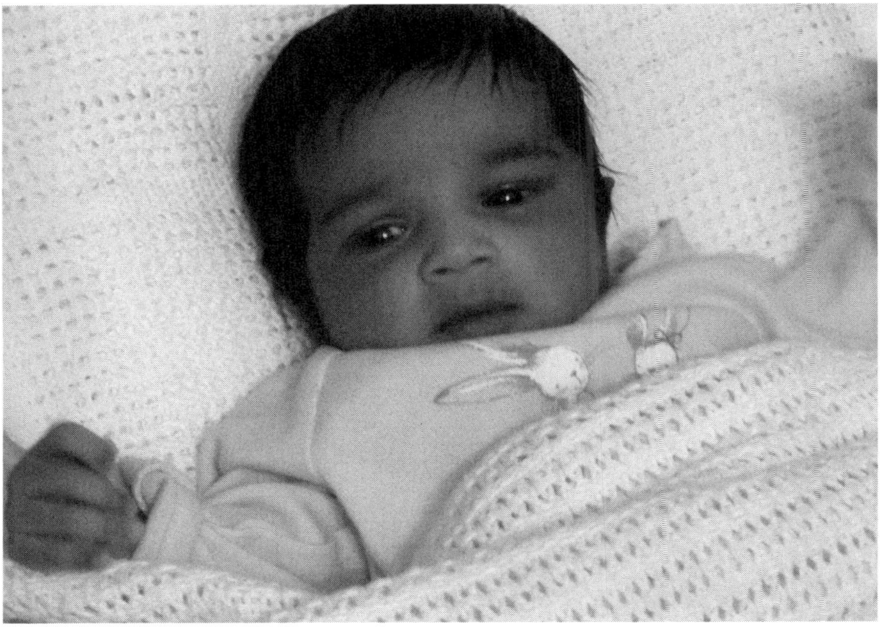

CHAPTER 19

Labour and delivery

Sanjana and Ranjith look forward to the birth of their child. It is the culmination of months of hopes and dreams. Finally the time has arrived to go through the process of labour and be rewarded with a baby. Sanjana is beset with mixed feelings. She is excited, but at the same time, filled with trepidation. After all, it is a mysterious process and the terms 'labour' and 'pains' evoke a sense of anxiety. It is important for her to understand the process so that she can undergo labour with the least amount of apprehension.

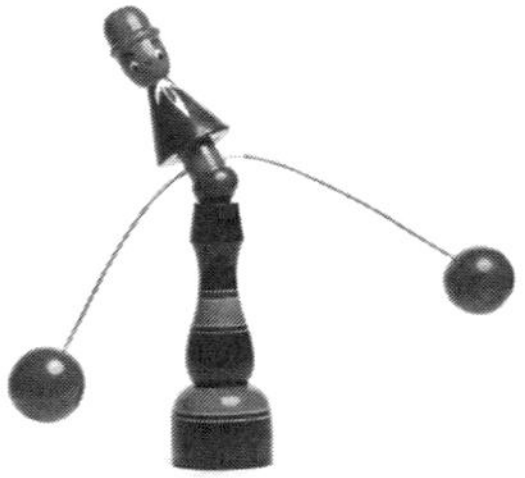

19

Labour and delivery: welcoming your baby into the world

These are the last few weeks of your pregnancy. At the office, you have been asking your friends who have had a baby about their experiences. Your mother tells you very little because she says 'she doesn't want to frighten you'. And that scares you even more! Your husband is very supportive and plans to be in the labour room with you, but he too is apprehensive.

It is normal for a couple to be concerned about the hospital stay, the pain of labour and about how long the whole process will take. This chapter will give you the information needed to make you feel you are in control of your own body. It will give you the confidence to go through the entire birthing process, with the least anxiety.

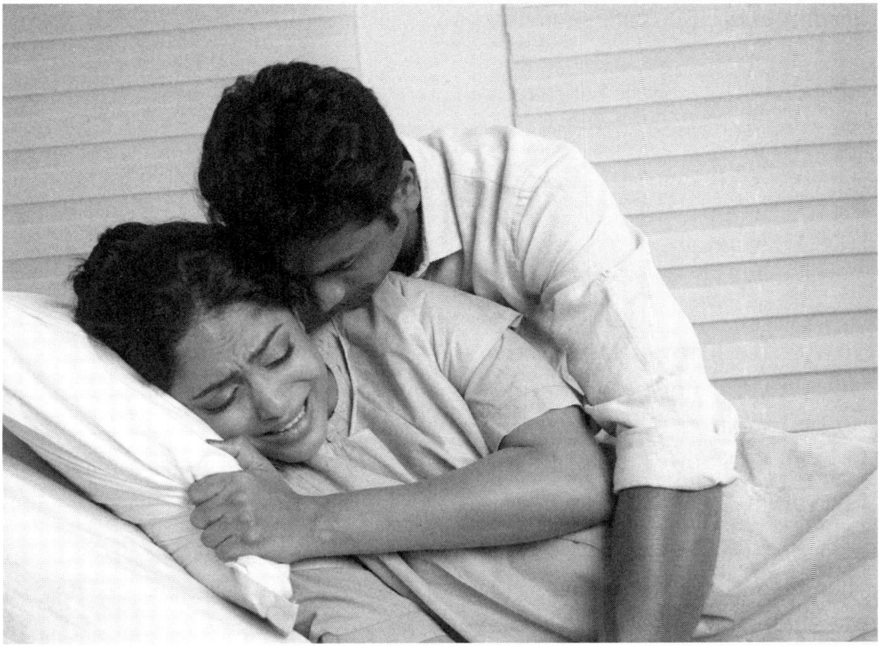

When will I deliver?

A human pregnancy usually lasts 280 days or 40 weeks. Once you complete the 37th week of pregnancy, you are considered to be at term. Most women will deliver between 37 and 40 weeks, though some may deliver by 41 weeks. Remember that only 5 per cent of women will deliver exactly on the given due date!

What triggers labour?

Many theories abound but no one really knows what starts off the process. It could be oxytocin released from the mother's pituitary gland or a hormone released by the baby.

If any signs of labour occur before 37 weeks of pregnancy, the labour is considered *preterm* or *premature*. You should see your obstetrician immediately if you have any signs or symptoms of labour before 37 weeks (see **Chapter 32**, *When the baby comes too early: preterm labour and birth*).

A normal pregnancy can also go beyond the due date that your obstetrician would have given you. There is no need to panic if you have not delivered by your due date. When the pregnancy goes one week beyond the due date, it is called postdated pregnancy. If your pregnancy is progressing well and your baby is healthy, your obstetrician will wait 7–10 days after the due date and then plan on delivering you (see **Chapter 33**, *When the baby is overdue: the postterm pregnancy*).

Labour is the process that starts with uterine contractions, enables the cervix to open, and assists your little one to be born.

Delivery is the passage of the baby and the placenta into the external world. A vaginal delivery happens through the birth canal and an abdominal delivery through an incision made into the uterus through the abdominal wall (caesarean section).

How will I know I am in labour?

Although it is not possible to know exactly when labour will begin, you can be prepared by knowing what to expect. Being prepared can make it easier for you to relax and focus on the arrival of your baby when the time comes.

Most first-time mothers are worried that they may not recognize labour when it starts. Even women who have had a baby earlier, may forget what it felt like when they went into labour the first time around!

Do not worry. It is almost impossible to go into labour and not know it. Most women can tell when they are in labour. Sometimes, however, it is hard to tell when labour begins. There are some signs that labour will start soon. As the body prepares for labour it sends out signals. You may or may not notice some of them before labour begins.

Signs that you are approaching labour

Sign	What is it?	When does it happen?
Lightening: feeling as if the baby has dropped lower down in your abdomen	This is known as 'engagement' or 'fixing' of the baby's head. The baby's head has settled deep into your pelvis	From a few weeks to a few hours before labour begins
Show: increase in vaginal discharge (clear, pink, or slightly bloody)	A thick mucus plug that has accumulated at the cervix during pregnancy is pushed out into the vagina	2–3 days before labour begins, or even at the onset of labour
Rupture of membranes: discharge of watery fluid from the vagina in a trickle or a gush	The fluid-filled sac (membranes) that surrounds the baby during pregnancy breaks	From several hours before labour begins to any time during labour

Signs that you are in labour

- *Contractions or pains:* When contractions start, you may have a regular pattern of cramps that may feel like a bad backache or menstrual cramps. These pains may occur every 15–30 minutes to begin with. Your uterus will tighten and relax. The frequency of contractions increases as labour progresses (from 20–15 to 10–8 to 5–3 minutes apart). The contractions become more painful as the cervix opens and the baby moves down the birth canal.

Timing your contractions

- Note how long it takes from the start of one pain to the start of the next one
- Keep a record for at least an hour
- If you are having regular pains that increase in intensity, labour may have started
- If the pains are very irregular and fizzle out in a short while, you are probably having Braxton-Hicks contractions, the 'practice contractions' that your uterus has from time to time

- *Discharge from the vagina:* As the cervix (mouth of the uterus) starts to open up, you will notice a thick mucus discharge. This is called the 'mucus plug' that had blocked the cervix. There can also be a blood stained discharge, called the 'bloody show'. This can vary between a slight stain on your underclothes to enough bleeding to necessitate a pad. The mucus discharge and the bloody show can happen anywhere between 48 hours before labour or even just as labour starts.
- *Membranes rupture:* The amniotic sac surrounding the baby may break even before pains start or this may happen during the process of labour. You will find water trickling down your thighs or you may have a sudden gush. Put on a sanitary napkin to monitor if the discharge is continuous. Once the water breaks, you must definitely get to the hospital as soon as possible, even if you do not have pains.

Greenish or dark water discharge

The amniotic fluid that surrounds the baby is usually a clear to yellowish liquid. Sometimes, when a woman's water breaks, it can be yellow-green or even a dark green colour. This means that the baby has passed motion (meconium) inside the womb. Though most of the time this is not of great significance, it may signify that the baby is facing some problem inside the womb.

As soon as you reach the hospital, the doctor will monitor the baby's heartbeat to check that the meconium does not indicate a problem.

Once labour starts, when should I leave for the hospital?

- ***Contractions:*** Wait for at least 1 or 2 hours till the pains are regular and are coming less than 10 minutes apart. Remember that it will be several hours before you deliver, especially if you are a first time mom-to-be
- ***Bloody show:*** There is no need to rush to the hospital till pains start. If the bleeding is heavy and you are changing your pad every 30-60 minutes, you should get to the hospital to check why you are bleeding more than usual
- ***Membranes rupture:*** If the water breaks (sometimes even before the onset of pains), it is important that you leave for the hospital immediately

How do I know it is not false labour?

Sometimes it can be hard to differentiate false labour from true pains. Usually, false contractions are less regular and not as strong as true labour. In true labour, progressive changes will occur in the cervix that will ultimately lead to delivery. False labour pains will usually subside if you walk around or rest, and may be continuous as compared to true pains that will come and go. False pains are usually in the front and in the lower abdomen, whereas true pains will travel from the top of the uterus to the lower abdomen or from the back to the front.

Sometimes, the only way to tell the difference is by seeing your obstetrician and having an internal examination done, to find changes in your cervix that signal the onset of labour. Occasionally, even after an examination, it might be difficult to tell whether you are in labour. You may then be admitted to the hospital and observed. If the pains go away and if your labour does not progress, you may be sent home.

Differences between false labour and true labour

Type of change	False labour	True labour
Timing of contractions	Often irregular and far apart. May be continuous without a break	Come at regular intervals and, as time goes on, get closer together. Each contraction lasts about 30–60 seconds
Change with movement	Contractions may stop when you walk or rest, or may even stop with a change of position	Contractions continue, despite movement
Strength of contractions	Usually weak and do not get much stronger (may be strong and then weak)	Increase in strength steadily
Pain of contractions	Usually felt only in the front, especially lower abdomen	Usually starts in the back and moves to the front. Moves from the top of the uterus downwards

What if you are sent back home?

If you thought you were in labour but the doctor sent you back home, then you were not in true labour. At home, your pains may continue to come on and off or your pains may disappear. You have to wait patiently for them to start again or get stronger.

Once labour pains start again, time them and see if they are getting more frequent and stronger. Don't rush to the hospital after just a few pains. You will have enough time to get to the hospital since labour usually takes several hours.

Don't forget to keep counting foetal kicks because that is a good indication that the baby is fine (see **Chapter 16**, *Tests of foetal well-being: is the baby tolerating pregnancy well?*).

What happens when I get admitted to the hospital?

When you reach the hospital, the obstetrician or the obstetric nurse will examine you.

- Your records will be checked to confirm your obstetric data
- Your blood pressure will be recorded
- The baby's heartbeat will be listened to and recorded
- The frequency and strength of the contractions will be noted

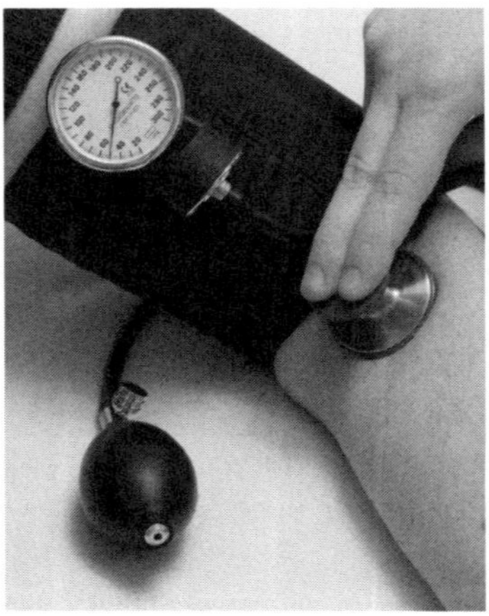

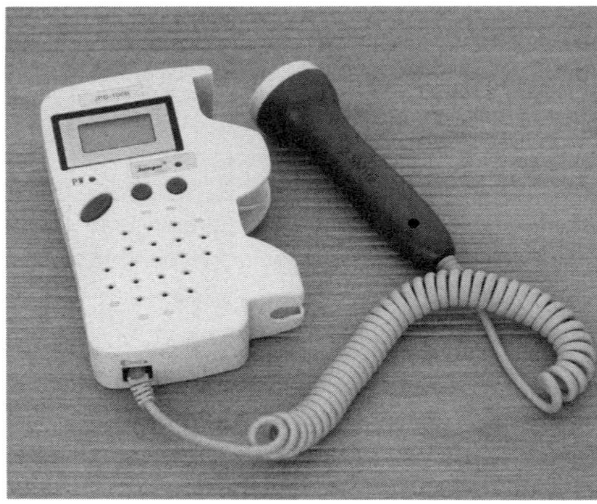

The most important decision that will be made at that time is whether you are in true labour. If it is difficult to determine whether you are in labour, you may be admitted for a few hours to see if the pains become regular and if labour progresses.

How will they know if it is true labour?

- You are observed to see if your contractions
  - Are occurring at regular intervals
  - Last for at least 45 seconds or more

- An internal examination is done to check the changes in the cervix. You are considered to be in labour if:
  - The cervix is thinned out (effaced)
  - The cervix is dilating progressively

Confirming that the baby's health is fine

In women who have a complicated pregnancy, the baby's heartbeat may be recorded using a cardiotocograph (foetal monitor). The amniotic fluid volume may also be checked using an ultrasound scan.

How will my labour progress?

Every labour is different. How long it lasts and how it progresses differs from woman to woman and from birth to birth. There are, however, general guidelines for labour that your obstetrician uses to decide whether it is progressing normally. If it is not progressing normally you may need medical assistance or a caesarean delivery.

Enema

An enema is not given routinely. If you have not had a good bowel movement, then an enema might be given.
A small amount of medication will be inserted gently into the rectum and this will make you pass motion. An empty rectum makes it easier for you when you have to push in the third stage of labour.

For the convenience of monitoring progress, labour is divided into three stages.

First stage of labour:
In the first stage of labour, cervical dilatation progresses from a closed cervix (0 cm) or a partially open cervix, to full dilatation (10 cm). The first stage is the longest stage of labour.

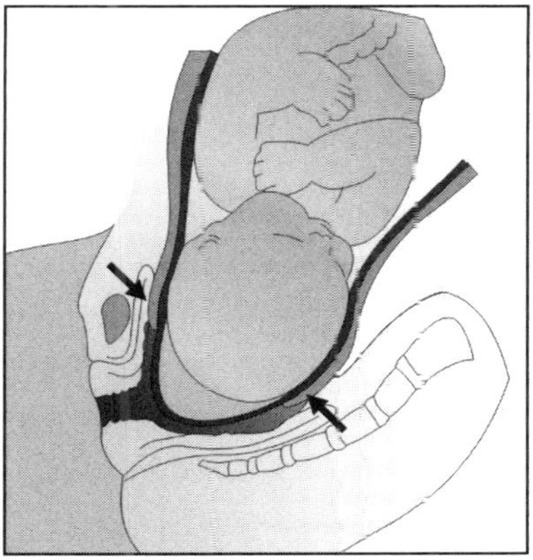
Fully dilated cervix (arrows) at the end of the first stage of labour

Second stage of labour:
The second stage of labour lasts from full dilatation of the cervix to the delivery of the baby. The second stage can last from 20 minutes to two hours. This time may vary from woman to woman.

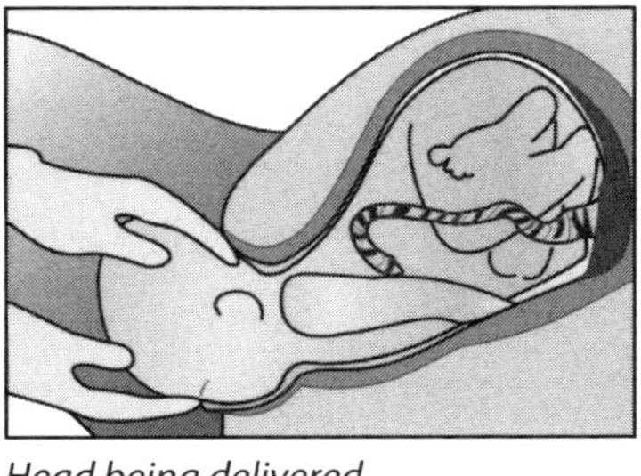
Head being delivered

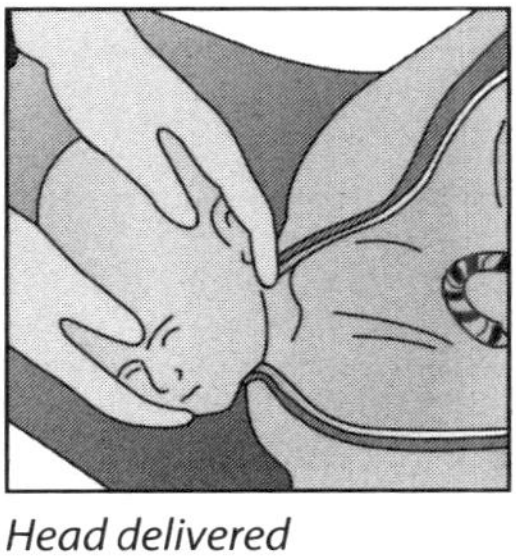
Head delivered

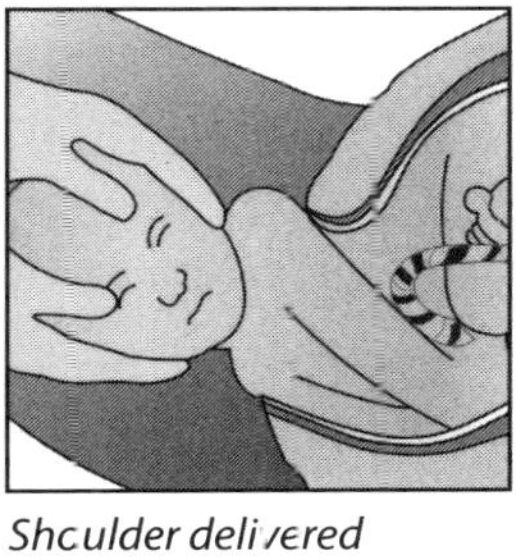
Shoulder delivered

Third stage of labour:
The placenta is expelled in the third stage of labour. This is the shortest stage of labour.

Arti asked: My mother asked me to sweep the house after my pains started. She said it would make the delivery easier. Is that true?

My answer: Not true at all. It will not make your delivery easier. It probably was a method to distract young women from the discomfort of the latent phase and then became a myth about 'easy delivery'!

Handling the three stages of labour

First stage of labour

At the beginning of labour, the cervix may be closed or partially open. In the first stage of labour, the dilatation progresses from a closed cervix (0 cm) or a partially open cervix, to full dilatation (10 cm). The first stage is the longest stage of labour.

The first stage of labour is divided into

- Latent phase (early labour): from onset of labour to 4 cm dilatation
- Active phase: from 4 cm to 10 cm dilatation

Latent phase (from 0–4 cm dilatation)

Contractions begin in the latent phase. Some first-time mothers experience a prolonged period of early labour with minimal or no change in their cervical dilatation in the first few hours. The contractions help with the thinning of the cervix (**effacement**) and start the process of opening up **(dilatation)**. The latent phase lasts till the cervix is dilated to 4 cm.

Signs

Pains may begin at irregular intervals but will gradually become regular, stronger and more intense. They usually start 15–20 minutes apart and increase in frequency to about 5 minutes apart. The pain can be concentrated in the low back or in the lower part of the abdomen. Look for contractions that continue even if you move around, that get stronger, and that start in your back and move around to the front.

How long?

The latent phase can last 6–8 hours if this is your first pregnancy and 4–6 hours for mothers who have had a baby before.

What you can do to handle it

If you are in early labour, try walking around, reading a book or watching a movie. This might make it easier to bear the pains. Support from your husband and the family will help you get through this frustrating part of early labour.

Active phase

The active phase of labour is when things really progress. Once the cervix has dilated to 4 cm, the active phase is considered to have started. You will definitely be in the hospital by now. During this phase of labour, the cervix will continue to thin (efface) and open up (dilate).

The process of thinning (effacement) and opening (dilatation) of the cervix (mouth of the uterus)

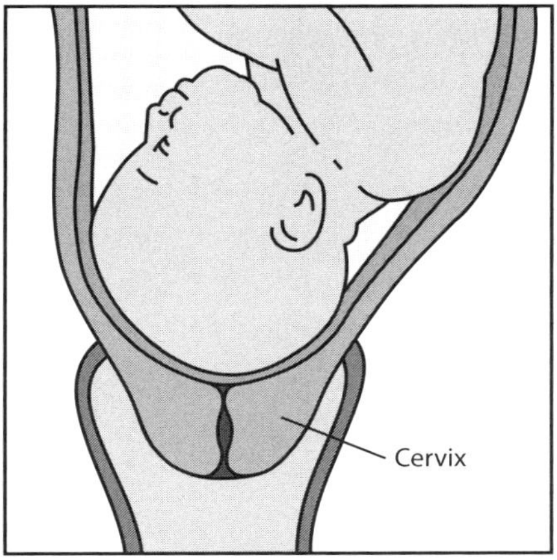

1. Cervix is not effaced or dilated

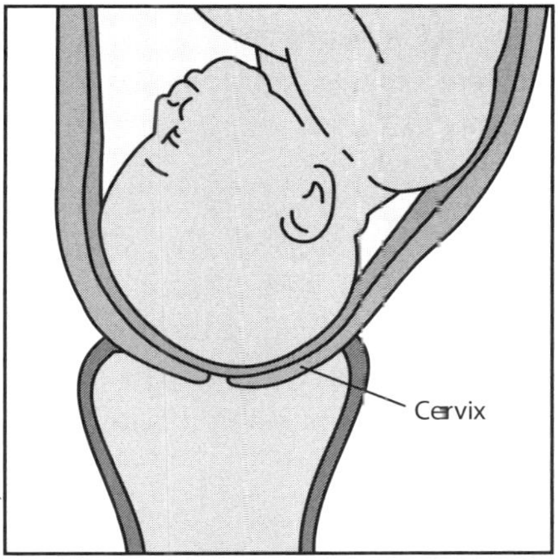

2. Cervix is fully effaced and dilated to 1 cm

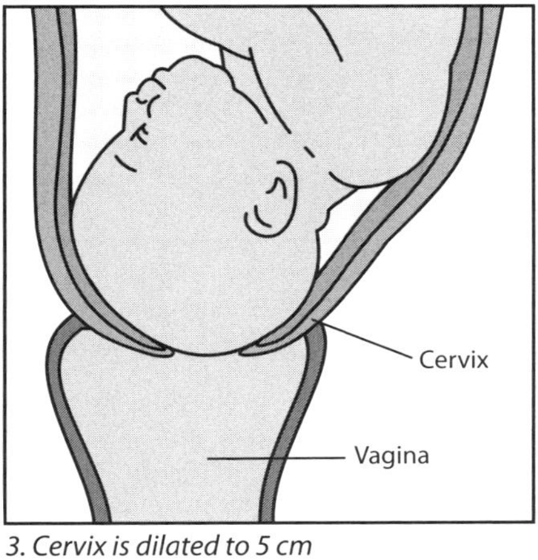

3. Cervix is dilated to 5 cm

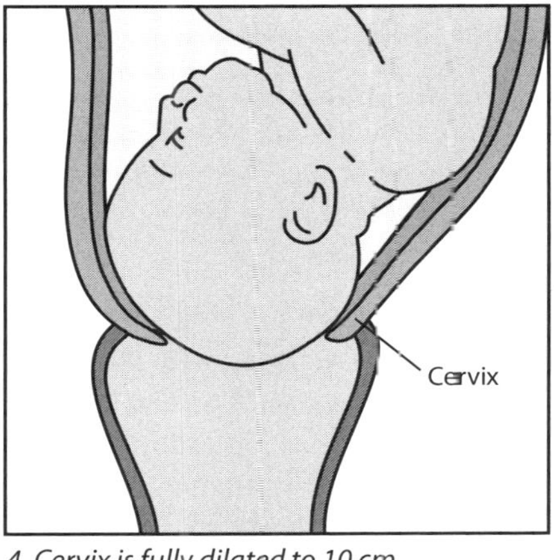

4. Cervix is fully dilated to 10 cm

Your obstetrician will examine you at regular intervals to assess how your cervix is dilating. The average woman in her first labour may dilate about 1 cm per hour during the active phase of labour. If you have had a baby before, you may dilate 2 cm per hour or more. When the cervix has reached 10 cm it is 'fully dilated'. Toward the end of active labour, the baby's head may begin to descend through the birth canal.

Tough stage for both of you

This is where you may find yourself losing your temper and wondering if labour will ever come to an end. Your partner should try to be prepared for your despair and anger. Pain relief is definitely advised in this phase.

The baby's heartbeat will be monitored with a stethoscope, a hand-held Doppler device or cardiotocograph (foetal monitor). Read more about it in **Chapter 23**, *Monitoring the baby's well-being during labour.*

Signs

As labour progresses, the contractions become more frequent, longer and stronger. They may occur every 3–4 minutes and last up to 60 seconds. The cervix begins dilating more quickly. This is the point when you might ask for pain relief, including an epidural (see **Chapter 22**, *Pain relief in labour and delivery*). Your membranes may rupture spontaneously or your doctor may rupture them.

Rupture of membranes

The membranes may also rupture spontaneously during active labour and you may be aware of a gush of fluid from the vagina.

If the membranes have not ruptured on their own, your obstetrician may decide to rupture them. This is called an *amniotomy*. The amniotomy serves two purposes.

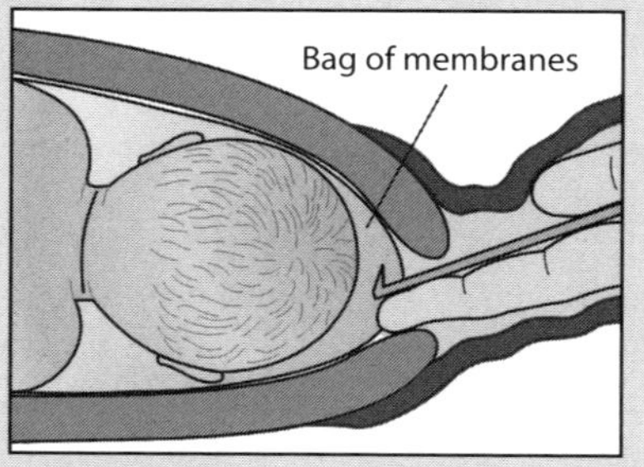

Amniotomy

- It may help make your labour progress faster
- It also allows the doctor to check the colour of the amniotic fluid. If it is clear, it is a good sign and indicates the baby is doing well. If it is greenish this may be an indication that the baby has passed meconium inside the uterus. This may sometimes be a sign that the baby is facing difficulty inside the uterus

As the cervix dilates, you may feel nauseous and you may retch, or vomit.

After the cervix is dilated to 8–9 cm, labour pains may ease off for a brief period of time. This is called the transitional phase of the first stage of labour. But soon, the contractions become stronger and come at frequent intervals of 2–3 minutes. As the baby's head drops well into the birth canal and starts impacting against the rectum, you may get a strong urge to push down. Without your own volition, you may start grunting and pushing down. Your obstetrician might ask you not to push till the cervix is fully dilated. You will have to breathe rhythmically and try to relax so that you do not push at this point.

How long?
The active phase can last 3–6 hours for a first-time mom and 1–3 hours for mothers who have had a baby before. Your doctor may augment labour to hasten the process (see **Chapter 20**, *Augmentation and induction of labour*).

What you can do to handle it
In the early stages of the active phase, you can walk around. As the pains get stronger, you might want to sit or lie down. Your partner can help by massaging your lower back. A hot water bottle may also be of use. If you have had a narcotic pain killer, you may feel sleepy and may be advised not

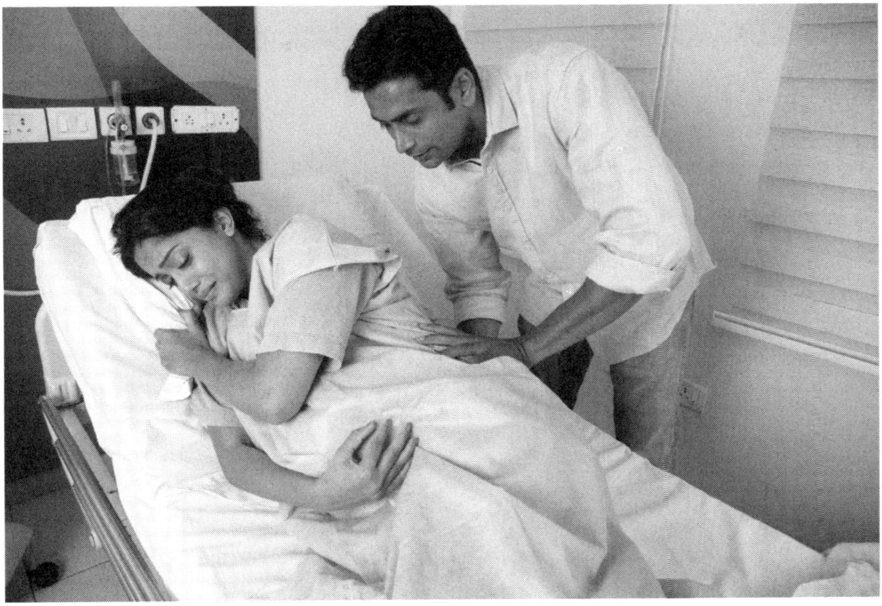

to walk around. If you have taken an epidural, you may sit or lie down and can turn from side to side.

This is also a good time to use the breathing techniques you learned in labour preparation classes (see the section on Breathing techniques in **Chapter 22**, *Pain relief in labour and delivery*). This is where your partner's presence next to you is invaluable for emotional support.

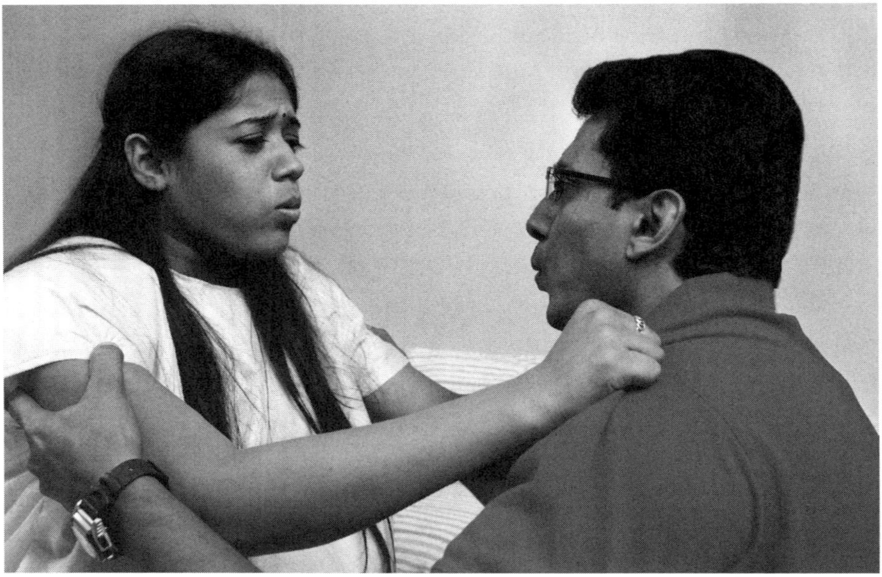

Keep yourself hydrated with liquids (tender coconut water, thin buttermilk and fruit drinks are good choices).

Bladder

Try to pass urine frequently. A full bladder can be very uncomfortable. Sometimes the baby's head is low and it may be difficult to pass urine. A small tube (catheter) may be passed into the bladder to empty it and to relieve your discomfort.

Second stage of labour

The second stage of labour lasts from full dilatation of the cervix to the birth of the baby. After the cervix is fully dilated, the baby moves down the birth canal aided by uterine contractions and your pushing efforts, and makes her grand entrance into the world.

What happens?

You will continue to feel pain with the contractions. The urge to push is uncontrollable (though you may not feel the urge if you have had an epidural). You will want to pass motion but it is actually your baby's head pushing against the rectum that gives you this sensation.

By now you may be exhausted but will need to pull out your last reserves of strength to push the baby out. There may be slightly more blood-stained discharge at this time. As the baby pushes its way out of the vagina, you may feel a stretching, burning sensation.

Crowning and delivery of the baby

When the mother has pushed for a while, the baby's head is seen at the opening of the vagina. This is called the 'crowning' of the baby's head. Soon, with a few more pushes, the baby will be delivered.

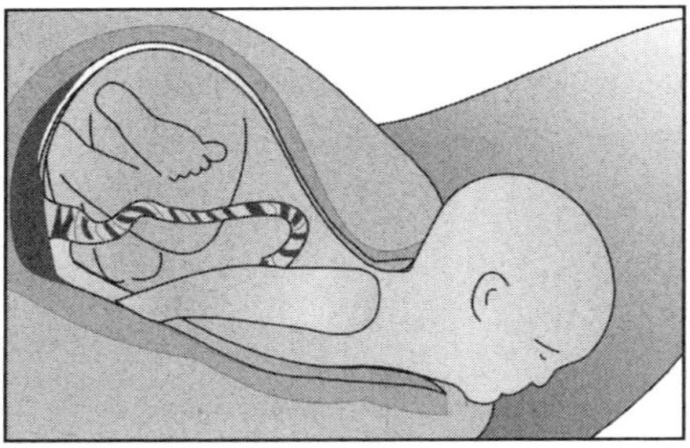

Crowning of the baby's head

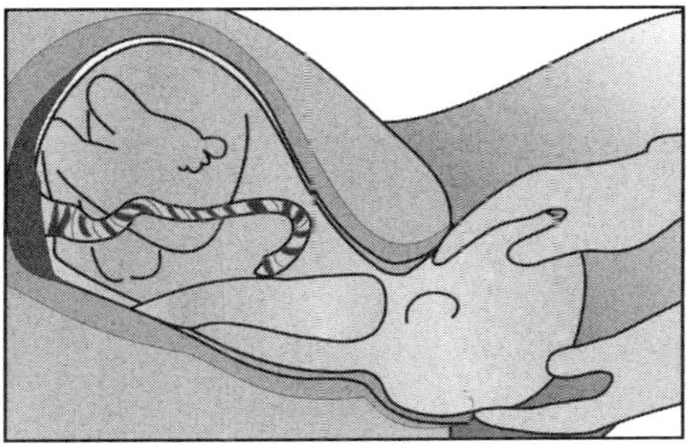

Delivery of the baby's head

At this point, your obstetrician will decide whether you require an episiotomy. The baby's head will then be gently helped out of the birth canal. The shoulders and the rest of the baby will then follow very quickly. The obstetrician will guide the baby out, trying to avoid injury to your tissues.

Cord clamping

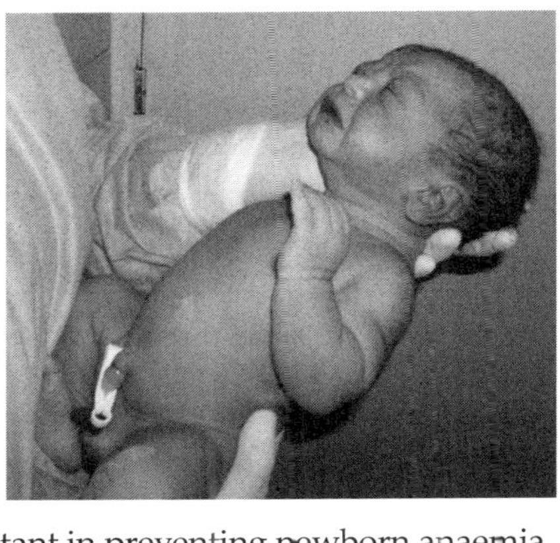

As soon as the baby is born, the doctor will ensure that she is crying and taking good breaths. If blood is being drawn from the cord for stem cell banking, the doctor will draw the blood before clamping the cord (see the section on *Cord Blood Banking* at the end of this chapter). The cord is usually clamped 1–3 minutes after the baby is born so that the baby gets the maximum amount of blood flowing into her from the placenta. This is important in preventing newborn anaemia.

How long?

The second stage of labour is significantly shorter than the first stage. The second stage usually lasts from 1–2 hours, averaging about 90 minutes. This time may vary from woman to woman and may be as short as 20 minutes.

What can you do to handle it?

You have to gather all your strength and concentrate on bringing the baby into the world. You will be amazed at how you find that last reserve of determination to get through this part of delivery.

Remember that there is always a gap of two to three minutes between each contraction. Just go limp, take deep breaths and relax during that time so you can gather up enough strength for the next push.

Pushing

This is the toughest part of labour. You have to use mechanical pressure to assist the uterine contractions in pushing the baby out. It is almost like being severely constipated and having to give terrific pressure to pass motion.

Your husband will be able to help you by supporting your head and neck as you push down. If you are lying on your back, the most effective way of pushing is to take a deep breath, put your chin on your chest and push down into your rectum. Many labour tables will have handles that you can hold to help you push. Some women find it comfortable to lie on their side and push.

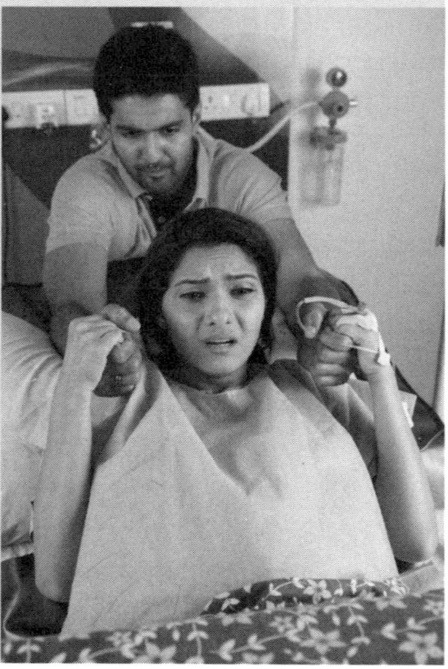

Make sure that you have spoken to your doctor (well before labour) about what positions you can adopt to help you push. Some women like to squat and some women like to go on their hands and knees to push. This requires great cooperation from every one in the labour room.

You have to listen if your doctor asks you to stop pushing for a couple of contractions. She may want you to do this so that she can ensure that the baby does not deliver too rapidly. To control the urge to push, you can pant or take deep breaths.

Episiotomy

What is an episiotomy?

An episiotomy is a surgical incision made through the perineum (the area below the vagina and just above the anus). This is usually done to enlarge the vagina and assist the delivery of the baby. It is one of the common medical procedures performed on women.

Routine episiotomies are no longer recommended. Still, the procedure is warranted in some cases. At present, most obstetricians will restrict episiotomies to 40-50 per cent of deliveries. If you have had a baby before, the vagina may be more lax and it might be easier to deliver without an episiotomy.

Your obstetrician might resort to an episiotomy if

- The perineum and vagina will have extensive tears without the episiotomy
- Forceps or vacuum delivery are being done
- Your baby is large (foetal macrosomia)
- Your baby needs to be delivered quickly due to problems arising during labour

In a first delivery, the tissue of the perineum may be not be very lax and may tear during the delivery. If your obstetrician feels that you will have more damage to your pelvic tissues if the cut is not made, she might perform an episiotomy. An episiotomy might also help cut short the second stage of labour.

An episiotomy is usually done under local anaesthesia. It is sutured after the delivery of the baby. Most women will not feel the episiotomy being done, especially if it is done during a contraction.

After care for the episiotomy

An episiotomy can be painful for a few days after the delivery. Usually, the pain will peak around the 4th or 5th day and then will gradually become less.

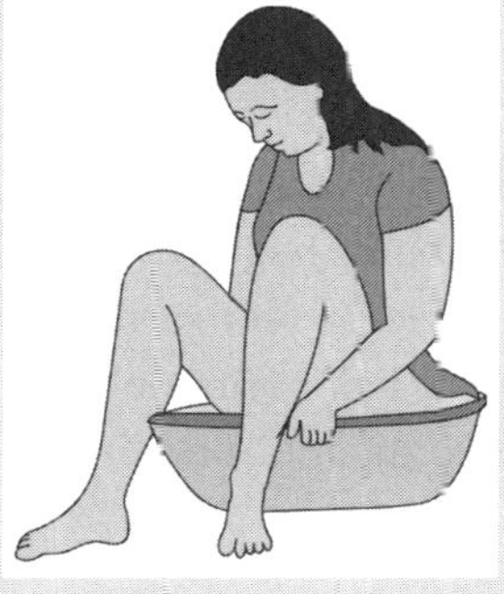

There is no need for any oral antibiotics to be taken just because you have had an episiotomy. You need not apply any ointment on the episiotomy.

For pain relief, you can take a pain killer like ibuprofen. You may also be advised a Sitz bath which is basically a basin filled with warm water in which you can sit. This is soothing for the pain. An infrared lamp can also be used on the episiotomy to relieve the pain.

APGAR score

When the baby is born, your obstetrician will assign him an APGAR score. This is a good way of measuring the baby's response to his first few minutes of life after birth. The scores are given at 1 minute, 5 minutes and 10 minutes.
A high score (8 and more) is indicative of a healthy baby that is responding well to birth. A low score at 5 and 10 minutes (less than 6) means that the baby has had trouble adapting to birth and may require admission to the newborn nursery.

A = Appearance (colour)
P = Pulse (heartbeat)
G = Grimace (reflex)
A = Activity (muscle tone)
R = Respiration (breathing)

Each of these is assigned a score of 2, 1 or 0, depending on the condition of the baby.

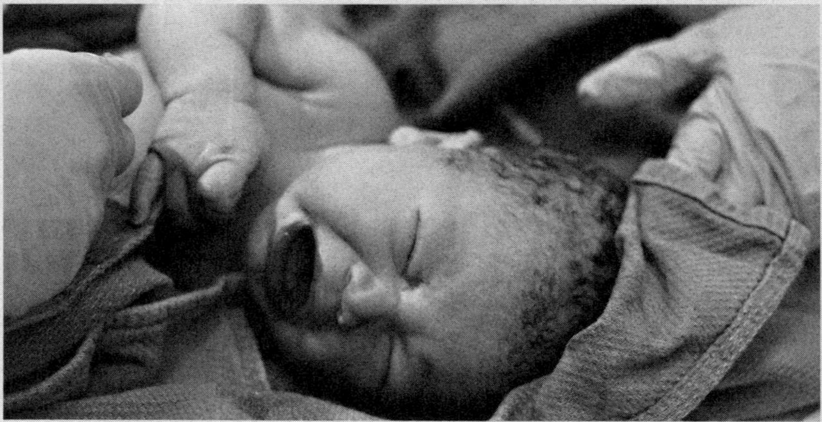

Third stage of labour

The baby has been born! You can't believe you are actually holding this miracle in your arms. You are almost done with the process of delivery. There is just one more thing to complete and that is the expulsion of the placenta and membranes. This is the final stage of labour.

What happens?

There may be some discomfort though you don't have to do any more hard work! You may or may not feel some contractions as your uterus tries to expel the placenta. When your doctor confirms that there are signs of the placenta having separated from the uterine wall, she may ask you to push gently to expel the placenta. In some cases, she may reach inside and gently help pull out the placenta.

As soon as the placenta is out, you will receive an injection to help your uterus contract. This is a preventive measure to avoid excessive bleeding from the uterus.

How long?
This stage generally only takes 5–15 minutes. Rarely, the placenta may not detach from the uterine wall and the third stage may last a little longer.

Chances are that you may not pay much attention to this stage of labour because you will be busy holding your little bundle of joy!

Your obstetrician will make sure that the uterus has contracted well and that you are not having any excessive bleeding. She will also check to see if there have been any cuts in the vaginal tissue. If there has been any tearing or an episiotomy has been done, the doctor will suture them at this time.

After the delivery

You have been through one of the toughest experiences in your life and have been rewarded with a beautiful baby. The excitement of holding your baby will bring smiles and tears of joy. Your husband will want to take photos of your little one and start posting them!

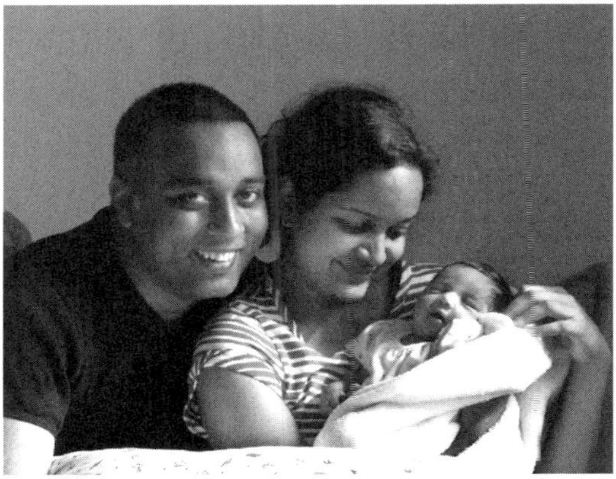

As soon as the baby is born and the doctor and nurses have made sure that the baby is breathing well, the baby will be placed on your chest for some skin-to-skin bonding. This is very important for both you and the baby. Your husband also will hold the baby.

Ensure that the baby is brought back to you for breastfeeding as soon as you and the baby are cleaned up, preferably within an hour of birth (see **Chapter 27**, *Breastfeeding*).

You shouldn't be surprised at some of the things you will experience after the delivery.

- Shivering and shaking is common immediately after the delivery. You may need a blanket for a short while to keep you warm
- You may feel like you have run a marathon. You know what, you actually have! You have been through quite a physical workout and you may ache all over
- You may have pain and soreness over the vaginal area. If you have had an episiotomy or stitches for tears, the discomfort will get worse after the local anaesthetic wears off
- You will have vaginal bleeding and will need to use sanitary napkins for 4–6 weeks after the delivery. The bleeding will decrease gradually over the next few weeks
- Your face may look puffy and red for a few days after the delivery because of the pushing you did during labour
- You might be surprised to see a few red spots in the whites of your eyes the day after the delivery. These are blood clots that form when small blood vessels rupture when you are pushing. They are absolutely harmless and will disappear after a few days

Cord Blood Banking

You may have heard about stem cell banking. One of your friends may actually have stored her baby's cord blood at the time of delivery. Should you also do this? Read this carefully before you make your decision.

What is umbilical cord blood banking?

Once considered a waste product that was discarded with the placenta, umbilical cord blood is now known to be rich in potentially life-saving stem cells. When used for stem cell transplantation, umbilical cord blood offers several distinct advantages over bone marrow or peripheral stem cells.

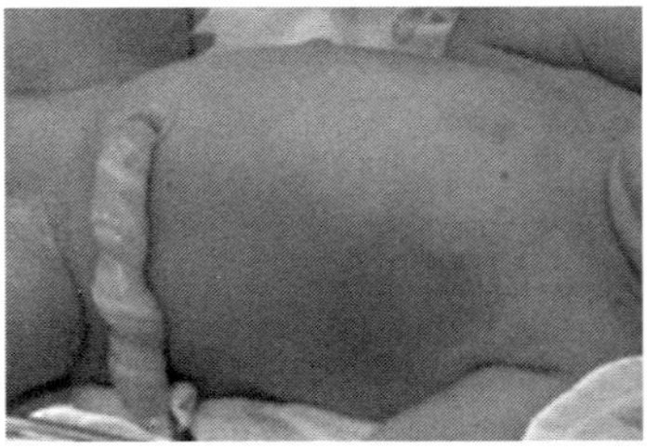

The commonest indication for the use of stem cells is in the cure of certain childhood blood diseases. Currently, stem cells from cord blood can cure 60 per cent of children with thalassaemia or blood cancers (leukaemia). The use of stem cells for other conditions is still in experimental stages.

Private vs. public cord blood banking

In many parts of the world, including India, private companies have aggressively marketed the need for the storage of umbilical cord blood. The marketing definitely plays on the guilt of parents and grandparents who feel that if they do not store their baby's cord blood, they have not done something essential to safeguard the baby's future.

On the other hand, **public cord blood banks**, like the Jeevan Stem Cell Bank, Chennai, (run by a not-for-profit public trust established in 2008), allow this valuable product to be stored and used by anybody, much like blood banks store units of blood that can be used to save anyone's life, not just the donor's.

Can't we get the stem cells from another country?

If we don't have a public cord blood bank of significant size in our country, can we import stem cells from another country to save the life of a dear one? Unfortunately, this is not always possible. Stem cell match (HLA) is highly dependent on the ethnicity of the donor and patient and therefore Indians alone can help Indians. It is only now that India has its first public stem cell bank. So, we have nowhere to go to get matching stem cells. Even if one is lucky enough to find a match outside India, one unit of stem cells will cost over Rs 20 lakhs!

How is cord blood collected?

Once the baby is delivered, the umbilical cord attached to the placenta is cleaned and a needle is inserted into a cord blood vessel. About 70–120 millilitres of blood is obtained. Once the cord blood is collected, it is sent for testing and processing. Lab technicians run the blood through a battery of tests, extract the stem cells from the sample, and prepare the sample for the freezer, where the cells remain until they are needed.

The sample cannot be used for stem cell transplant if it has a volume of less than 70 ml and contains less than 750 million stem cells. In that case the unit is discarded. Many private stem cell banks do not disclose this requirement to patients.

Should all parents store their baby's cord blood?

The Indian National Stem Cell Guidelines were released in 2013: **'There is no scientific basis for preservation of cord blood for future self-use and this practice is not recommended.'**

They also mentioned that there are ethical concerns about the promotional advertisements by private banks offering storage of cord blood for possible future use. Such advertisements are often misleading for the public and lack comprehensive and accurate information to the consumer. **Parents should be encouraged for voluntary donation to public cord blood banks for allogeneic transplantation.**

In India, collection, processing and storage of cord blood in a **private** company can cost between Rs 80,000 and Rs 1 lakh to the parents. On the other hand, **donating your baby's cord blood to a public cord blood bank is free**!

Approximately 10,000 stem cell transplants have been done around the world till now. The vast majority of cord blood stem cell transplants have been done using cells from **unrelated donors** from public banks. About 300 transplants have involved sibling donors while **less than 50** have been done using a child's own cells.

Will your child need its own cord blood in the future?

Most parents are terrified that their child might develop a condition in the future that might be only curable with its own stem cells. They are particularly concerned about genetic diseases or leukaemia (blood cancer). Unfortunately, if a child has a genetic disease or childhood leukaemia, his or her own cord blood would be useless in treating it because the cells will be chromosomally or genetically abnormal. A sibling's cord blood or an unrelated donor's cord blood might help.

No accurate estimates exist of the likelihood that children will need their own stored cells, but estimates range from 1 in 2,700 to 1 in 200,000.

For marketing purposes, many companies say that cord blood stem cells will be useful in the future for treating diabetes, heart disease, nerve diseases and arthritis. **There is no scientific basis for this at present**. Healthy families should not succumb to marketing ploys because the likelihood of ever using the blood is rare, and future medical uses for it are uncertain.

What is more concerning is that the amount of stem cells present in the unit of cord blood stored will not be sufficient for treating an adult. Using two or three units from a public cord blood bank might be more efficient.

Stem cell transplants from a donor are as effective as from the same individual. Donating the cord blood to a pubic blood bank will be more useful and cost-effective than storing it for one individual.

Let your baby start its life with a charitable act

Donate your baby's cord blood to a public cord blood bank instead of throwing it into the bucket. It may save the life of another child. Don't forget to inform your obstetrician that you want to donate the blood so that arrangements can be made well before the actual delivery.

If you want more information, contact Jeevan Stem Cell Bank (a public not-for-profit cord blood bank) at **stemcell@jeevan.org** or visit their website **www.bethecure.in**

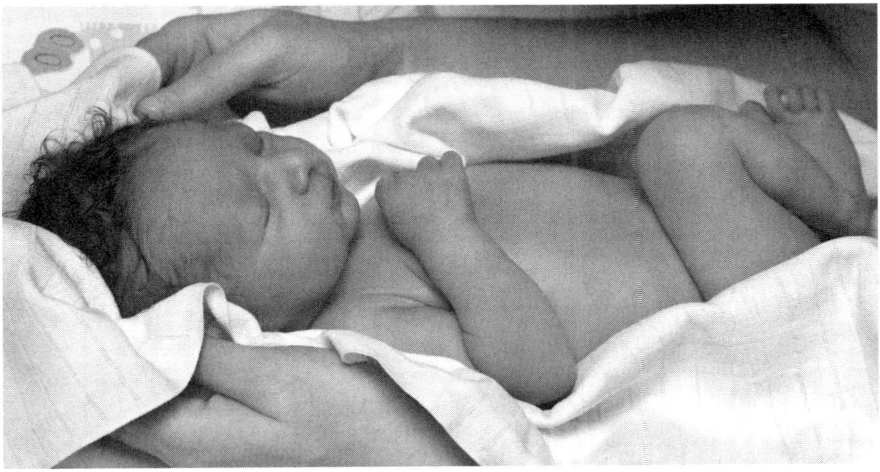

CHAPTER 20

Augmentation and induction of labour

Shivani has been in labour for seven hours. Her pains have become weak and are not effective. The cervix has not dilated further in the past two hours. She will be given medication to augment labour so that she can deliver without further delay.

Sangeetha is 41 weeks pregnant. Her obstetrician has advised her to get admitted to the hospital. She will be undergoing induction of labour.

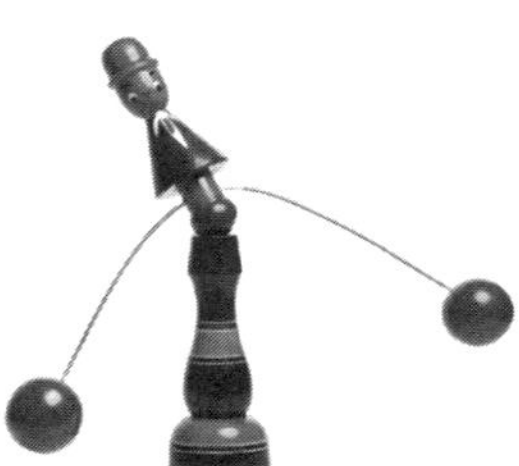

20

Augmentation and induction of labour

Though it is the expected thing for contractions to start when they should, and labour to progress as it should, things don't always go smoothly according to plan. Sometimes labour pains don't become strong enough and need a little help from the doctor. This is called augmentation of labour. Sometimes, labour does not start on time or may need to be started because certain situations dictate that the baby should be delivered as soon as possible. This is called induction of labour.

Augmentation of labour

If you are in labour but the progress of labour has slowed down or come to a halt, labour is hastened (augmented) by rupturing membranes (amniotomy) or by administering oxytocin. This gentle push to the slightly 'lazy' uterus will ensure stronger, more effective contractions so that you deliver your baby safely and within a comfortable timeframe.

Induction of labour:

If you are not in labour but the baby needs to be delivered (for example, you are beyond your due date), labour is started artificially (induced) by using mechanical means or medications. This is an attempt to avoid a caesarean section. Globally, almost 25 per cent of women will have their labour induced.

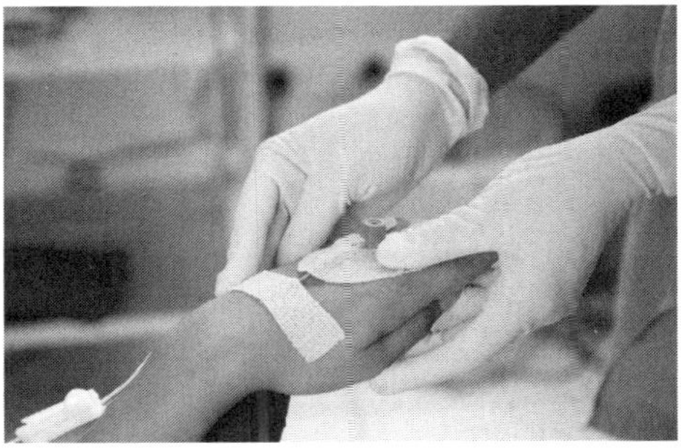

Labour augmentation: when and how?

Reasons for augmentation

Occasionally, labour may not progress as rapidly as it should. You may have gone into active labour (see **Chapter 19**, *Labour and delivery*) but contractions may have slowed down or completely stopped. The doctor may have examined you but is not happy about the slow rate of dilatation. There's no need to be concerned. Sometimes the uterine contractions just seem to take a small break!

When the contractions continue to be irregular and are not effective in dilating the cervix and moving the baby down the birth canal, steps need to be taken to help the process along. Augmentation increases the frequency, duration and intensity of contractions.

How is labour augmented?

Your obstetrician will carefully assess

- The pattern of the contractions
- How much your cervix is dilated
- How far your baby has descended into the birth canal
- If the baby is not too big for you to deliver vaginally
- That the baby's heart rate stays normal both during and immediately after contractions

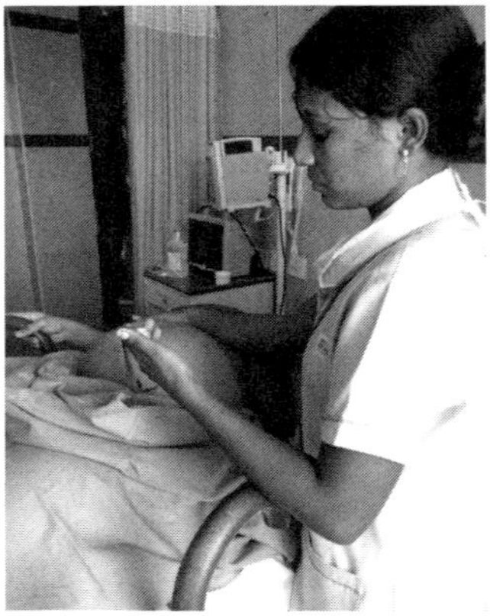

Contractions being timed

Once your doctor has determined that there is no reason to worry that either you or your baby will have a problem with augmentation and stronger contractions, she will choose one of the following methods for augmentation.

Amniotomy

This is a common form of augmenting labour. If the membranes have not ruptured on their own, your obstetrician may decide to rupture them.

An amniotomy has the advantage of allowing the doctor to check the colour of the amniotic fluid.

- If it is clear, it is a good sign and indicates that the baby is tolerating labour well
- If it is greenish in colour, this may be an indication that the baby has passed meconium inside the uterus. Though most of the time the baby will do well, occasionally it may be a sign that the baby is not receiving adequate oxygen through the placenta. In this case the doctor will monitor the baby's heart rate pattern (see **Chapter 23**, *Monitoring the baby's well-being during labour*)

Oxytocin

Amniotomy by itself may not be very effective in hastening labour. The most common drug that is used for augmentation is a synthetic form of the hormone **oxytocin**. You will receive it through an intravenous (IV) drip.

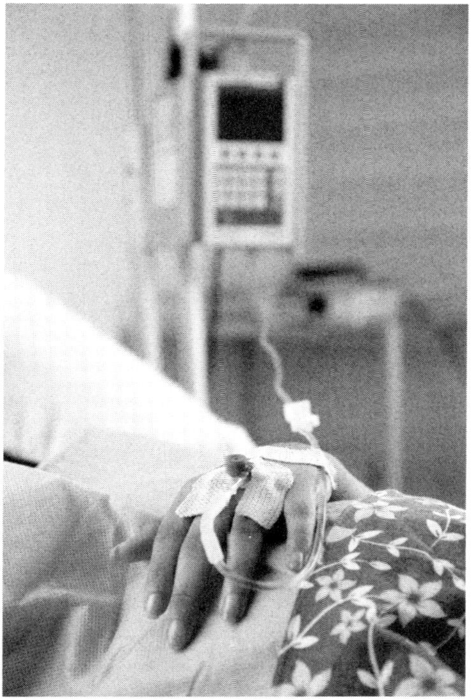

Augmentation is usually started with a small dose, and the dose is gradually increased until your uterus responds appropriately. The aim is to have about three contractions in ten minutes.

Your pains will be monitored till you are having effective contractions. It is also important to make sure that your pains are not too frequent or too strong. Effective contractions will cause your cervix to dilate and will help the baby's head descend into the birth canal. While your labour is being augmented, the baby's heartbeat will be monitored regularly to make sure the baby is tolerating labour well.

Labour induction: when and how?

You have been waiting for labour pains to start. Your doctor has examined you and said that the baby's head has dropped into the birth canal, the cervix has started to thin out and the cervix has actually dilated a bit (common in first-time moms, even before labour). Now it is one week beyond your due date and your doctor feels she has to induce (in other words, kickstart) your labour.

This means that the obstetrician may use medication or other methods to make you go into labour so that you can have a vaginal delivery. This is only done if vaginal delivery poses no threat to you or the baby. Whether the labour will be induced also depends on the condition of the mother and the baby, the week of pregnancy, the status of the cervix and the size of the baby.

Common reasons for inducing labour

Labour is induced if the health of the mother or baby is at risk.

- Postterm pregnancy i.e., pregnancy that has continued at least 7–10 days past the due date
- Rupture of membranes before labour has started
- You have a condition (such as high blood pressure, preeclampsia, or diabetes) that may jeopardize your health or the health of your baby if the pregnancy continues
- If the baby has growth restriction and is not growing as well as she should
- Infection of the amniotic sac (chorioamnionitis)
- Separation of the placenta (abruption) from the inner lining of the uterus
- Logistical reasons (for example, the pregnant mother lives too far from a hospital or there is a history of fast labour)
- Death of the baby before birth (intrauterine foetal demise)

Will induction be safe and successful?

To determine that the induction will have a good chance of success and that it will be safe for mother and child, your doctor will confirm that the conditions are right for induction. If it is suspected that induction may jeopardize either the mother or the baby, she will proceed directly with a caesarean section.

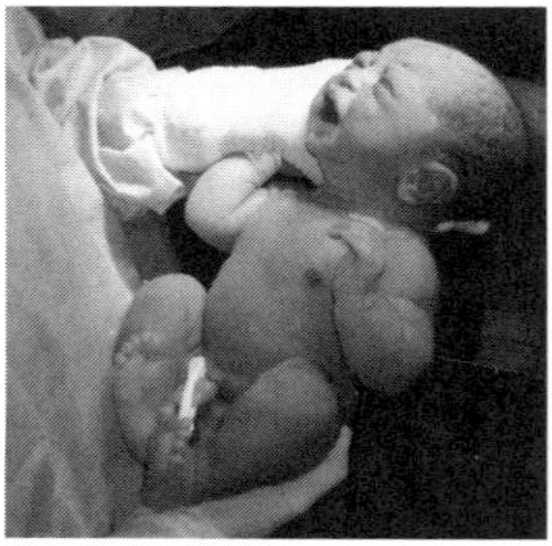

Signs for success—mother	Signs for safety—baby
The cervix has thinned out	Adequate amniotic fluid volume as confirmed by ultrasound*
The cervix has started to dilate	Good reserves to tolerate labour as confirmed by non-stress test*
The baby's head has descended into the birth canal	The baby is not too big to be delivered vaginally

* See **Chapter 16**, *Tests of foetal well-being*: is the baby tolerating pregnancy well?

Increasing the success rates of induction

If the cervix is not ready for induction i.e., it is not effaced or dilated, the chances of the induction failing are high. In other words, the chances for a vaginal delivery are low. A cervix that is still thick and closed is said to be **unfavourable** or **unripe**. To improve the chances for a successful induction, the obstetrician will proceed with ripening of the cervix.

Najma asked: I have been told that my labour needs to be induced. I am scared that these pains will be worse than natural labour. Should I be worried?

My answer: Women worry that induced labour is not 'natural' and is therefore more painful. Unfortunately there is not much to choose between the two– both will be difficult without some form of pain relief. If an induction is done properly, care will be taken to mimic natural labour as much as possible. This means that first the cervix is 'ripened'. This is a process where the cervix is softened and gently helped to open up. Medications are also started at low doses initially so that it feels more like natural labour. The pains will start off slowly and then pick up in frequency and strength. Of course, just as in spontaneous labour, the response will differ from woman to woman and even from one pregnancy to another.

Do inductions lead to an increased chance of caesareans?

Earlier, medical research seemed to support the theory that inductions lead to more caesareans. However, with the availability of newer ripening agents, and the ability to follow a more 'natural' course of labour even with induction, recent studies show the rate of caesarean to be the same as for spontaneous labour.

To increase the success rate, the induction must be done for a definite medical indication. The doctor will also choose indications that will not jeopardize you or the baby. It is important for you (and your doctor) to believe in the process and not give up too quickly.

Ripening of the cervix

Stripping or sweeping of the membranes

This is a procedure where the obstetrician inserts the examining finger through the opening of the cervix and gently sweeps the finger around the inside edge, thereby detaching the membrane of the amniotic sac from the wall of the uterus. This may help start the process of ripening. This is done in the doctor's clinic. You go home and wait for pains to start. It works more effectively in women who have had a baby before.

Prostaglandins

Prostaglandins are hormones that are part of the spontaneous process of labour. Therefore using them for cervical ripening has a high degree of success. Ripening of the cervix is achieved by using

- **prostaglandin gel** placed in the cervix
- **prostaglandin tablets** placed in the vagina or given orally

Balloon catheter

A Foley catheter is a narrow silicone tube with a small balloon at the tip. The doctor inserts it into the cervix and inflates the balloon with saline. This helps the cervix efface and dilate. The catheter is left in place (usually for 24 hours) until pains start or the cervix has opened enough for the balloon to fall out.

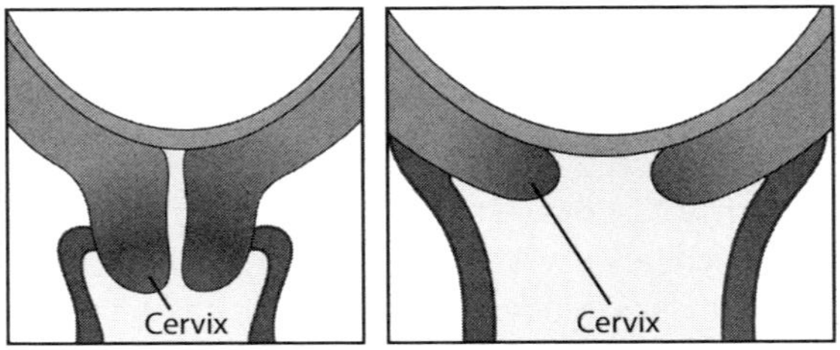

Unfavourable or unripe cervix *Favourable or ripened cervix*

Methods used for ripening sometimes lead directly to the start of labour. If that happens, no further intervention is required. Your labour and delivery are managed the same way as a spontaneous labour.

Methods of inducing labour

If the cervix is ripe (thinned out and dilated) either spontaneously or after cervical ripening, it will be time to start induction.

Oxytocin

The commonest drug used for induction, the world over, is oxytocin. Oxytocin is the hormone that the body produces in spontaneous labour. It makes the uterus contract. For induction, a synthetic form of the drug is given intravenously (IV).

The dosage of oxytocin is always low to begin with and then gradually increased till adequate and effective contractions set in. The contractions are monitored carefully to make sure that they are not stronger than what is safe for the mother and baby.

As with any procedure, induction of labour with oxytocin must be done according to standard protocols. This will help avoid any risk to the mother and baby.

Amniotomy

Rupturing the membranes (an amniotomy) may not be an effective method for labour induction by itself, but it works well in combination with oxytocin.

During an internal examination, the obstetrician identifies the membrane lying over the baby's head and ruptures it with a special instrument.

When the membranes are opened, you may feel the amniotic fluid leaking, especially when you are having a contraction.

Amniotomy is avoided if the baby's head is too high and has not descended into the birth canal.

Prostaglandin tablets

As an alternative to oxytocin, prostaglandin tablets (misoprostol) may be given orally. They are more useful for cervical ripening than induction of labour in a term pregnancy.

> Prostaglandin tablets (misoprostol) should be avoided if the mother has had a previous caesarean section. Their usage can result in the previous scar giving way and leading to a dangerous condition: uterine rupture.

What are the risks of labour induction?

When monitored properly, induction of labour is safe. But as with any procedure, induction of labour may carry some risk for the mother and baby. To minimize these risks, the contractions are monitored carefully. The amount of drug given is only increased gradually. The medication is reduced or stopped completely if there is any problem.

In some cases, there is a small risk of complications such as:

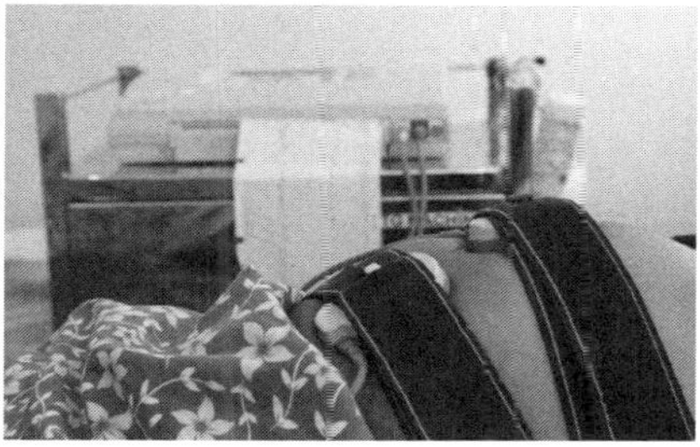

- **Foetal distress:** If contractions are too strong or frequent, they may result in an abnormal foetal heart rate due to decreased oxygen reaching the baby. If this happens, the oxytocin infusion will be turned off and the baby's heart rate will be monitored carefully. If the baby's heart rate is back to normal, the oxytocin may be restarted at a lower dose. If the baby's heart rate does not return to normal, an emergency caesarean section may be done.
- **Tear or rupture of the uterus:** If the pains are too strong and frequent, there is a small risk of the uterus tearing. If the labour is monitored carefully, the chance of this complication is minimal. The risk is increased if there has been a caesarean section in a previous pregnancy. That is why induction is only attempted with great caution in a woman with a previous caesarean section.

- **Caesarean section:** An induction may lead to a caesarean section if the pains do not result in a vaginal delivery. A caesarean may also be required if there is foetal distress.

When should labour not be induced?

Induction of labour is not attempted when:

- There is a placenta praevia i.e., the placenta lies very low in the uterus, and is lying in front of the baby's head. The opening of the uterus is partially or completely covered by the placenta
- The baby is lying in an abnormal position like breech, transverse position or shoulder presentation
- The mother is a diabetic and the baby has been diagnosed to be larger than 3.8–4 kg (macrosomia)
- The fluid around the baby is abnormally low
- The umbilical cord has prolapsed i.e., it has entered the birth canal in front of the baby and is in danger of being compressed. This emergency requires an immediate caesarean section
- There is a deep scar on the uterus because of a previous surgery like a caesarean or removal of a fibroid

Can you induce labour 'naturally'?

The baby seems comfortably ensconced inside you. It is almost the due date and there is no sign of labour. Can you do something to nudge your uterus into labour?

- 'Have sex!' says your best friend. Theoretically, having sex should make you go into labour because semen contains prostaglandins, the same hormone that makes your uterus contract. However, **there is no scientific evidence that this works.** Moreover, it may be quite uncomfortable to have intercourse at this stage of pregnancy.
- 'Sweep and mop the house', says your mother. Sadly, you might end up with a clean house but no nearer labour. **This too will not help.**
- Your grandmother wants you to have castor oil as a surefire method of inducing labour naturally. I will warn you right away: castor oil tastes and smells vile and can cause uncontrollable diarrhoea that may dehydrate you. Again, there is **no scientific evidence that this works.** It is just an old wives' tale.

Terms you will hear in the labour room

Amniotic fluid

Amniotic fluid consists mostly of foetal urine and water, and fills the sac surrounding the foetus.

Breech presentation

When the foetus has not turned to the head-down position and is coming through the birth canal with its buttocks or feet first.

Cephalopelvic disproportion (CPD)

The baby is too large to safely pass through the mother's pelvis. Conversely, the mother's pelvis may be too small to let even an average-sized baby through.

Caesarean section

An incision through the abdominal and uterine walls for extraction of the baby.

Contractions

There is tightening and relaxation of the uterine muscle at regular intervals. These contractions push the baby through the birth canal.

Dilatation

The cervix (mouth of the uterus) opens to let the baby through. This opening of the cervix is called dilatation. It is measured in centimetres, with full dilation being 10 centimetres.

Effacement

This refers to the thinning of the cervix in preparation for birth and is expressed in percentages. The cervix will be 100% effaced and fully dilated when you begin pushing.

Epidural

An excellent method of pain relief used during labour. Pain medication is given through a catheter that is threaded through a needle, into the dural space near the spinal cord.

Episiotomy

An incision made on the perineum (the space between the vagina and anus), to widen the vaginal opening for delivery.

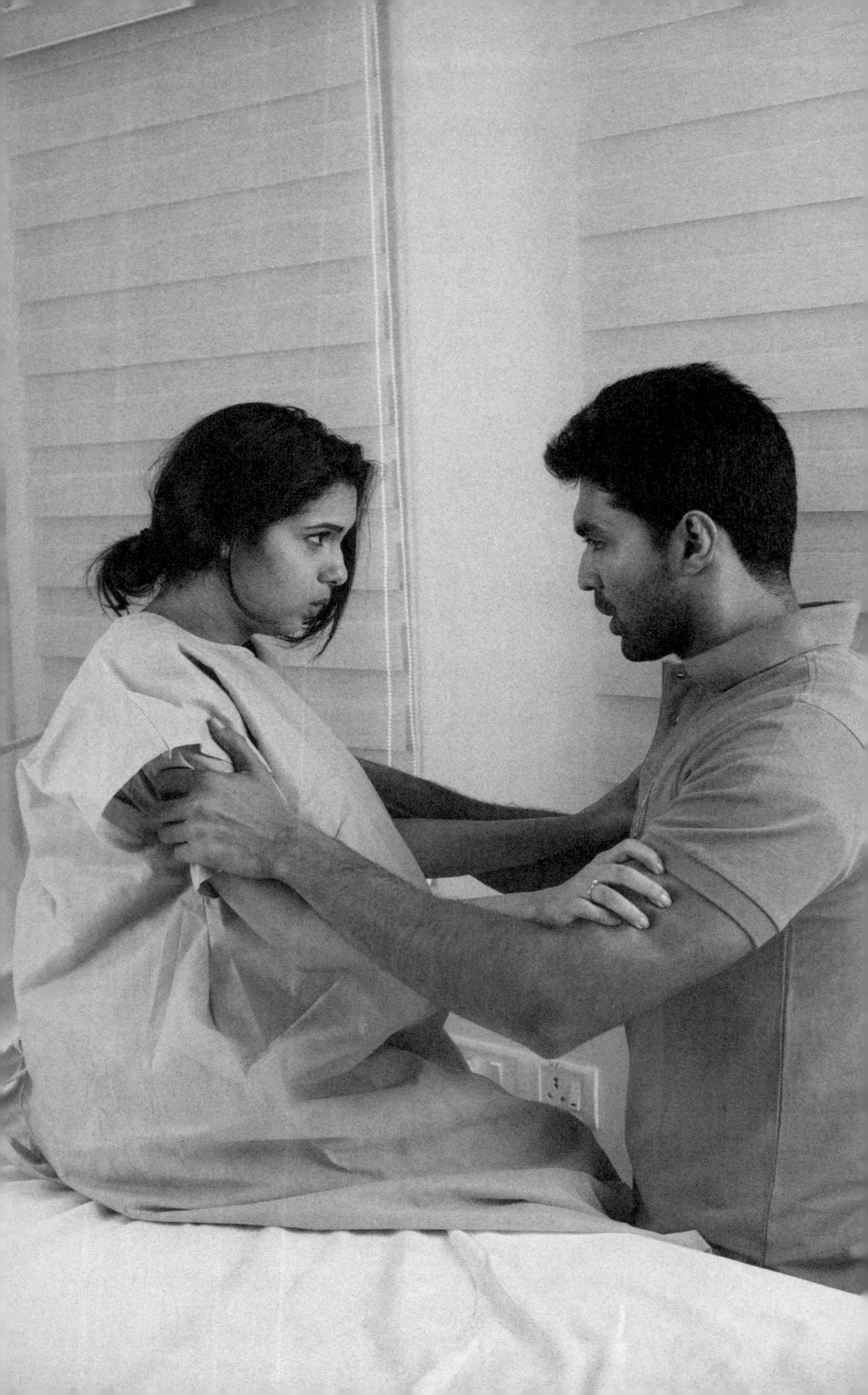

Foetal distress

This is a condition when the baby is not receiving enough oxygen. It is recognized by abnormalities in the baby's heartbeat.

Forceps

Stainless steel instruments which may be placed gently on either side of the baby's head and used to help guide the baby's head out of the birth canal during delivery.

Meconium

This is the greenish-black substance that is present in the bowels of a growing foetus and is normally discharged shortly after birth as the baby's first few bowel movements. Occasionally, this is discharged during labour and may suggest that the baby is having foetal distress.

Neonatologist

A paediatric specialist who cares for newborns.

NICU

Neonatal Intensive Care Unit.

Oxytocin

Hormone secreted by the pituitary gland that stimulates contractions and the milk reflex. In the synthetic form, this hormone is used to induce or augment labour.

Placenta

The tissue that connects the mother and baby to transport nourishment and take away waste.

Vacuum cup

A vacuum cup is an instrument used to assist the delivery of the baby.

CHAPTER 21

Forceps delivery and vacuum-assisted birth

Sudarshana has been in labour for five hours. For the past one and a half hours, she has been trying to push the baby out of the birth canal. She is exhausted. She needs help. Her obstetrician will assist her birth by applying a vacuum cup to the baby's head and easing it out of the birth canal.

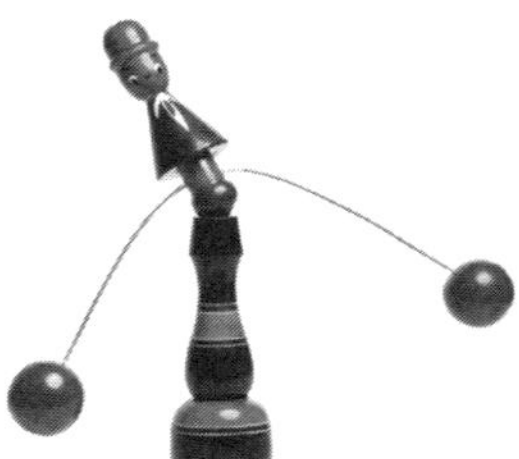

21

Forceps delivery and vacuum-assisted birth

Occasionally, your obstetrician may use a forceps or vacuum cup to help you deliver the baby. These instruments are placed on the baby's head so that she can be gently eased out with the least trauma to you and her. This is called an instrumental delivery. Instrumental deliveries are less common in women who have had a spontaneous birth before.

Instrumental deliveries, when done well and in properly selected cases, increase vaginal delivery rates and decrease caesarean births.

Will I have an instrumental delivery?

About 10–15 per cent of women may need instrumental delivery. Both vacuum cups and forceps are safe, and are only used when necessary for you and your baby.

Vacuum delivery or forceps might be required when:

- You are having a difficult time pushing the baby out through the birth canal
- You have been trying really hard but have become too tired and exhausted to continue pushing
- You have had an epidural and may not have a strong urge to push
- Your baby needs to be delivered as soon as possible because it is showing signs of foetal distress. The baby may have changes in the heart rate that might suggest that it is receiving less oxygen thereby requiring immediate delivery

Other uncommon reasons for instrumental delivery are:

- If a woman is delivering twins, the second twin might require assistance in delivery
- The labouring mother has a medical condition that will deteriorate if she pushes too long (for example, heart disease)

What is a vacuum-assisted birth?

The vacuum cup is attached by a flexible rubber tube to a small vacuum pump. The cup, which fits on top of the baby's head, may be made of metal or silicone plastic. The soft silicone cups are less likely to cause damage to your baby's head, and are more commonly used now. The chances of vaginal tearing are also less with a vacuum cup than with forceps.

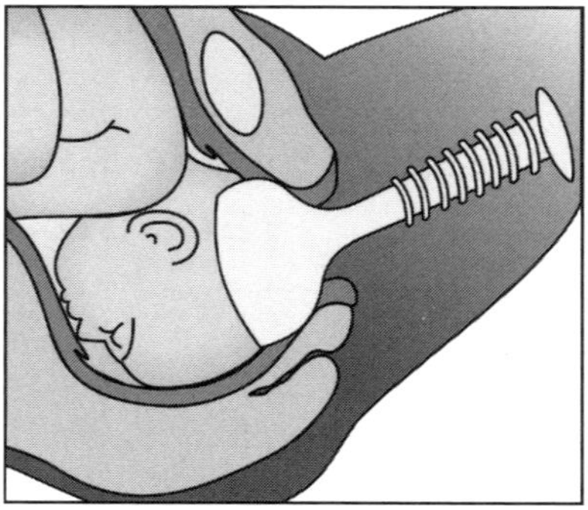

Vacuum-assisted birth

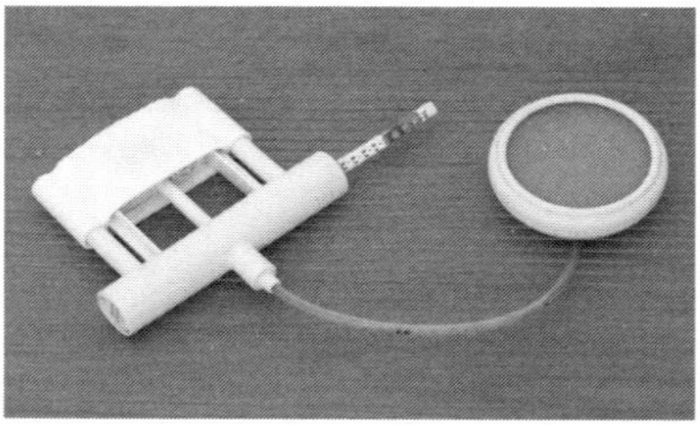

Vacuum cup with hand-held pump

During a contraction you will be encouraged to push and the obstetrician will apply gentle traction on the tube attached to the cup. During the next few contractions, the baby will be lifted out of the birth canal. Don't be concerned if you see a small, soft swelling on your baby's head after it is born. This is called a *chignon* and occurs where the cup created a vacuum. This will disappear in the next day or two. The cup may also leave a bruise on your baby's head called a *cephalhaematoma*. Though a cephalhaematoma may last a little longer than a *chignon*, it will disappear over time. It is not a major complication but it may result in newborn jaundice (see **Chapter 46**, *Your new baby*).

What is a forceps-assisted birth?

Forceps are stainless steel, spoon-shaped instruments that are placed gently on either side of the baby's head and are used to cradle the head. The forceps are placed in position between contractions. Your doctor might ask you not to push while she applies the forceps. During a contraction, while you push, the obstetrician will apply traction on the forceps and lift the baby out of the birth canal.

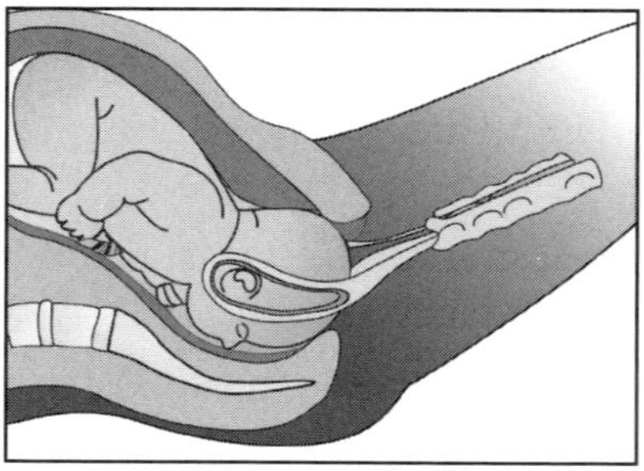

Forceps-assisted birth

Forceps are more successful in delivering the baby than a vacuum cup but may cause greater vaginal tearing.

After the baby is born, you might notice some marks from the forceps on your baby's face. These will usually disappear within 48 hours. Ten per cent of babies born with forceps may have small cuts on the face or scalp. These will heal very quickly.

Anaesthesia for vacuum-assisted and forceps-assisted birth

If you have not taken an epidural, you will receive a local anaesthetic to numb the skin and tissue between the vagina and the anus.

Episiotomy

Though episiotomies are not done routinely, you may have one if you undergo an instrumental delivery.

After your baby is born

Even after a normal vaginal delivery, the baby's head may be a little elongated and conical. This happens because the baby has to mould itself to the shape of the birth canal. In babies born with the help of a forceps or a vacuum cup, the head may be a little more conical or there may be a prominent bulge where the vacuum cup was applied. This will usually subside in a few days. There is no need to massage the head—it will get back to a normal shape on its own.

Gurpreet asked: I am worried that I may require forceps during delivery. My friend had a baby delivered by forceps and that baby has some intellectual disability.

My answer: I understand your concern. Some women do worry that a forceps delivery or a vacuum-assisted birth can harm the baby. Except for very minor marks due to the mild pressure used to apply the forceps or vacuum cup, there are no major complications. When a child is born with cerebral palsy or intellectual disability, parents are sometimes quick to blame the use of instruments. In reality, instrumental deliveries cannot result in a baby being born with intellectual disability.

CHAPTER 22

Pain relief in labour and delivery

Shraddha is due to deliver in another week. She is very apprehensive. She has heard tales of horror from many of her friends and dreads the pain of labour. Though her mother has reassured her that labour pains are tolerable, she is still concerned. Shraddha should talk to her obstetrician about the options available for pain relief in labour.

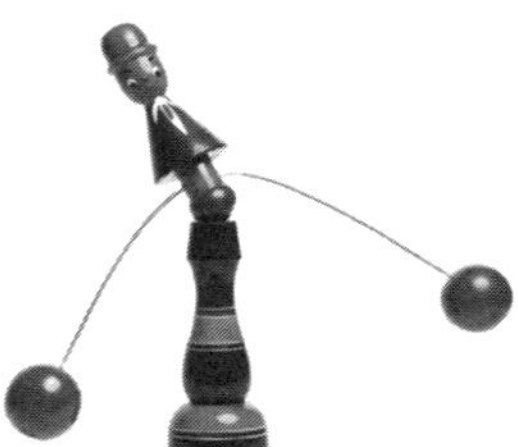

22

Pain relief in labour and delivery

> Labour is a very difficult time for most women. All women, therefore, deserve to be supported in their decision to have as painless a delivery as possible.

In every language in the world, the words childbirth and labour are synonymous with pain. The joy of giving birth is always coloured with the fear of pain during labour. Pain is a natural part of labour and every woman is unique in the ability to handle the level of pain. Pain tolerance varies from woman to woman. Some women dread childbirth to the extent of demanding a caesarean section instead of going through natural childbirth.

You may be filled with apprehension. Your friends and relatives may have used some ill-chosen words to describe the travails of labour. You may be really frightened about going through labour. You need not worry. Modern obstetrics offers you many choices for pain relief in labour and delivery.

Why is labour painful?

There are several reasons for pain during labour and delivery.

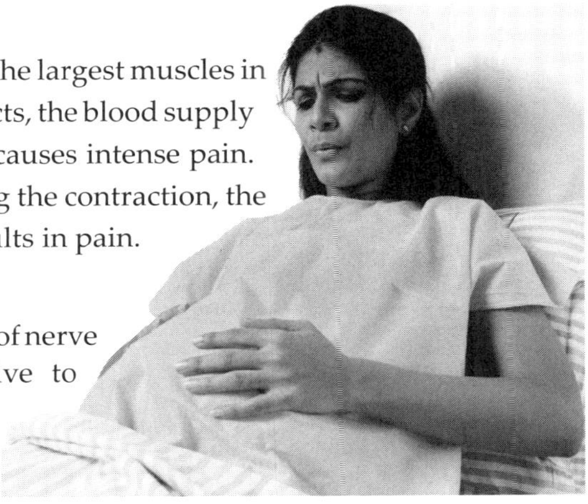

Uterine contractions

The pregnant uterus is one of the largest muscles in the body. As the uterus contracts, the blood supply to the muscle is cut off. This causes intense pain. The other reason is that during the contraction, the muscle stretches and this results in pain.

Cervical dilatation

The cervix has a large number of nerve endings and is very sensitive to pain. As the cervix dilates in active labour, the stretching causes pain.

Pressure on the pelvic nerves

As labour progresses, the descending head of the baby causes pressure on the pelvic nerves, causing pain.

Dilatation of the vaginal and perineal tissues

As the baby's head descends through the vagina and pushes against the skin at the opening of the vagina, the stretching results in pain.

Pain management in labour

Pain relief offered during labour is safe for both the mother and the baby. There are many ways to lessen pain during labour and the birth of the baby. Being prepared with knowledge of the birth process is the first step towards being able to handle labour pains. Labour preparation classes for the couple are, therefore, important.

The type of pain relief that is right for you depends on your pain threshold. Some women can tolerate pain to a greater extent than others. Some women have a low threshold for pain and this, combined with the fear of labour pains, can make them very intolerant of even the slightest pain. A woman's physical fitness, attending labour preparation classes, the length of labour, the intensity of labour pains and the size of the baby play a role in the ability to handle the pain of labour.

Ganga asked: This is my second pregnancy. Funnily, I don't quite remember the pain during the last delivery but the one thing I remember is that I kept asking for painkillers and was told that pain is part of labour and I should just put up with it. Is there no safe way of reducing the pain of labour? I have heard of 'painless labour'. Why not for me?

My answer: You absolutely deserve a pain-free childbirth, as does every woman. Of course, the ability to give you a relatively pain-free childbirth depends on the attitude of the obstetrician and the facilities available at the hospital you are delivering at. Check on this before you choose your hospital.

You must, however, remember that there is never a completely painless delivery. There definitely are methods to decrease the pain you feel. An epidural helps the most in relieving the pain of labour. The first step towards a pain-free childbirth is to attend a good birth preparatory class. Many hospitals are offering this now. Fear of the unknown always makes it seem worse that it actually is. These classes will help you understand the process of labour and allay your anxiety.

The common methods of pain relief are

- Breathing and relaxation techniques
- Pain-relieving drugs that can be given as an injection
- Newer methods include epidural analgesia and pain relieving gas mixture

Breathing and relaxation techniques

When that first strong pain hits, most women are taken by surprise at its intensity. It is important to learn and practise breathing techniques ahead of time so that you can use them when the pains start becoming uncomfortable. If you can attend a labour preparation class with your husband, both of you will be ready to handle labour.

> Music has been shown to have a great effect on mood and emotional well-being. Playing music in the labour room can distract the mother's mind from the pain and help her cope better.

Breathing techniques give you something to focus on. When the pains get stronger, many women lose control. Breathing rhythmically enables you to feel in control. Most importantly, proper breathing ensures that you and your baby get an adequate supply of oxygen in labour.

Different breathing exercises can be useful during the different stages of labour.

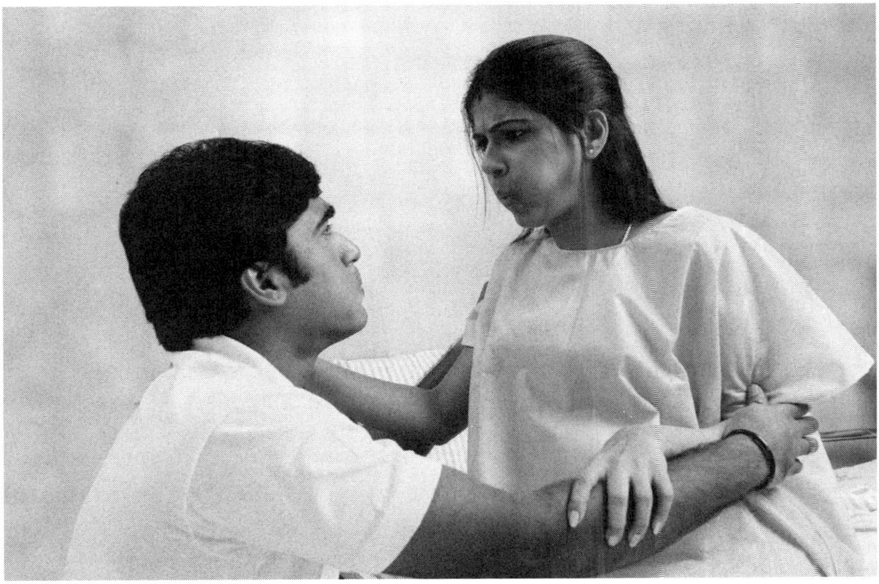

Breathing techniques in early labour

During the initial stage of labour, you should focus on slowly inhaling and exhaling throughout your contraction. Inhale through your nose and then exhale slowly through your mouth. When you are exhaling, it helps to purse your lips and blow out your breath. Face your husband, focus on his eyes or mouth and hold his hands as you go through the rhythmic breathing together.

Breathing in the active stage of labour

With the beginning of each contraction, continue to inhale through your nose and exhale through your mouth as you were doing during the earlier part of labour. As the intensity of the contraction increases, you can start to take shallower, quicker breaths. As the contraction reaches its peak, it may help to breathe in and out through your mouth as if you were panting. When the intensity of the contraction begins to lessen, resume rhythmic inhalation: in through your nose and out through your mouth.

Closer to delivery, you may get a strong urge to push. If you are not fully dilated, your doctor may ask you not to push. Concentrate on your breathing and try not to push at this time.

Breathing and pushing

Once your cervix is fully dilated, you will be asked to push the baby through the birth canal. For effective pushing, use the following method:

Take a deep breath and hold it. Push down into your rectum, as if you were severely constipated. After a good push, take a deep breath again and push again if the pain is still there. Once the pain subsides, take a few deep breaths and then relax.

Practise the breathing techniques

Start practising the breathing techniques with your husband, in the last month of pregnancy. Once you are in labour, it will be difficult to follow rhythmic breathing unless you have practiced it before.

Drugs for pain relief

Narcotics (such as pethidine or tramadol) may be used during the first stage of labour to help you relax. In a hospital setting, drugs to reduce pain should be available and offered to all women in labour who desire medication.

Narcotics are usually injected into a muscle (IM). These drugs generally take about 20 minutes to start working. Narcotics lessen the pain and can help you feel less tense or anxious.

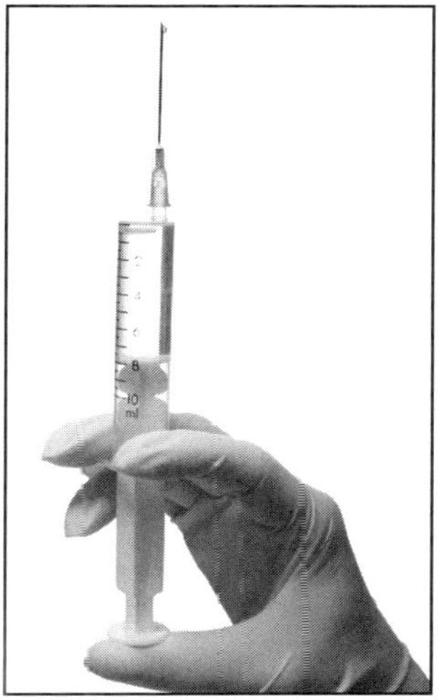

Pethidine

You may actually feel drowsy with pethidine. Some women may also develop nausea or vomiting with pethidine. The effects usually last for about two to four hours. If needed, the injection can be repeated. The effects of the drugs, such as drowsiness, can be passed on to the baby. It is, therefore, not given if it appears that the baby will be delivered within 2–4 hours after the injection.

Remember, an injection of pethidine will not eliminate the pain completely. It will only take the edge off the pain so that you can deal with it more easily.

Tramadol

Though an analgesic, it is not as effective as pethidine. Its efficacy in relieving pain is only 10 per cent of pethidine. Pethidine is not easily available in all hospitals due to a requirement for a narcotic license, so tramadol is used in its stead. It has no side-effects for the baby.

Pain relieving gas mixture

Pain relieving gas (Entonox®, a mixture of oxygen and nitrous oxide) is often used to relieve labour pain. Gas mixtures will help to relieve pain but will not eliminate it completely. It provides good pain relief without causing undue sleepiness. You breathe in the gas and air through a mask or mouthpiece, which you hold yourself. The gas works quickly, but takes about 30–45 seconds to have the pain relieving effect. It is best to start breathing it in just as a contraction begins. It is advisable to take slow, deep breaths.

You have total control of how much you want to inhale and how much pain relief you are comfortable with. The gas mixture crosses the placenta but is not known to have any effect on your baby. Since nitrous oxide is an anaesthetic gas, you may feel a little dizzy. Some women may have nausea.

Regional analgesia

A regional block lessens or completely blocks the pain in a specific part of the body. The goal of regional analgesia is to reach a balance between easing the pain and still feeling the urge to bear down, to actively participate in delivering your baby. The regional analgesia commonly used in labour is **epidural**. Spinal anaesthesia is also a regional block but is used only for a caesarean and not for pain relief during labour.

Epidural analgesia

The epidural block is a commonly used type of regional analgesia during labour. In labour, you may reach a point where narcotics are no longer giving you adequate pain relief. At this point, you may opt to go ahead with epidural analgesia. With epidural analgesia, there is no loss of consciousness, so you can actively participate in the process of delivery. An epidural block is a great way to actually enjoy childbirth without having to feel the pain of contractions.

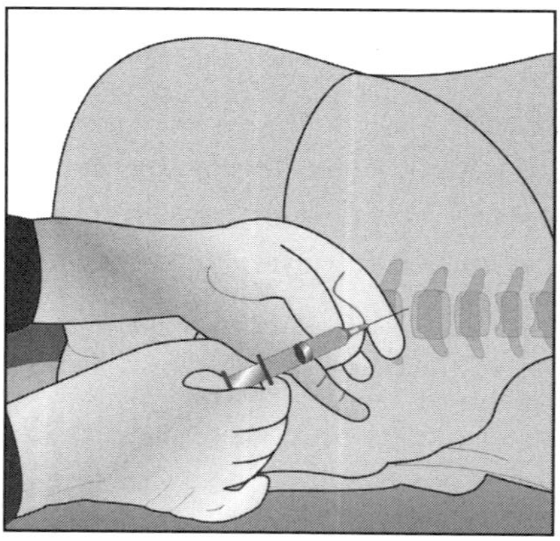

Epidural needle being inserted

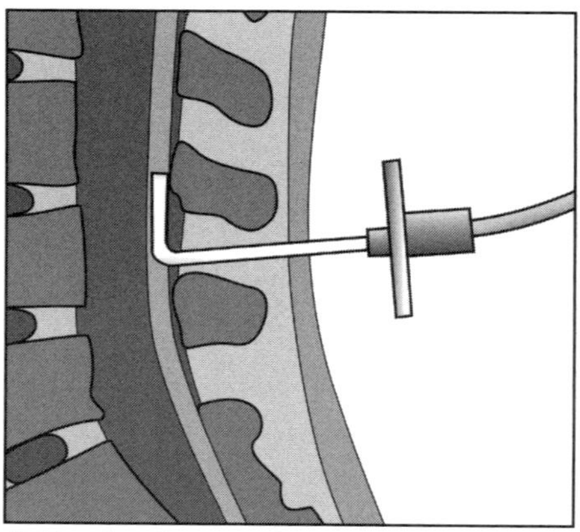

Epidural catheter in place

Your doctor will make sure you are in active labour before giving the epidural. Usually it is a good idea to take the epidural when you are 3-4 cm dilated.

What is an epidural block?

An epidural block is given in the lower back into a small area (the epidural space) below the spinal cord. You will be asked to sit or lie on your side with your back curved outward and to stay this way until the procedure is completed. The position may be a little uncomfortable but it is only for a short while.

After the epidural block is given, you can lie down and still move from side to side. You may not be allowed to walk around.

Before the block is performed, your skin will be cleansed with an antiseptic solution. Local anaesthesia will be used to numb the area of your lower back where the needle will be inserted. After the epidural needle is inserted, a small tube (catheter) is introduced through it, and the needle is withdrawn. In some cases, the catheter may touch a nerve, at which point there may be a brief tingling sensation down one leg. You might notice a bit of temporary numbness, heaviness or weakness in your legs.

Small doses of the medication are then given through the catheter to reduce the discomfort of labour. The medication can also be given continuously.

The effect of the epidural may take a few minutes to be felt because the medication needs to be absorbed. Pain relief will begin within 10–20 minutes after the medication has been injected.

In low doses, an epidural block eases the pain of contractions and numbs the birth canal during labour and delivery. Low doses are used because they are less likely to cause side effects for you and the baby. The pressure of the contractions is still felt with an epidural block, but the pain component will be minimized. In higher doses, an epidural may be used for caesarean sections. An epidural will almost completely take away the pain. Even with an epidural, you will feel some pressure and discomfort during the actual delivery of the baby, but this will be only 10 per cent of what you would feel if you had no epidural at all.

Pushing with an epidural block

Although an epidural block will make you more comfortable, you still may be aware of your contractions. You will also continue to have some degree of discomfort when you are examined to see if the cervix is dilating. The anaesthetist will adjust the degree of numbness for your comfort. When it is time to push, the epidural will be allowed to wear off a little bit so that your urge to push is not suppressed.

What are the side-effects of an epidural?

The medicines used in epidural analgesia are less likely to pass to the baby or affect the baby because they do not enter the blood stream.

- An epidural block may cause the mother's blood pressure to drop. This may in turn cause the baby's heartbeat to slow down. To help prevent

> **Esther asked:** My doctor spoke to me about taking an epidural during labour. My friends are frightening me about this. They say that I will have back pain as a result of this procedure.
>
> **My answer:** Many women are apprehensive that an epidural can cause back pain that will persist for years. This is an unfortunate myth. Taking an epidural DOES NOT increase the chance of low back pain after the delivery. Recent studies have shown that you are no more likely to get a backache after having an epidural for labour than if you deliver without an epidural.

this from happening, fluids are given to the mother through an IV drip before the epidural block is given.

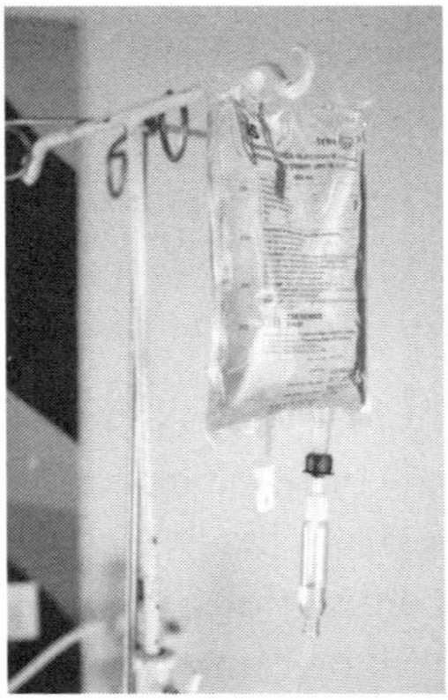

- Very rarely, a slow leak of spinal fluid can occur after an epidural and this may lead to a pounding headache. You might be advised to lie flat for a day or so until the leak seals itself. If needed, a second injection may be given to seal the leak.

Pain relief during labour without drugs

Each woman has a different threshold for pain. How a person deals with the pain depends on her attitude to labour. Attending labour preparation classes helps relieve the anxiety about labour. Methods that do not involve drugs help you cope with labour pain rather than directly lessen the pain.

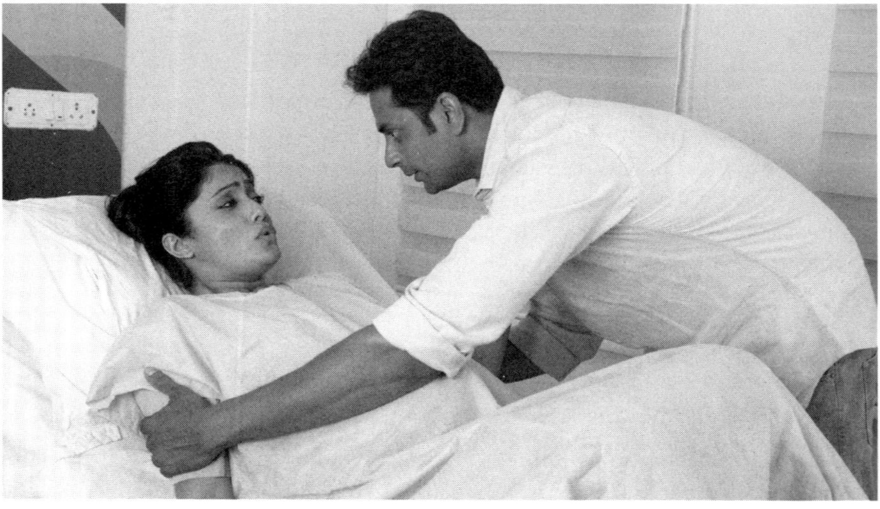

- *Breathing exercises* are an important part of pain relief during labour (see section on *Breathing techniques* above).
- *Continuous labour support:* Your husband's presence in the labour room is also important. Your husband can encourage and support you as you go through labour. It is a strong bonding experience. You and your husband can take classes to learn about childbirth, body conditioning exercises and methods of relaxation. All of these techniques can be used with other treatments for labour pain. If your husband will not be available at the time of delivery, ask your doctor if a close female relative of yours can be with you through the process.
- *Touch and massage:* When you are feeling helpless in labour, a caring and reassuring touch by another person can be very comforting. Massage of the low back and thighs also helps relieve some of the pain.

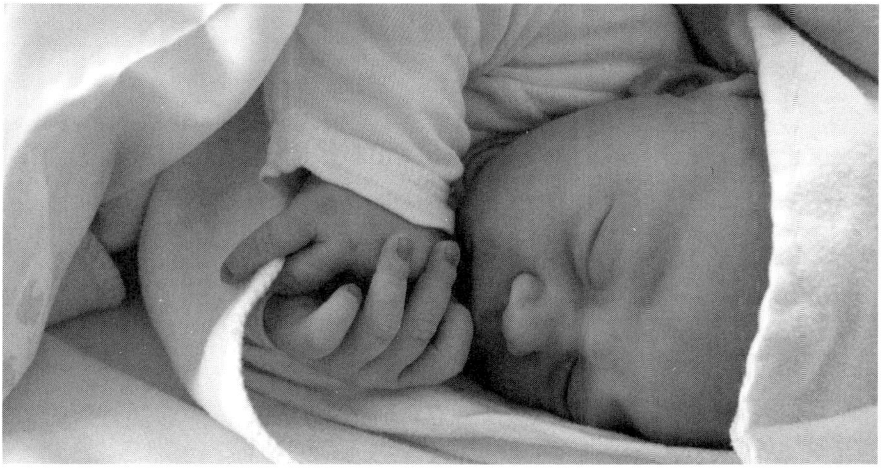

CHAPTER 23

Monitoring the baby's well-being during labour

Sanjana has been in labour for the past four hours. She has high blood pressure that began in the seventh month of pregnancy. She is concerned. Will her baby tolerate labour well?

It is important to monitor the baby's well-being during the process of labour and checking on his or her heart rate is an important way of doing that.

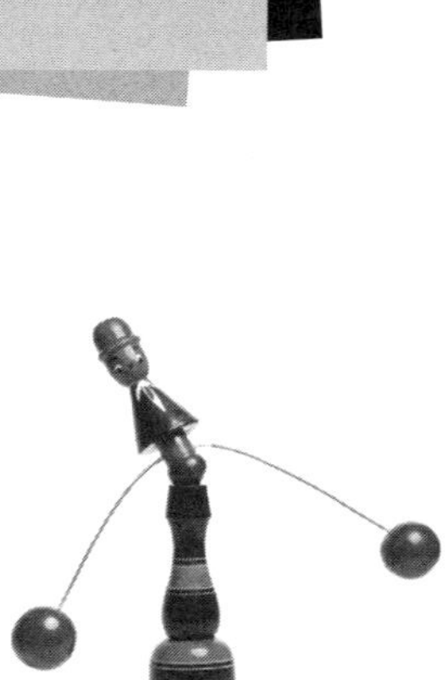

23

Monitoring the baby's well-being during labour

When you are in labour, your obstetrician has to take care of two individuals, you and your baby. While checking how your labour is progressing, she will also constantly check to see if the baby is tolerating labour well.

In labour, women are encouraged to lie on their sides rather than on their backs. This helps increase the blood flow to the baby.

During labour, the baby will continue to receive oxygen through the placenta. During a contraction, the uterine muscles tighten and temporarily cut off the blood flow to the placenta. A healthy placenta will have enough oxygen reserves to supply the baby during the contraction. A healthy baby also can handle a slight decrease in the oxygen supply for a short period of time.

Conditions that can cause decreased oxygen supply

A compromised placenta

The placenta can be unhealthy or inefficient if

- The mother has high blood pressure in pregnancy
- The mother has diabetes in pregnancy
- The placenta has not developed well
- The placenta has separated from the uterine wall (abruption, see **Chapter 31**, *Bleeding in pregnancy*)

A compromised umbilical cord

During labour, the umbilical cord can get compressed. This can happen by being pressed against the uterine wall, or by being wound around one of the baby's limbs. If the amniotic fluid around the baby is low, there are greater chances of the cord getting compressed.

A compromised baby

The baby may be unable to handle even the slight decrease in oxygenation during a contraction if she has no reserves. This can happen if the baby is growth restricted (which means that the baby has not grown as much as she should have). A growth restricted baby may also have decreased amniotic fluid that may increase the chance of cord compression (see **Chapter 34**, *Foetal growth problems: too small or too big*).

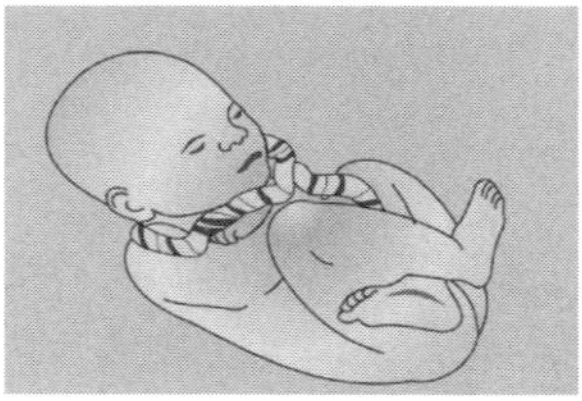

Madhuri asked: My friend said I should have an ultrasound scan to check out whether my baby's cord is wrapped his or her neck. She said that in that case my baby might have trouble during labour.

My answer: Remember that 1 out of 3 babies born vaginally have the umbilical cord wound around their neck. This is completely normal. It is an erroneous belief (among women and some doctors too) that if you identify the cord around the neck on an ultrasound scan, it predicts that the baby will face problems during a vaginal delivery. There is no medical reason to check the position of the cord by ultrasound.

There is an old wives' tale that you should not reach above your head with your arms or you should not turn from side to side while lying down because this may cause the cord to wrap around the baby and jeopardize the baby. **This is not true!**

The baby's response to decreased oxygen in labour

When the baby gets less oxygen than it should in labour, it will respond by

- Abnormal changes in the heart rate
- Passing meconium (motion) into the amniotic fluid

That is why the baby's well-being in labour is monitored by looking for abnormal heart rate patterns and change in the colour of the amniotic fluid.

Foetal heart rate

How do we know the baby is doing well?

We know that the baby is tolerating labour well if her heart rate

- Stays between 110–160 beats per minute
- The heart rate increases every time the baby moves
- The heart rate does not drop during or after a contraction

How do we know the baby is having a problem?

There are specific abnormal heart rate patterns that will alert your doctor that a problem may be present and the baby is not receiving enough oxygen.

If there is a serious change in the foetal heart rate pattern, the baby is said to be having **foetal distress**. At this point, the doctor will take steps to help the baby.

We know the oxygen supply to the baby is getting compromised if the heart rate

- Drops below 110 beats per minute for a prolonged period of time
- Increases above 160 beats per minute for a prolonged period of time
- Drops during or after a contraction

How often is the baby's heart rate checked?

Listening to and checking the foetal heart rate in labour is an important component of good obstetric care.

First stage of labour (when your cervix is dilating to 10 cm): The foetal heart rate is monitored at least every half to one hour in the first stage of labour.

Second stage of labour (from complete cervical dilatation to when your baby is born): In the second stage, the nurse or doctor will listen to the foetal heart every 5–15 minutes. The heart rate will be particularly monitored during and immediately after the contraction so that any stress to the baby is picked up.

Methods of checking the foetal heart rate

The common methods of observing foetal heart rate include:

- Auscultation using a foetoscope or a hand-held Doppler device
- Cardiotocograph (CTG) or electronic foetal monitoring

Auscultation

Auscultation simply means periodically listening to the baby's heartbeat during labour. As mentioned earlier, the number of times that the baby's heartbeat is listened to depends on which stage of labour you are in, the frequency and strength of your contractions and any risk factors for the baby. If abnormal patterns are found with auscultation, cardiotocography (electronic monitoring) may be done.

Foetoscope or stethoscope

A special instrument called a foetoscope is commonly used to listen to the foetal heartbeat. A stethoscope may also be used. The broad end is pressed on your abdomen and the nurse or doctor can hear the baby's heartbeat and will be able to count the heart rate.

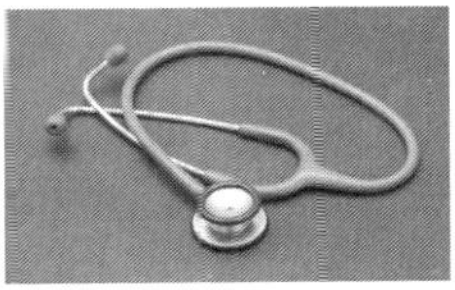

Hand-held Doppler device

This is a small electronic device that is placed against the abdomen to hear the baby's heartbeat. It uses a form of ultrasound to convert sound waves into signals of the baby's heart. The heartbeat can be heard clearly because it is amplified—you can hear it too! Most hospitals now use this for listening to the baby's heartbeat.

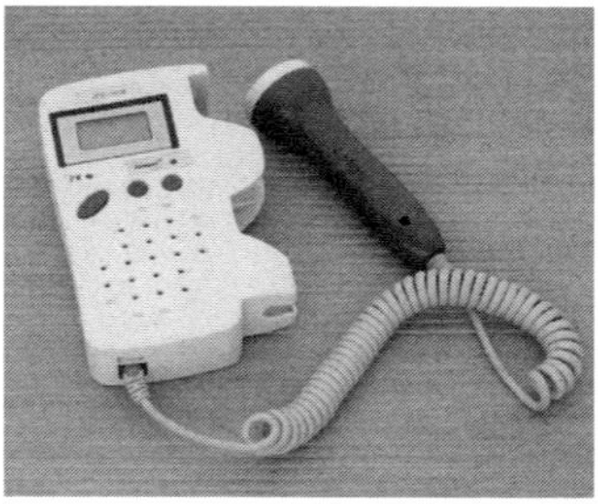

Cardiotocograph (CTG) or electronic foetal monitoring

Most uncomplicated labours are monitored with auscultation. When the foetal heart rate is found to be slow or too fast with auscultation, the doctor will want to confirm if the baby is having foetal distress. For this she might monitor the baby's heart rate with an electronic monitoring device.

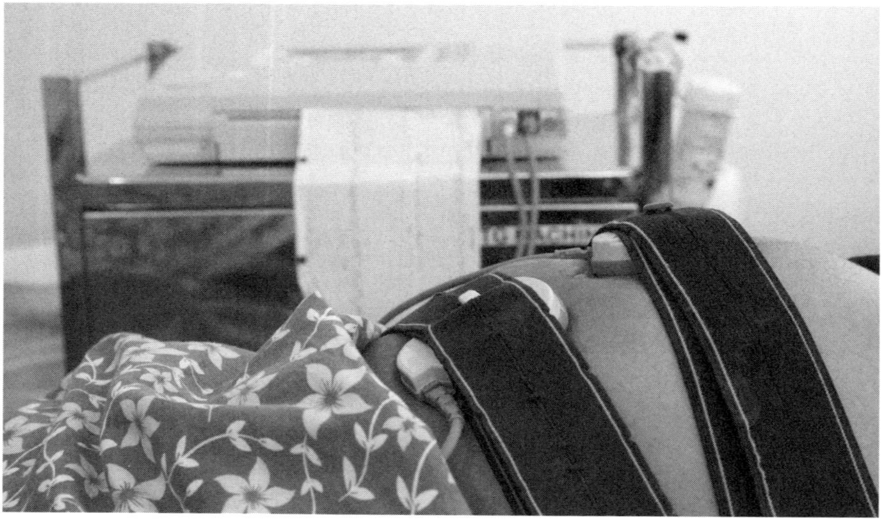

If you have a complicated pregnancy you might be monitored with an electronic monitoring device from the time you start having regular, strong contractions. Some hospitals use CTG monitoring for the entire duration of labour, even if you have no complications.

What is it?

Just like adults have an ECG taken to diagnose abnormalities in the heart, electronic foetal monitoring uses special equipment to provide a record of the foetal heart rate. A graph records the baby's heartbeat and the doctor or the nurse reads this record. A normal foetal heart rate pattern can reassure the doctor that the baby is tolerating labour well. On the other hand, abnormalities in the heart rate pattern can alert the obstetrician that the baby is in distress. This equipment also records the contractions of the mother's uterus during labour.

How is it done?
A pair of elastic belts is wrapped around your abdomen. To one is attached a device which uses Doppler to detect the foetal heart rate. This information is transmitted to the machine and the heart rate pattern is recorded. The other device records the frequency and duration of the uterine contractions.

Admission test

When you are admitted to the labour room, your doctor might do an admission test. This means that you will be monitored with a CTG (or electronic foetal monitor) for 20–30 minutes. If the baby's foetal heart tracing is normal, the doctor may decide to follow your labour with auscultation (hearing the heartbeat with a foetoscope). If there is any suspicion that the baby may develop a problem during labour, a decision may be made to monitor you continuously with the CTG.

Managing abnormal foetal heart rate patterns (foetal distress)

If there is an abnormal foetal heart rate pattern, certain steps may be taken to help the baby.

If it does not look like the delivery will happen soon, or if a vaginal delivery may worsen the condition, then the doctor may proceed with an immediate caesarean section (see **Chapter 24**, *When things go wrong in labour*).

Colour of amniotic fluid

Another indicator of foetal well-being is the colour of the amniotic fluid which surrounds the baby. When the membranes rupture, either spontaneously or are ruptured by the obstetrician, the colour of the fluid is always noted and documented. When it is clear (like water) or a yellowish liquid, then the baby is usually not having any problems.

When is foetal distress suspected?
When the fluid is greenish, it means that the baby has passed motion inside the uterus. This can be indicative of decreased oxygenation to the baby.

The decision to continue with a vaginal delivery or proceed with a caesarean section at this point depends on a number of factors (see **Chapter 24**, *When things go wrong in labour*).

CHAPTER 24

When things go wrong in labour

Sunanda and her husband have been looking forward to a normal vaginal delivery. They both attended the labour preparation class and have practiced relaxation techniques. Unfortunately, she has developed a complication in labour. The baby's heartbeat has started slowing down and her doctor is worried.

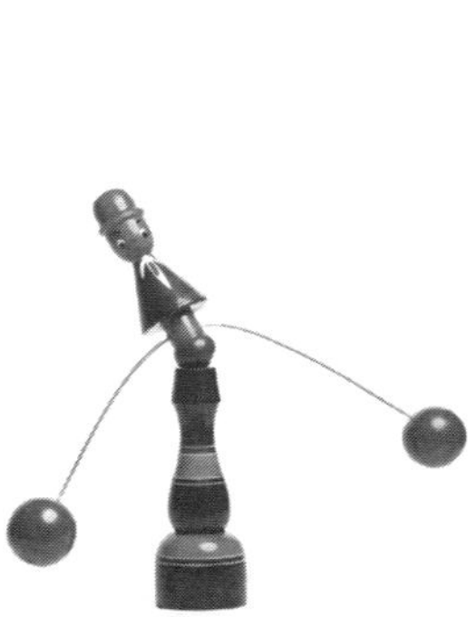

24

When things go wrong in labour

You have meticulously undergone all your antenatal check-ups. You did the scans and the blood tests as instructed. You have followed all the advice your doctor gave about diet and exercise. You look forward to a reasonably comfortable and smooth labour and delivery. Unfortunately, not every woman has an uncomplicated labour.

Some problems may be anticipated before labour starts. For example, your obstetrician may suspect that the baby may be too large for your pelvis and you may have trouble delivering. Sometimes, the baby is too small and may face problems during labour.

On the other hand, you and your obstetrician may be expecting a vaginal delivery but a complication might crop up during labour that may result in your having a caesarean section (see Emergency caesarean section in **Chapter 25**, *Caesarean section*).

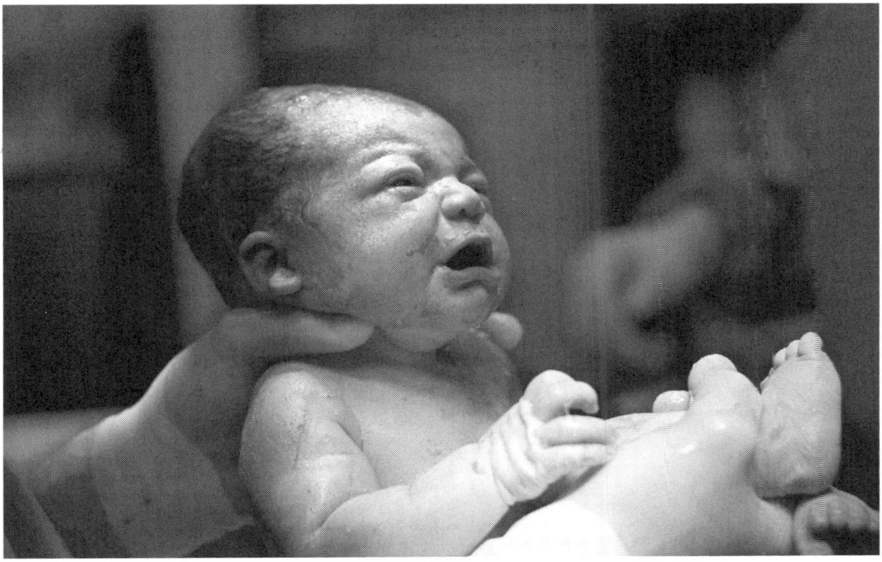

Mallika asked: My sister had been in labour for 8 hours and then suddenly her doctor told her she needed a caesarean section. Can that happen to me too?

My answer: Even when we expect a vaginal delivery, some unanticipated problem may occur during labour. Anywhere from 20–25 per cent of women who go into labour may require an emergency caesarean section. Of course it does not mean that because your sister had an emergency caesarean section you too will end up with one.

When can problems be anticipated?

- *Large baby (macrosomia):* On examination, your obstetrician may suspect that the baby is large. In Indian women, a baby is considered large if it is expected to weigh more than 3.5–3.8 kg at birth (depending on your height and weight). An ultrasound scan may also be done to calculate an estimated birth weight (though it may not be completely accurate). If your baby is large but your obstetrician thinks that your pelvis will allow a vaginal delivery, you may be allowed to labour. If the labour does not progress normally, she may then opt for a caesarean. This is known as a 'trial of labour'
- *Small baby (growth restricted):* On the other hand, babies that are much smaller than expected for that stage of pregnancy (growth restricted) may also develop problems during labour that may result in a caesarean section (see **Chapter 34**, *Foetal growth problems: too small or too big*). In such cases, your doctor may not allow you to labour and may schedule you directly for a caesarean section

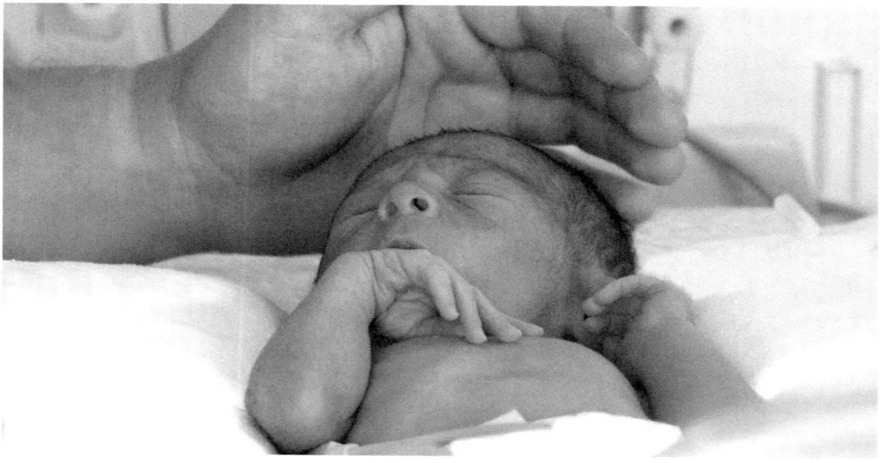

- If you have gone more than one week beyond your due date, then problems may be anticipated (see **Chapter 33**, *When the baby is overdue: the postterm pregnancy*)
- If you have hypertension or diabetes complicating your pregnancy, there may be an increased chance of having a caesarean section (see **Chapter 37**, *High blood pressure in pregnancy* and **Chapter 38**, *Diabetes in pregnancy*)
- Women older than 35 and younger than 18 also have a higher chance of caesarean section due to complications arising during labour (see **Chapter 40**, *Pregnancy after 35*)
- If the labour has been induced for certain medical reasons, then the chance of undergoing a caesarean section increases

What are unanticipated problems?

Failure of labour to progress

When labour lasts much longer than it is supposed to, it may indicate a problem. Prolonged labour is called failure to progress and can be due to

- Contractions that are not strong enough (your doctor may try to give you medication to make the contractions stronger)
- The cervix not dilating, a condition called cervical dystocia
- The baby lying in a slightly abnormal position that does not allow it to descend through the birth canal

Failure to progress in labour is the commonest cause for undergoing a caesarean section.

Cephalo-pelvic disproportion

When the foetus is too big to fit through your pelvis or if your pelvis is too small for your baby to pass through, it is called cephalo-pelvic disproportion (CPD). Cephalo-pelvic disproportion can cause a failure of descent (when the head of the baby is unable to come down the birth canal) or failure of dilatation (when the cervix does not dilate).

Foetal distress

This can be an unexpected problem in labour that may lead to a caesarean section. When the foetus shows signs that indicate it is not getting enough oxygen, the foetus is said to be in distress (see **Chapter 23**, *Monitoring the baby's well-being during labour*).

The two common signs of foetal distress are:

- Changes in the baby's heartbeat
- The passage of meconium inside the uterus

Abnormal changes in the baby's heart rate

The normal heartbeat of the baby is between 110–160 beats per minute. If the heartbeat drops to 110 or below, foetal distress is suspected. Occasionally, the lack of oxygen can cause the baby to push up its heartbeat, so a heart rate above 160 can also be a sign of foetal distress.

Managing abnormal foetal heart rate

If there is an abnormal foetal heart rate pattern, certain steps may be taken to help the baby. If you are receiving oxytocin to make your pains stronger, it will be stopped.

You may be

- Asked to lie on your left or right side—this may take the pressure off the cord if it is getting compressed
- Given oxygen through a mask or a small tube in the nose—this increases the oxygen reaching the baby
- Given intravenous (IV) fluids (this indirectly increases blood flow to the placenta)

What happens if the abnormal foetal heart rate pattern persists?

If in spite of all these steps the baby's heart rate does not improve, your obstetrician will make a decision depending on:

- The severity of the abnormality
- How close you are to delivery
- The size of the baby
- The colour of the amniotic fluid

If conditions are favourable and delivery is expected soon, then the obstetrician may proceed with a forceps delivery or a vacuum-assisted birth (see **Chapter 21**, *Forceps delivery and vacuum-assisted birth*).

If it does not look like the delivery will happen soon, or if a vaginal delivery may worsen the condition, then the doctor may proceed with an immediate caesarean section.

Passage of meconium

The baby normally does not pass meconium (motion) inside the uterus.

When the baby's oxygen supply through the placenta and the umbilical cord are compromised, then the baby may pass motion as a reflex. Meconium is greenish coloured and can turn the amniotic fluid green. When meconium is seen during labour, the heartbeat of the baby is carefully monitored. Your obstetrician may take a decision to deliver the baby by caesarean.

Managing meconium-stained amniotic fluid

The decision to continue with a vaginal delivery or proceed with a caesarean section at this point depends on a number of factors. The foetal heart rate is recorded and abnormalities in the pattern are looked for.

A caesarean section might be considered if

- There is foetal heart rate abnormality along with the greenish fluid
- The meconium-stained (greenish) amniotic fluid is very thick

Cord prolapse

Foetal distress may also occur if the umbilical cord slips out of the cervix ahead of the baby's head. This is a rare occurrence and is called cord prolapse.

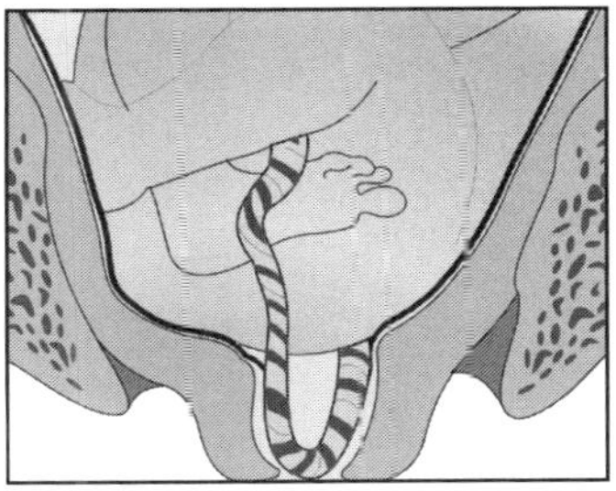
Cord prolapse

A cord prolapse is an emergency situation and can cause problems to the baby if not recognized and treated immediately. Compression of the cord can occur leading to foetal asphyxia i.e., the baby does not get enough oxygen to its brain. It occurs most commonly in the following situations:

- When the fluid around the baby is abnormally increased (polyhydramnios)
- During delivery of the second baby in a twin pregnancy
- The baby is lying crosswise in the uterus (transverse lie)
- The baby is in the breech position
- When the membranes rupture spontaneously or when the doctor ruptures the membranes during a vaginal exam before the baby's head has descended into the pelvis

Shoulder dystocia

When the baby has broad shoulders, the baby's head will deliver but the shoulders may get caught in the birth canal and cause difficulty in delivery. This is called shoulder dystocia.

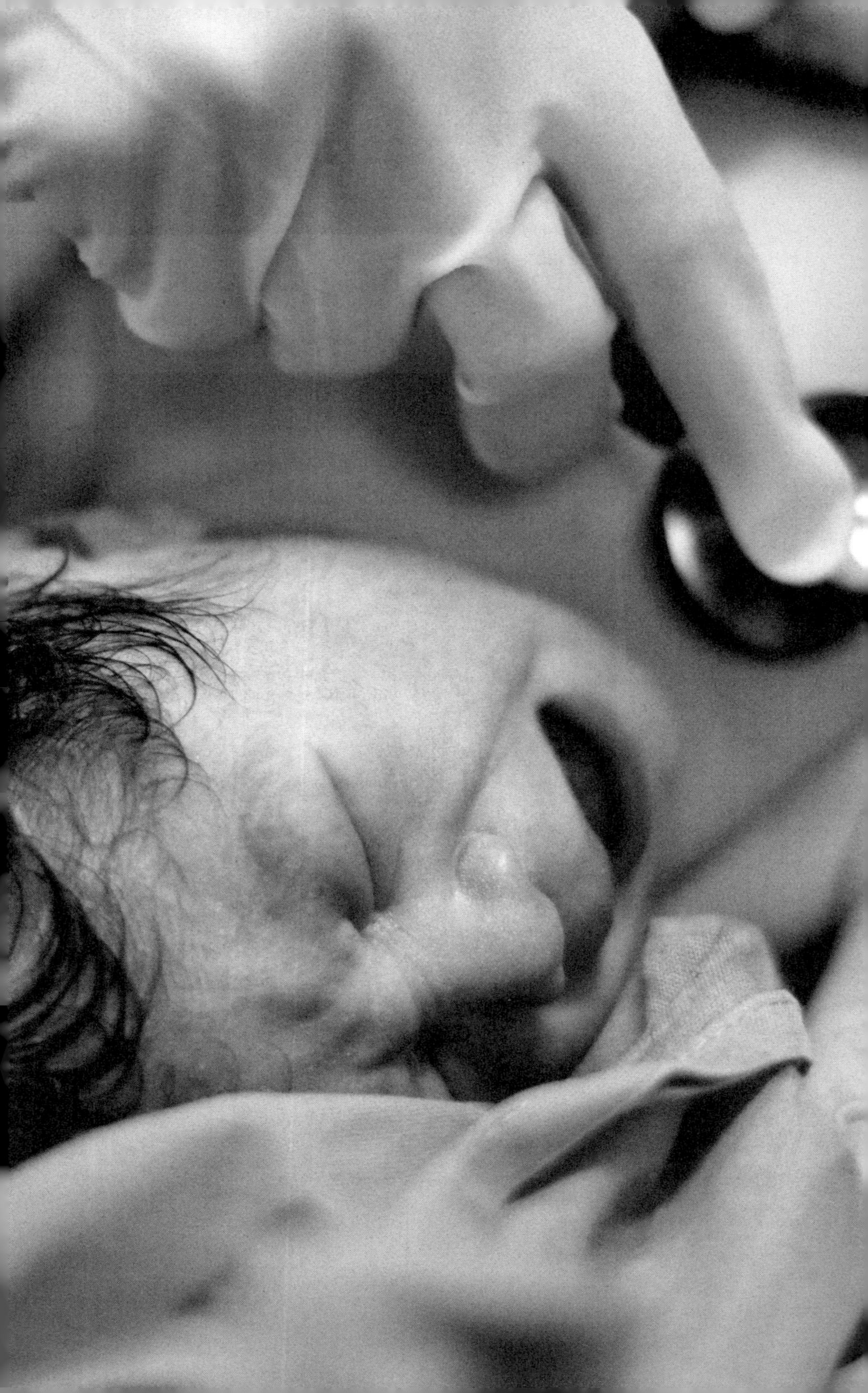

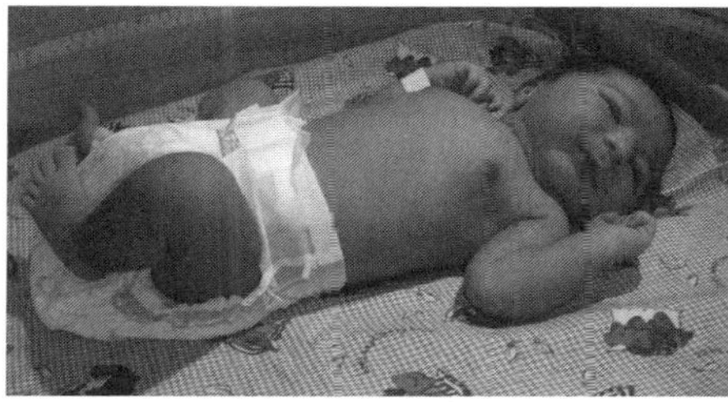

Large baby of diabetic mother

After the baby's head is delivered, the obstetrician may find that it is very difficult to deliver the rest of the baby. With the shoulders stuck in the birth canal, the baby may have trouble breathing because the chest is compressed. As a result, oxygen levels in the baby's blood decrease. This complication is more common with large babies, particularly those of diabetic mothers (see **Chapter 38**, *Diabetes in pregnancy*).

When this complication occurs, the obstetrician quickly tries various techniques to free the shoulder so that the baby can be delivered vaginally. In extreme circumstances, the baby may be delivered by caesarean section.

Postpartum haemorrhage

Postpartum haemorrhage is excessive bleeding following the birth of a baby. The average amount of blood loss after the birth of a single baby by vaginal delivery is approximately 500 ml. The average amount of blood loss during a caesarean section is approximately 1,000 ml. When the blood loss exceeds these amounts, you are considered to be having postpartum haemorrhage. Most postpartum haemorrhage occurs immediately after delivery, but it may occur after a few hours or even days.

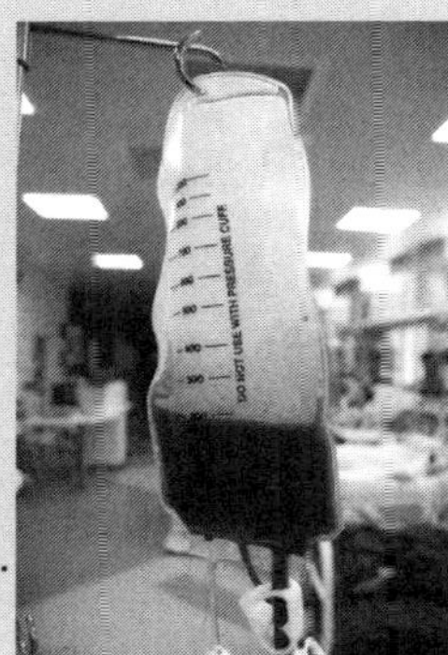

Causes of postpartum haemorrhage

Once a baby is delivered, the uterus contracts to compress and control the bleeding from blood vessels. Medications are given to help the uterus contract. Occasionally, in spite of these medications, the uterus will not contract. This is called **uterine atony**. This is the most common cause of postpartum haemorrhage. Sometimes the bleeding occurs if there are pieces of placenta left behind in the uterus or if there are cuts or abrasions in the vaginal area due to the baby passing through.

CHAPTER 25

Caesarean section

Shameem is in her eighth month of pregnancy. Her best friend just had a baby and underwent a caesarean section. Shameem is keen on having a normal, vaginal delivery. She wants to know if there are ways to ensure that.

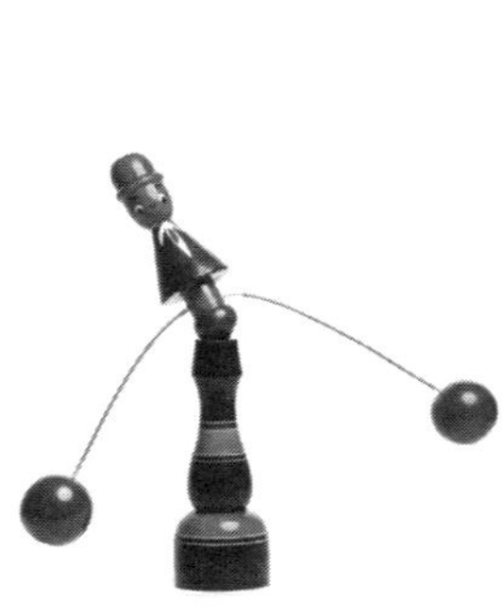

25

Caesarean section

There are various reasons why a caesarean section is done but the aim is always the same: protecting the baby or the mother, and sometimes both, from harm. At times, the baby will not fare well if put through the stress of a vaginal delivery. At other times, the caesarean is done to protect the mother from unnecessary physical complication or injury.

It cannot be disputed that a caesarean birth can save the life of a mother and/or a baby. However, it is important for both parents-to-be and their doctors to acknowledge that there are no benefits to mothers and babies when a caesarean is done when it is not required.

Many parents have been brainwashed into thinking that a vaginal delivery is risky and a caesarean is safer. This is very far from the truth when it comes to an uncomplicated pregnancy.

In India, there is also unwarranted emphasis placed on delivering the baby at an auspicious time. This leads parents to submit themselves to an unnecessary caesarean that has risks for both mother and baby.

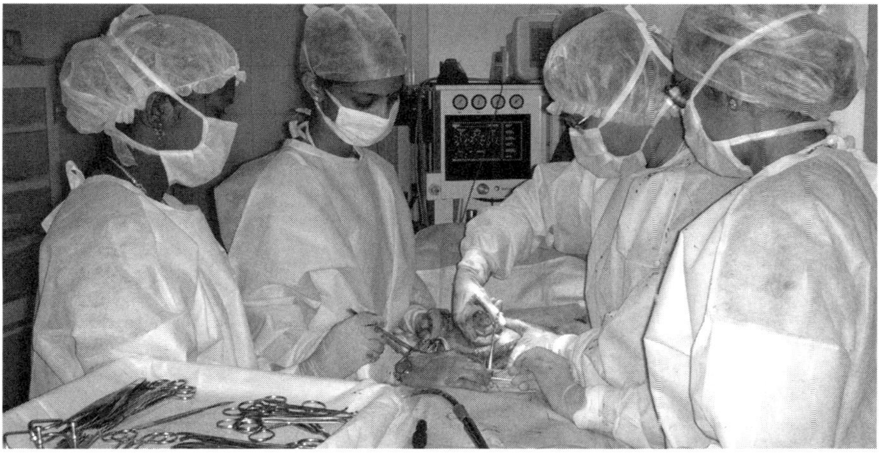

Why is there controversy about caesarean rates?

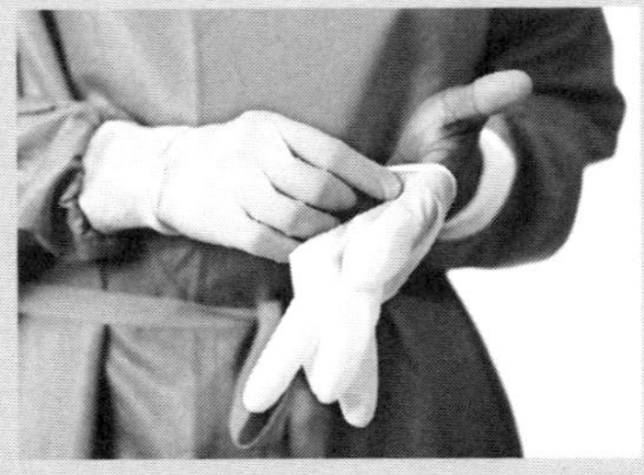

In a petition (started in January 2017), to the Ministry for Child Development, Ms Subarna Ghosh has collected close to 150,000 supporters who want to make it mandatory for all doctors and hospitals to declare the percentage of caesarean delivery rates. The Ministry of Women and Child Development has taken note of this and will hopefully be taking steps to staunch this epidemic of caesareans in this country.

According to Ms Ghosh, there is an indiscriminate trend of conducting caesareans, and she felt that women need to be made aware of caesarean section rates of different hospitals and maternity homes, so they can choose their hospital carefully.

What are your chances of having a caesarean?

For the past three decades I have always emphasized that one of the ways you can ensure that you have the best chances for a normal, vaginal delivery is to ask for the caesarean section rates for the hospital or obstetrician you are consulting. It is important to know that caesarean section rates may vary from hospital to hospital. On an average, an overall rate of 20–25 per cent is acceptable. The World Health Organization recommends a caesarean birth rate of 10–15 per cent. In a hospital that deals both with complicated and low-risk pregnancies, it may be difficult to keep the rate that low. Recent studies have confirmed that 20–25 per cent is a more reasonable rate to adhere to.

Robson classification

In 2001, Michael Robson proposed a system that classifies women into 10 groups, based on their obstetric characteristics (number of previous deliveries, previous caesarean, weeks of pregnancy, onset of labour, whether the baby is in a head-down or bottom-down position and the number of babies). In 2015, WHO suggested that Robson classification be used worldwide as an audit tool. This means that every hospital should review their caesarean rates based on these criteria.

In simple terms

Your chances of a normal, vaginal delivery should be 82–85 per cent, if it is

- Your first pregnancy
- You have crossed 37 weeks of pregnancy
- The baby is lying in a head-down position
- Your labour pains started on their own

What is a caesarean section?

A caesarean section is an abdominal operation performed to deliver a baby when vaginal delivery is not possible or safe. A cut is made through the mother's abdomen and then the uterus, to deliver the baby. This procedure is also called a C-section. Caesarean sections can save the lives of newborns and their mothers or prevent the potential complications of a delayed vaginal birth.

Planned (or elective) caesarean section

A caesarean section may be performed before labour begins if there are medical reasons for not allowing labour or a vaginal delivery. For example, the health of the mother or the baby may be in jeopardy if the pregnancy continues, or vaginal delivery might be impossible or unsafe. This is called a planned or elective caesarean section.

Emergency caesarean section

A caesarean section may be done when labour begins or during labour if certain problems occur, either for the mother or the baby. This is called an emergency caesarean section.

Radhika asked: My cousin was in labour for more than 8 hours and then ended up having a caesarean section. The mother and baby are doing well but why was it not known that she would land in a caesarean? Did she have to suffer for so long?

My answer: Your cousin had an **emergency caesarean section**. This refers to a caesarean that is done after labour has begun or during labour, if certain problems occur. For an onlooker, it might seem that she was made to suffer unnecessarily but I feel the reality is that the doctor would have been trying to make sure that she had a safe and normal vaginal delivery.

Sometimes there are indications early in labour that things are not going to go smoothly. It is then easy to make a decision to go ahead with a caesarean without waiting too long. However, sometimes you have to give the labour pains a chance to act so that the end result is a vaginal delivery. In the end, it is always better to have given the mother an opportunity for a normal delivery without rushing into a caesarean. Of course, the doctor will make this decision based on how well the baby and mother are tolerating labour.

Reasons for doing a planned (elective) caesarean

Complications in the mother

- Did you have a caesarean birth with your last pregnancy? You have a 50–60 per cent chance of another caesarean. Discuss with your doctor whether you are a candidate for a successful vaginal delivery and whether you can have a trial of labour

Vaginal birth after caesarean (VBAC)

Many women who have had a caesarean birth before may be able to give birth vaginally in the next pregnancy. This depends on the reason for which the caesarean was done the first time. If the reason does not exist in this pregnancy, your obstetrician might suggest trying for a vaginal delivery, also known as *vaginal birth after caesarean* or VBAC. A vaginal delivery after a previous caesarean delivery may not be a good option for a woman when the baby:

- Is very large
- Not in the proper position
- The interval between the previous caesarean and this pregnancy is less than two years

- If the placenta is lying in front of the baby's head (placenta praevia, see **Chapter 31**, *Bleeding in pregnancy*), it will block the baby's exit from the womb. A caesarean birth is the only option
- Are you older than 35 and have conceived after extensive infertility treatment? You may be offered a planned caesarean delivery
- If the mother has an infection like HIV or active genital herpes, a caesarean birth is mandatory to minimize transmission of infection to the baby

Complications in the baby

- *Small baby:* If your baby has been diagnosed to be smaller than he or she should be, (see **Chapter 34**, *Foetal growth problems: too small or too big*) and the amniotic fluid is significantly reduced, you may undergo a caesarean delivery to prevent problems for the baby
- *Large baby*: If the baby is large (estimated to have a birth weight more than 3.5–3.8 kg), especially in diabetic mothers, a caesarean is done to avoid trauma to the baby and/or mother
- *Breech*: If your baby is still in a breech position close to the due date, an elective caesarean section may be done. This means that instead of the

baby's head proceeding towards the birth canal, the baby's buttocks or feet are coming first. This happens in 4 per cent of pregnancies. The breech position is not always safe to deliver vaginally. Some problems might occur which can cause complications for both mother and child (see **Chapter 35**, *Breech delivery*)

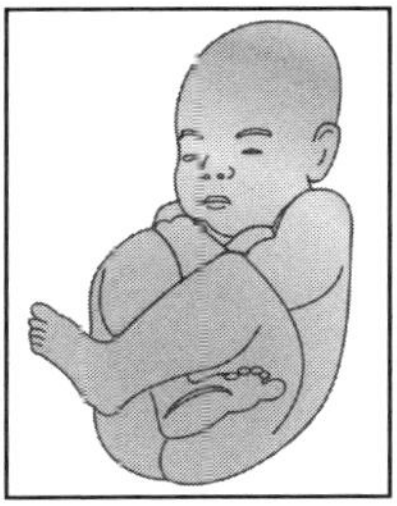

Breech baby

- *Twins*: In a twin pregnancy, if the first baby is not in the head-down position, then a caesarean will be required (see **Chapter 36**, *Twins: double trouble*)
- *Triplets*: If you are carrying triplets or more, you will almost certainly have an elective caesarean birth
- *Previous problems*: If the mother has had a difficult vaginal delivery or unfortunately had a stillbirth earlier, an elective caesarean delivery will be offered

Having a twin pregnancy does not automatically mean a caesarean birth. As long as the baby that is going to come out first is in the head-down position, a vaginal delivery is possible. In this situation, there is no scientific evidence that a caesarean birth is better.

Thendral asked: I am really worried that a vaginal delivery may be tough to bear. I also feel it may be better for the baby to have a safe caesarean birth. Can I request a caesarean delivery?

My answer: This is a complex decision that should be carefully considered and discussed with your doctor. Remember that a vaginal delivery is the best way to have a baby. Recovery from a vaginal delivery is almost immediate, as compared to a caesarean that may take a week or two. With the options for pain relief that are available now, labour is definitely easier to bear.

Having a caesarean does not guarantee that the baby will not have any problems. So, if you are under the impression that a caesarean section wil prevent all risks for you or the baby, and are requesting a planned caesarean section based on this, remember that this is not true. Though it is an excellent option when done to save the baby or the mother, like any surgery, a caesarean also carries some risk.

Reasons for doing an emergency caesarean

Failure of labour to progress

About one-third of caesarean sections are done because labour does not progress normally (see **Chapter 24**, *When things go wrong in labour*). In a

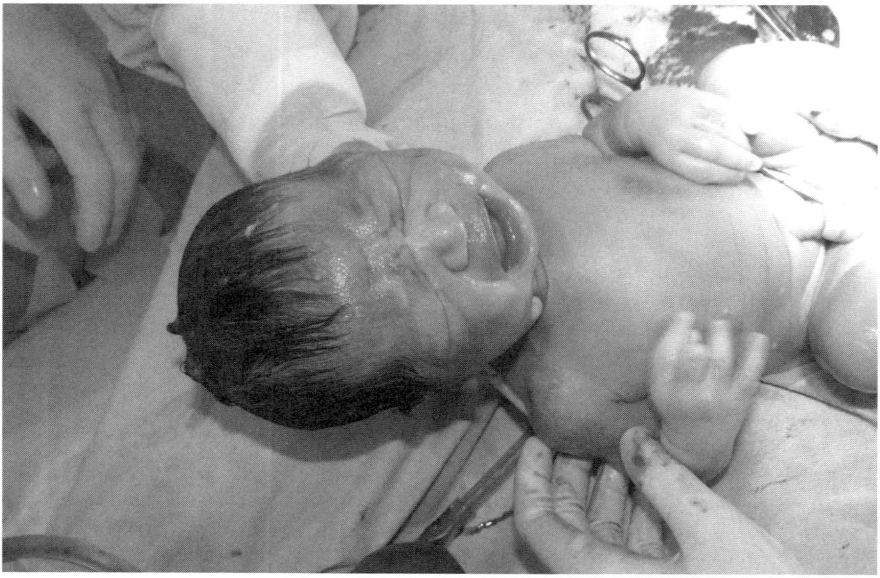

normal labour, as the pains get more frequent and stronger, the cervix will gradually open till the baby can pass through. In some women, there may be a failure of labour to progress. This means that the cervix does not open normally. If this is because of poor contractions and labour is progressing slowly, the obstetrician can speed up labour with medication. You will be monitored carefully to determine whether labour is progressing well or not. Your obstetrician may watch for several hours before deciding on a caesarean section.

Foetal distress

This is one of the common reasons for a caesarean section (see **Chapter 24**, *When things go wrong in labour*). The heart rate is monitored periodically during labour. When there is an abnormal change in the baby's heart rate, it could indicate that the baby is having trouble during labour and may need to be delivered by caesarean birth. A slow heart rate can be caused by compression of the umbilical cord. Sometimes, not enough blood flows to the baby from the placenta. This is particularly possible in a postterm baby or where the baby is smaller than it should be.

Mismatch between baby's size and the mother's pelvis

When there is a mismatch between the size of the baby and the size of the mother's pelvis, it can result in cephalo-pelvic disproportion (CPD). In simple terms, this means the baby is too large to fit through the birth passage. Occasionally, the baby may be of average size but the mother may be small-built and may not have enough space for the baby to fit through.

Being prepared for a caesarean

When do you need to go to the hospital?

If you have been scheduled for an elective caesarean section, you may be admitted to the hospital on the afternoon or night before the date of surgery. Sometimes you are advised to get admitted at least a day or two prior to the caesarean in case you need to be observed and treated for complications of pregnancy. This is particularly true with diabetes or hypertension complicating pregnancy.

You will be instructed to eat a normal meal before admission. Once you are admitted, you will be given instructions about what you can eat in the hospital. You should have an empty stomach before an operation. You will be instructed not to eat or drink anything for at least 6–8 hours before surgery.

Leave jewellery and other things of value at home. If you wear jewellery, you will be asked to remove it before the operation. You can choose to keep your *mangalsutra* on.

What happens after admission?

After admission, the admitting nurse will take you to your room and check your temperature, pulse and blood pressure. She will also record your baby's heartbeat. You will be advised not to eat or drink for 6–8 hours before the scheduled time of surgery. This will ensure that you have a smooth surgery and recovery.

Your obstetrician or one of her team will come and see you on admission. The size and position of your baby as well as your baby's heartbeat will be recorded. Your medical record file will be checked. Some blood tests may be done if necessary. A sample of blood will also be drawn so that blood can be reserved for you in case you require blood transfusion during or after the caesarean section. The doctor will also discuss the caesarean section with you.

The **anaesthetist** will be informed about your admission and will be told about the time of the caesarean. At caesarean, since your doctor will be scrubbed up and cannot take care of the baby if there is a problem, in most hospitals a **paediatrician** (or **neonatologist**) will be present in the theatre or waiting just outside the theatre. The same paediatrician will take care of

Informed consent

You will be asked to sign a consent form before surgery. The consent form will explain what operation you will be undergoing and who will be performing the operation. You should make sure you understand this information. Don't be afraid to ask questions. Have the doctor go over something if it isn't clear to you. This process is called ***informed consent***.

As part of informed consent, your doctor or someone at the hospital will talk to you about:

- What will be done during the surgery
- Why you need it
- Risks of the surgery
- Risk of not having any treatment
- What other choices you may have

If it is an emergency caesarean, you may be in too much pain or may be too anxious to understand. Let your partner understand the consent though you will be the one who has to sign the form.

your newborn during your stay in the hospital. You may opt to follow up with him or her after discharge.

What happens on the day of the caesarean section?

You may be given an enema to empty your bowels. You will also be asked to take a bath with a medicated liquid soap. Avoid using any creams, talcum powder or cosmetics after the bath.

If there is hair over the abdominal skin that may interfere with the incision, it might be shaved just before being taken into the operation theatre. Complete shaving of the pubic hair is not required.

You will be asked to remove the following items if you are using them:

- Dentures and bridges
- Hearing aids
- Contact lenses/glasses
- Jewellery (you can keep your *thali/magalsutra* on)

You will be given a special gown and a cap to put on. You will be taken to an area in the operation theatre where you will wait until the surgical team is ready for you.

An intravenous (IV) line may be started to supply your body with fluids, medication, (or blood, if needed) during and after the surgery.

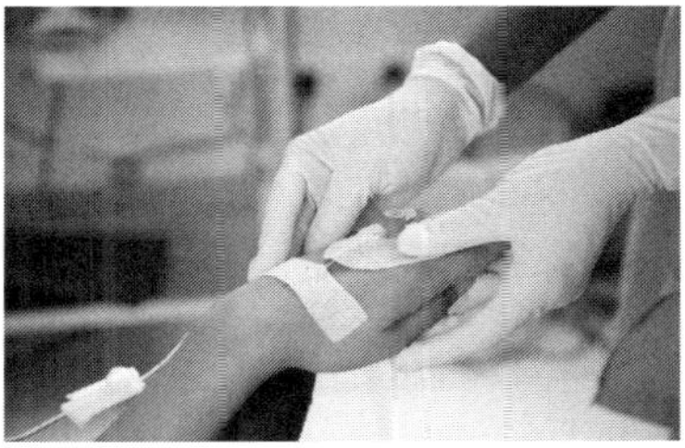

You may be given medication to help you relax. These pre-anaesthetic medications will make you feel a little drowsy and they will ensure smooth anaesthesia and recovery for you.

You may also be given any other medications that your doctor has ordered. If the doctor has prescribed any medication for the morning of the operation, the nurse will give it to you with a sip of water.

What happens in the operating room?

You will lie down on the operating table. You won't have much space to move and turn on this bed, but you will be comfortable. A blood pressure cuff and other devices will be attached to you so that your heartbeat and blood pressure can be monitored throughout the procedure.

A small tube (catheter) will be passed through the passage where you pass urine, to empty your bladder. This tube may be kept in place for 12–24 hours.

You will get a single dose of antibiotic in the operation theatre, just before the caesarean section is started. This is all you require to reduce the risk of infection in the wound. The majority of women undergoing a caesarean section do not require more than a single dose.

What sort of anaesthesia will be given?

You are given a spinal or epidural anaesthetic. This numbs the lower part of your body, preventing you from feeling pain during surgery. With spinal or epidural, you will stay awake. You will feel the doctor touch you but there will be no pain. Once the baby is born, you may be given a mild sedative that will make you drowsy.

If you are having an emergency caesarean and already had an epidural during labour, the epidural will be continued with a higher dosage.

Occasionally, a general anaesthetic is used. A general anaesthetic relaxes your muscles, puts you to sleep and also prevents you from feeling pain. Discuss this with your obstetrician/anaesthetist.

What is the difference between epidural and spinal anaesthesia?

- A spinal delivers the medicine directly into the cerebrospinal fluid that bathes the spinal cord. An epidural delivers the medicine outside the dura and acts only on the nerves that come out from the spinal cord
- Along with pain relief, spinal anaesthesia will also temporarily paralyze your legs so that you will not be able to move them for an hour or so. This effect is not seen with epidural analgesia. That is why a spinal is not given for labour
- A spinal is a single dose of medication and will last only for a short time. The dose cannot be repeated. An epidural is given through a catheter that is left in place. Drugs can be injected repeatedly into the catheter so that pain relief can be prolonged. That is why an epidural is excellent for labour

What happens during the procedure?

The obstetrician makes a cut below your navel. Usually, a transverse (side-to-side) incision is made on the skin. This is commonly called a 'bikini cut'. Occasionally a vertical (up-and-down) incision is used.

If you are considering a permanent birth control method (you both are sure that you do not want another baby), you can speak to your doctor beforehand and can undergo tubal ligation at the same time as the caesarean (see **Chapter 49**, *Methods of birth control*).

A cut is made in the lower part of the uterus to deliver the baby. After the baby is born, the placenta and membranes are removed. The cut in the uterus and abdomen are then closed.

Once the doctors have started your caesarean, your baby is usually born within 2–3 minutes of making the initial cut. The whole operation will take between 30–45 minutes. Soon after birth, your baby will be examined by a paediatrician or neonatologist and will be kept in the nursery for an hour or two, till you are ready to start breastfeeding.

What happens after the procedure?

You may stay in the hospital about 3–5 days, depending on your condition. You will be encouraged to get out of bed a day or two after the surgery. The catheter will be removed within 12–24 hours and you can use the toilet on your own.

Breastfeeding after a caesarean section

Having had a caesarean will not have an adverse effect on breastfeeding. Even the initiation of breastfeeding need not be delayed. Though there will be some discomfort because of the pain of the stitches, you will be encouraged to start breastfeeding as soon as possible.

Once you are fully conscious and alert and able to hold the baby, you can begin breastfeeding. You will, of course, need assistance the first few times.

Having the baby's father or another person staying with you in the hospital room can be a great help in lifting the baby, changing position, changing diapers, and so forth. This can help establish breastfeeding early (see more in **Chapter 27**, *Breastfeeding*).

After you get home

Care of the incision

The incision should be kept clean and dry. You may wash the incision with soap and water after the dressing is removed. It is recommended that you wear cotton underwear and no tight fitting clothing. The incision itself will heal in a few days, but it takes 6–8 weeks for the complete healing of the uterus and all the layers of the abdomen.

Do not be surprised if you have pain or a pulling sensation in your incision every time you laugh, sneeze or cough. Just place your palm firmly on your incision when you do any of these things. This discomfort will disappear in a few weeks.

Bathing

You can bathe every day. Let the water run over the suture line. You can gently apply soap over the wound. There is no need to apply any lotion or cream over the wound. You can wash your hair once a week for the first few weeks and then more often after that, if that is what you routinely do.

Activity

Your activity level should be gradually increased. In the first week after you get home, you can walk around the room and take care of your baby. Over the next week, you can start walking around the house. In the third week, you can start resuming small domestic chores, like cutting vegetables and making coffee or tea. A month after you are home, you can resume your normal work—that includes cooking and washing.

Stairs

You can start climbing stairs two weeks after the caesarean section. If you live on a higher floor, and don't have a lift, when you get home from the hospital you can walk up the stairs a few steps at a time. Once you are in your home, avoid coming down for two weeks.

> **Rekha asked:** Is there a special diet after a caesarean birth? Are there any restrictions? My grandmother told me not to eat 'cold' items to prevent me from getting pus in the wound.
>
> **My answer:** You will be on a normal diet a day or two after the operation. There are no food restrictions. You should concentrate on taking a balanced diet with a good amount of proteins. Drink plenty of fluids to avoid dehydration. Make sure you are not consuming unnecessary calories like large quantities of rice, sugar, and fat (ghee and butter). The weight that is gained during pregnancy and immediately afterwards is difficult to shed. Eating fish, or 'cold' food like curds (yogurt), fruits, juices and certain vegetables like ladies' fingers cannot cause pus in the wound. These are simply food-related myths. Bacteria, not food, cause infections.

Lifting things that are heavy

Avoid lifting heavy things (heavier than 4 kgs) for six weeks. This does not include your baby! You can carry your baby comfortably without having to call for help. You can start lifting anything after 6 weeks but let your body dictate how much you can. You may also need some assistance caring for your older child. Do not lift your toddler—have someone lift him on to your lap when he needs some cuddling.

Sex

Intercourse should be avoided for at least six weeks. When you do resume sex, the abdominal wound may still be a little tender but you will not harm it in any way. Remember that even if you have not resumed menstruating or are breastfeeding, you can still become pregnant. Birth control should be used once you resume intercourse. Make sure that you have spoken to

> **Raghav asked:** My wife just underwent a caesarean. We are not yet sure if we want another baby but if we do decide to have another one, how long do we need to wait?
>
> **My answer:** It is advised to wait for another pregnancy for **at least two years (or even three years)** after a caesarean. That is why it is important to use reliable birth control after a caesarean birth.

your doctor about birth control. See **Chapter 48**, *Methods of birth control*, for the right option for you.

Exercise

After 4–6 weeks, you may begin an exercise programme to regain abdominal muscle tone. Join a fitness programme that will help regain your muscle tone, especially of your abdominal muscles. There is absolutely no need for an abdominal belt. Read more of what you can and cannot do, in **Chapter 26**, *Taking care of yourself after birth*.

What are the risks associated with the surgery?

Most caesarean sections are safe. Occasionally, there can be complications that are inherent in any surgery.

- You may have excessive bleeding during or after the caesarean section
- You may develop an infection
- Rarely, the cut in the wall of the abdomen may leave a weak part in the wall. This may result in an incisional hernia
- You may still be allowed to have a vaginal delivery with your next pregnancy. However, chances for a repeat caesarean section increase depending on the reason the caesarean was done in the first place

Old wives' tales

- If you sweep and swab and do heavy physical labour during your pregnancy, you can avoid a caesarean. **Not true!** Just be active; it is important in any pregnancy.
- Eating fish, or 'cold' food like curds (yogurt) and fruit juice can cause pus in the wound. **Not true!** Bacteria, not food, cause infections.
- You should not lift anything heavy for six months after the caesarean. **Not true!** You can be completely normal in 3–4 weeks and can lift anything heavy six weeks after a caesarean section.

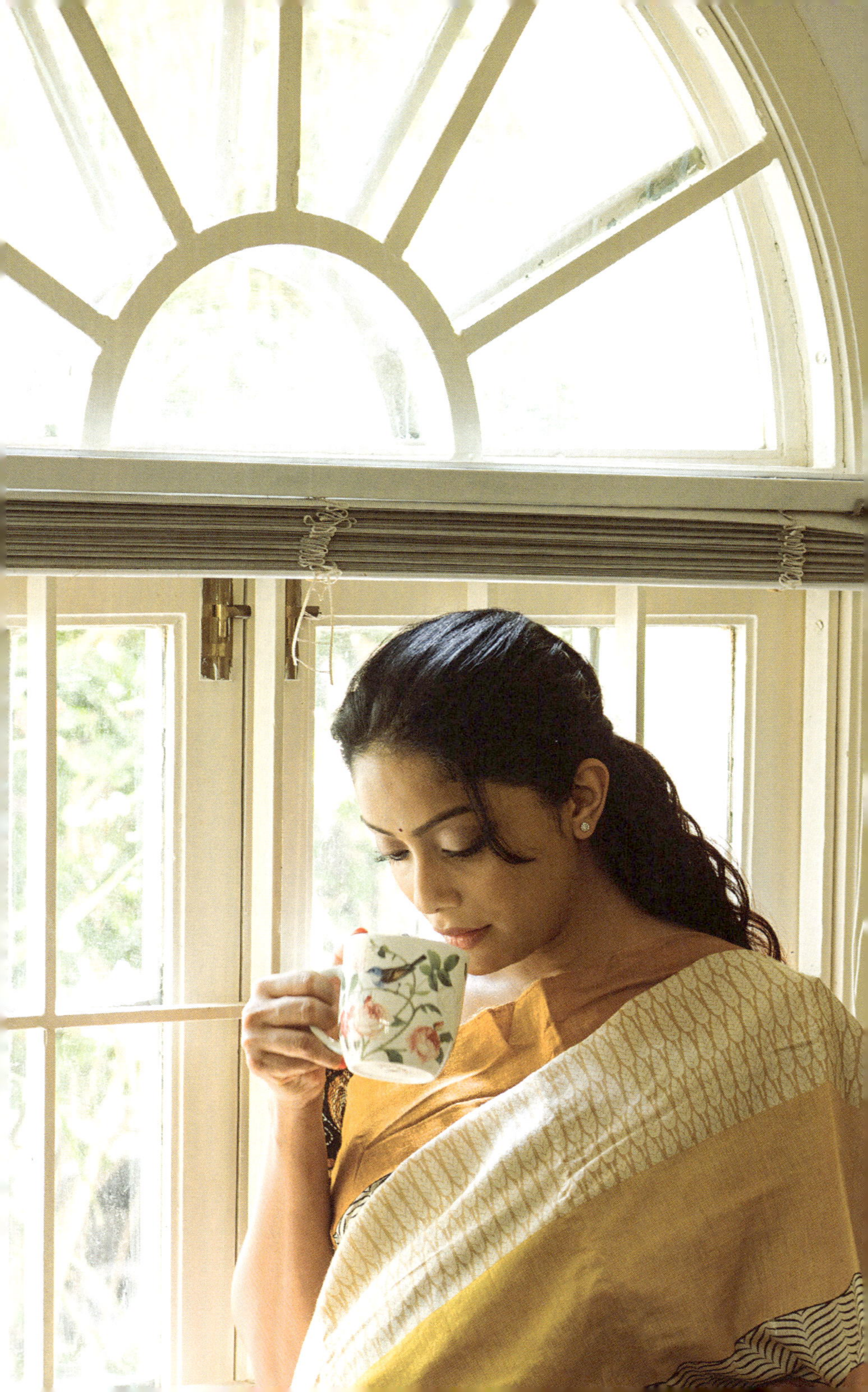

After the delivery

CHAPTER 26

Taking care of yourself after birth

Whether you have had a vaginal delivery or a caesarean section, it is important to get back to normal as early as possible after childbirth. Your new baby will make physical and emotional demands on you. Taking care of yourself by eating the right food and starting exercises early will go a long way in bringing you back to your pre-pregnancy state.

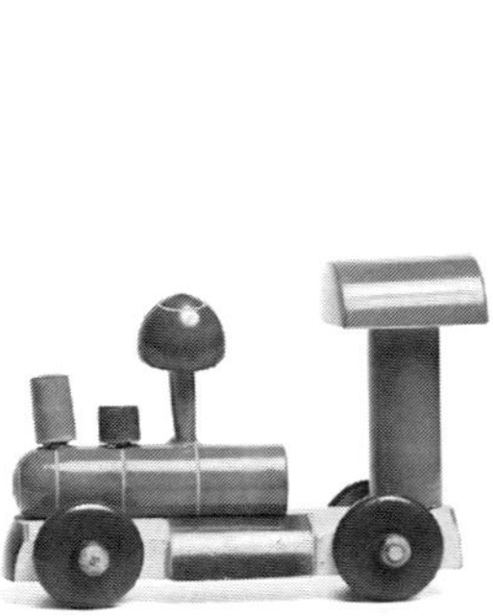

26

Taking care of yourself after birth

Most women have an uncomplicated and smooth recovery after delivery but the first 6 weeks after childbirth can be stressful, both physically and emotionally. Though it is a time of great joy for both of you (and your families), at times you may feel overwhelmed and inadequate. Adjustment to parenthood can strain your equanimity and patience. With the introduction of a demanding new member, the family dynamics change, with the focus almost entirely on the baby.

You need to take good care of yourself. To rebuild your strength, you will have to focus on plenty of rest and good nutrition. You will also have to exercise to regain your muscle tone and stamina.

Dealing with exhaustion and lack of sleep

Ask any new mother what she wants the most and she will surely say, 'Sleep!' Babies have a completely different biological clock than adults and it takes time for them to synchronize their sleep cycles to a more manageable one (see the section on Sleep in **Chapter 47**, *Your new baby*). Your baby may wake up every two to three hours to be fed, changed, and comforted. Her needs seem to be most demanding when your energy levels are the lowest and your sleep requirements are the highest. Most babies are up and crying between midnight and the early hours of the morning.

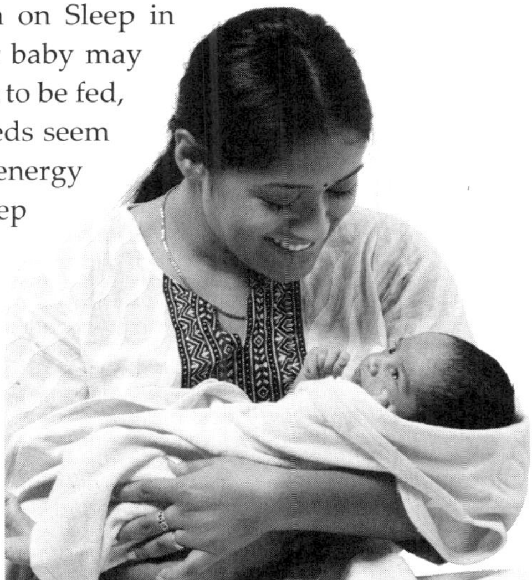

Although you may not get a solid seven to eight hours of sleep for several months, you can work out strategies to grab some sleep.

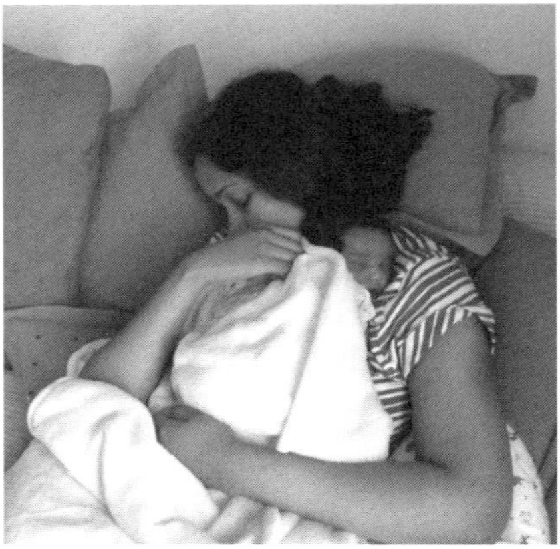

- Sleep when the baby sleeps. This is not the time to clean the house or do other chores. This is your chance to catch up and even small naps of 15–30 minutes can be enough to beat complete exhaustion
- If you can have someone to help you out for a few hours each day when you can get uninterrupted sleep, it would be very useful. In India it is possible to have your mother, mother-in-law, a sister or an aunt step in to help out. A responsible baby helper is not always easy to get but can be a boon
- Give yourself 15–30 minutes each day to stretch, walk, do yoga or exercise. It may seem impossible at times, but it will give you a boost of energy. You will also get relief from muscle aches

Your husband can be invaluable in handling the baby in the first chaotic weeks. He can help at nights by walking the baby to calm her, and burping the baby after a feed.

- After the baby is a month old, start taking small outings to the park or shops. It's good (and safe) for the baby and certainly will help you get over the cooped-up feeling

Changes in the uterus

Your uterus was stretched to accommodate your baby during the pregnancy. Now it has to contract and reach its normal size. In the first few days after delivery, you might find a hard round lump in the lower part of your abdomen—this is the uterus that has contracted to half the size it was just before your delivery. The uterus will shrink rapidly in the next few weeks.

You might have some cramping occasionally, especially when you breastfeed. That is why breastfeeding is good for you: it helps the uterus contract.

'After pains' is the term used to describe the pain that you experience as the uterus shrinks. 'After pains' occur with any delivery but may be mild with a first delivery and can be worse after subsequent deliveries. These cramps can be relieved with a painkiller like ibuprofen. A hot water bag can also be used.

Bleeding

It is normal to have vaginal bleeding for 2–6 weeks after the delivery. The discharge from the vagina after a delivery is called 'lochia'. The amount of bleeding may vary from day to day. It's not unusual to pass small blood clots as well. The colour will change from bright red to watery red/pink. After a few weeks, it will change to a yellow/white/clear colour. The type of sanitary napkin you use will depend on the amount of bleeding you have. You cannot use tampons.

Diya asked: I had a sudden gush of bleeding 4 days after the baby was born. I had to change 3 big pads within 2 hours and had to go to the hospital. Why did this happen?

My answer: Occasionally, you might have heavy bleeding immediately after the delivery (while you are in the hospital). This might be due to your uterus not contracting properly. You might be given medicines to help the uterus contract.

If the bleeding became heavy after you got home, especially if it did not stop or if you passed large clots (bigger than a large lemon), it is called late postpartum hemorrhage. A uterus that didn't contract normally, possibly because small bits of placenta or membrane remained in the uterus after birth may have caused this. If there had been fever or a foul-smelling discharge accompanying the bleeding, it could have been caused by a uterine infection.

Handling pain after delivery

Perineal pain (area between the vagina and anus)

It is common to have pain near the vagina and over the episiotomy. In the first 24 hours after delivery, you may be given an injectable painkiller if you find the pain unbearable. After that, you should be able to manage with oral painkillers like ibuprofen.

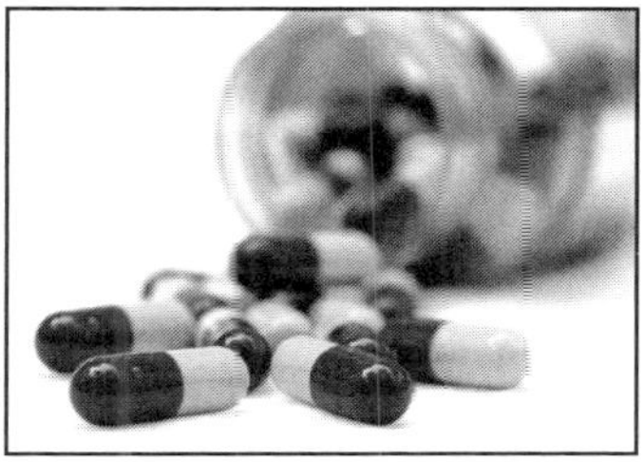

Sitz baths and infrared lamps can also help in relieving the pain of an episiotomy (see **Chapter 19**, *Labour and delivery*).

Incisional pain (after a caesarean)

You will get injectable painkillers for the first 24–48 hours after a caesarean. After the first 48 hours, you will be able to manage with an oral painkiller. You may find that you can get off painkillers within four to five days after the surgery. The pain may get aggravated if you are very active.

Bladder and bowel function

Bladder function

For months, the uterus was pushing on the bladder. During delivery too, there would have been pressure on the bladder. This can cause the bladder to lose sensation or become 'numb'. You might not always have the sensation that your bladder is full even though it is. It is important for you to pass urine at least every two to three hours. Drink plenty of fluids.

Atonic bladder

Sometimes, the bladder becomes so 'numb' after the delivery that it might keep filling up without your realizing it. After a few hours, your bladder might be overdistended. You might need to have a catheter inserted to empty your bladder. The best way to avoid an atonic bladder is to make sure that you pass urine within six hours after your delivery and then at least every 2–3 hours after that.

Bowel function

You might have your first bowel movement two to three days after your delivery. If you had a vaginal delivery, you might be scared that passing motion will be painful because of the episiotomy. There is nothing to be worried about. Make sure you take food high in fibre and drink plenty of fluids so that your stools are not hard. If needed, your obstetrician may give you a stool softener. After a caesarean too, you might pass your first stool two to three days after the surgery.

Haemorrhoids or 'piles'

In pregnancy, it is common to develop haemorrhoids. Haemorrhoids are distended veins of the rectum that can get worse in the third trimester. Due to the pushing during vaginal delivery, they may become bigger and painful. Make sure that your stools are soft after the delivery. If the haemorrhoids are large and painful, Sitz baths (sitting in a basin of warm water) will help. You can also take stool softeners and use a local anaesthetic ointment. Remember that most haemorrhoids will shrink after a few weeks though you may continue to have a small, painless swelling near your anus.

Eating healthy after a delivery

As Indians, we have a lot of misconceptions about the food that can be eaten after a delivery. It is important to remember that there are no dietary restrictions after a delivery. No particular food will prevent the healing of the uterus, the episiotomy or the incision in case of a caesarean.

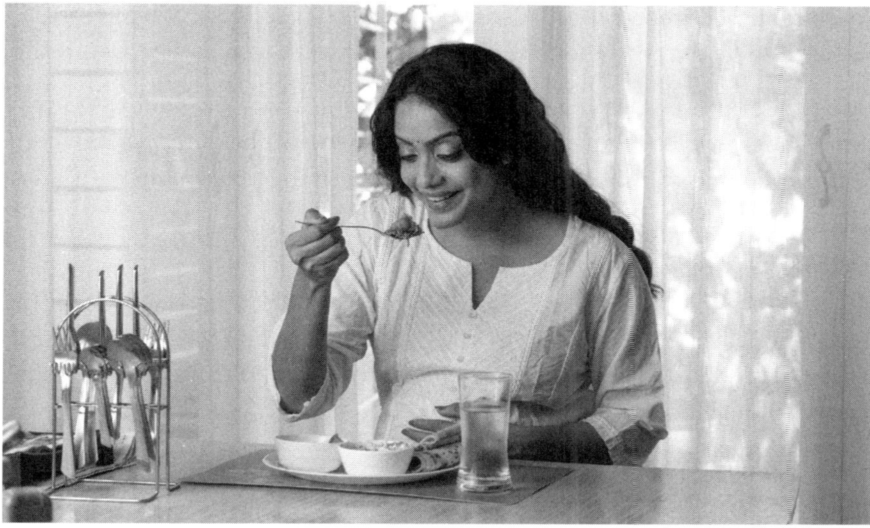

Overeating is a definite danger after a delivery. It is important to remember that if you put on too much weight after the delivery, you will find it difficult to shed the extra kilos. The excess weight gain after a delivery may lead to lifelong obesity. Discuss weight management with your obstetrician at your postnatal check-up.

Eat foods from the four food groups, especially those with iron (meat, beans, green leafy vegetables, dried fruit), calcium (milk, curds, cheese) and protein. Fats like ghee and butter should be had only in moderation, if not avoided all together (see **Chapter 28**, *Your diet after delivery*).

Drink plenty of fluids to satisfy your thirst. Keeping yourself well hydrated will also help in breastfeeding.

Continue taking the prenatal vitamins and iron supplements prescribed by your obstetrician. Since there is a certain amount of blood loss in childbirth, it makes sense to continue your iron supplement for at least three months after delivery.

Resuming normal activity

After a vaginal delivery

You can start moving around your room in the hospital as soon as you feel up to it. You can walk to the bathroom. You can have a bath the very next day after your delivery. You can wash your hair in a few days and as often as you want after that.

You might feel tired and exhausted after the delivery because you are still not used to the baby's schedule. Rest whenever the baby is sleeping.

Once you are home, you can resume normal activity gradually. You can climb stairs. A month after the delivery, you should be able to completely resume all your normal activities, including driving your vehicle.

After a caesarean birth

While you are in the hospital

You will be encouraged to get up and try to go to the bathroom within the first 24 hours after surgery. When you get up for the first time, you may feel a little dizzy. Sit up for a few minutes and then get up from bed only after the dizziness has passed.

Urinating after the catheter is removed can sometimes be uncomfortable—the nurse attending on you will help you.

You may need help in changing your sanitary pads soon after the surgery because of the incision pain. After 1 or 2 days, you will be able to manage by yourself.

Soon you will be able to stroll in your room and in the hospital corridor. Walking helps in relieving the gas pain that you may experience.

After you get home

After you return home, you can gradually resume normal work so that by the end of one month after the operation, you should be able to perform most of your normal housework. See **Chapter 25**, *Caesarean section* for instructions on how to increase your activity in weekly increments.

Anamika asked: I have heard that one can get a hernia after a caesarean. How do I avoid that?

My answer: A hernia is a weakness in the abdominal wall through which the bowel can push against the skin. It is seen as a bulge in some part of the abdominal incision. After a caesarean the chance of getting a hernia is only 2 per 1000. However this depends on using the correct suture material and technique. You can avoid a hernia by not lifting anything heavy (4 kg or more) for 6 weeks after the surgery.

Exercise after childbirth

Four weeks after a vaginal delivery and six weeks after a caesarean, you may begin an exercise programme that will help you regain your pre-

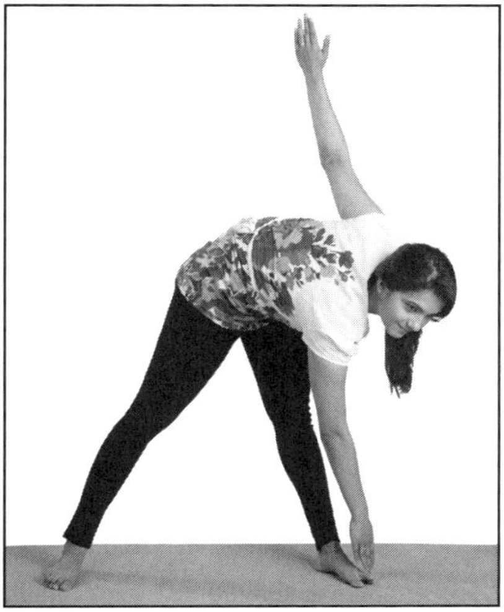

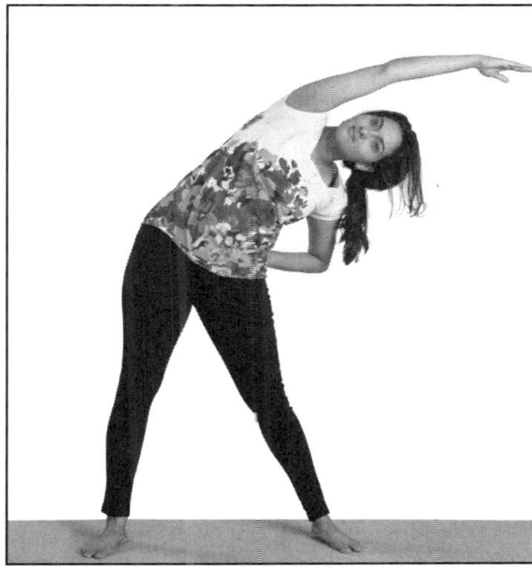

pregnancy figure. Join a fitness programme that will help you get back your muscle tone, especially of the abdominal muscles (see **Chapter 29**, *Getting fit after delivery*).

Mahima asked: Do I need to wear an abdominal belt after delivery?

My answer: Immediately after delivery, the abdominal muscles are flabby and without any tone. Most women are very concerned that they will never regain their muscle tone. Somebody might advise you to bind your abdomen tightly with a piece of cloth or to buy an expensive abdominal belt. **These methods are completely worthless.** The only way you can regain the tone of your abdominal muscles is by exercising, with special emphasis on toning up your abdominal muscles. Regular abdominal exercises can be started 4 weeks after a vaginal delivery and 6 weeks after a caesarean section.

Fluid retention

It is normal to see an increase in the swelling in your legs during the first one or two weeks after delivery. Remember that the body can retain up to 6 litres of water during a pregnancy! After delivery, this might tend to collect in your legs. In a few weeks, this swelling will come down by itself. Do what you did to reduce swelling during pregnancy: sleep with your feet propped on a cushion or a pillow to help the fluid drain faster.

Hydrate yourself

Drink plenty of fluids because as you lose all the excess fluid, you need to make sure you are well hydrated, especially since that will help with the breastfeeding.

You will find that you are passing urine much more frequently and in larger volumes after delivery. This is your body getting rid of the excess fluid.

Sexual intercourse

It is usually safe to resume intercourse six weeks after a vaginal or caesarean birth. By that time, you would have had your postnatal check-up and your obstetrician would have made sure that you have healed well. You may be a little apprehensive about pain the first few times but you will be comfortable soon.

Remember that even if you have not resumed your periods or are breast-feeding, you can still become pregnant. Birth control should be used when you resume sex. Talk to your obstetrician about the safest and most suitable birth control option for you (see **Chapter 49**, *Methods of birth control*).

Kegel's exercise

Kegel's is a specific type of exercise for the muscles that support the rectum, vagina and the urethra. Strengthening these muscles can help bladder control after a vaginal delivery, and decrease the risk of getting a prolapse. These are the same exercises that you were doing in the third trimester (see **Chapter 8**, *The third trimester*).

To learn how to contract the right muscles, try to stop the flow of urine when you are urinating. Do this several times. Once you know how to squeeze the muscles to stop the flow of urine, you know how to contract the right muscles.

You can then start doing these exercises anytime, anywhere, preferably while sitting down. Squeeze the pelvic muscles for 10 seconds and repeat 20–30 times. You can do this 3 times daily. Make sure you empty your bladder before doing the exercises. Check with your obstetrician, if you are not sure how to do them.

Reasons to call your doctor after delivery

- You should not have a fever after you get home. If you have a fever of more than 100°F (38°C), for more than 24 hours, you should call your doctor
- Sudden onset of pain over the abdominal incision, accompanied by redness and tenderness
- Foul-smelling vaginal discharge
- Burning urination or blood in the urine which may be indicative of a urinary infection

- Extremely heavy bleeding that soaks a maxi pad within an hour or the passage of large clots
- A sore, red, painful area on the breast that may be accompanied by fever. This might be the beginning of mastitis or a breast abscess (see **Chapter 27**, *Breastfeeding*)
- Feeling anxious, panicky, and/or depressed may be a sign of mild post-partum depression ('postpartum blues'). Mild anxiety and 'feeling down' is common. If this feeling persists and worsens and you are unable to cope, you might require professional help (see box below)
- Severe headache that begins right after birth and does not let up in intensity. This is rare but might be an indication of a blood clot in the brain

Post-partum depression

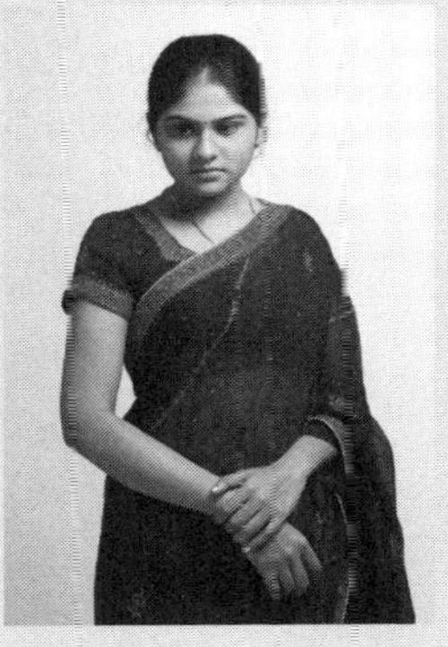

Most women experience 'postpartum blues' to some degree or the other. Soon after the delivery it is common to feel overwhelmed by the responsibility of taking care of the newborn baby. Exhaustion and sleeplessness can contribute to this feeling of helplessness.

In some women, this condition may not be temporary. It can progress to severe post-partum depression with frequent bouts of crying and irritability, no desire to see or touch the child and uncontrollable anger. This period could last from a few days to a few months. This is the time for strong family support and understanding. In severe cases, professional counselling may be required. Your doctor will refer you to the right professional.

CHAPTER 27

Breastfeeding

Stella is in the final weeks of her pregnancy. She is very keen on breastfeeding her baby because she knows that mother's milk is the best for the baby. She wants to do whatever is necessary to make sure that her baby gets enough milk from her.

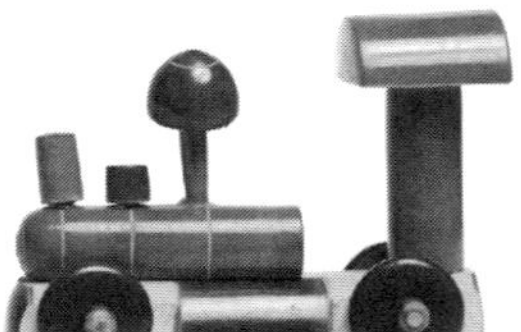

27

Breastfeeding

One of nature's miracles is the ability of a woman to nourish and sustain her baby with breast milk. It has been proved without a doubt that breast milk is the best form of nutrition for your baby. Breast milk has unique properties and is composed of a combination of nutrients essential to a child's health. In the first six months, the baby should be nourished exclusively by breast milk. It is recommended that mothers breastfeed for at least the first year of a child's life.

Most mothers are so anxious when they start breastfeeding that it will seem as if everything is going wrong. The baby keeps crying, does not seem to latch on and does not seem to be getting enough milk. Sometimes, overzealous relatives try to convince the mother that she does not have enough milk and should give milk supplements.

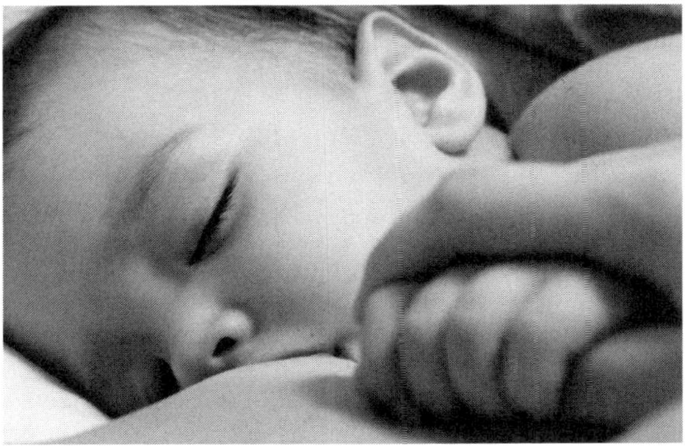

It is quite surprising that even when everything seems to be optimal, the baby's first attempts at breastfeeding are such a hit-and-miss experience. You and your baby need to learn the best breastfeeding positions that work for both of you. In a few days you will both get the hang of it and from then on it will be smooth sailing (most of the times!).

Breastfeeding the baby up to a year after birth provides the baby with good nutrition. If you are a working woman, and have to get back to work, try to feed the baby for as many months as possible. You can also pump your breasts and store the milk in the fridge so that it can be used when you are at work. Discuss this with your doctor.

Breast milk is best milk

- For the human baby, only human milk is a perfect composition of every thing he or she requires to thrive. It is rich in the nutrients that are essential for brain growth and nervous system development. Breastfed babies perform better on different kinds of intelligence tests as they grow older. They also develop better eye function. Certain fatty acid chains present only in human milk and which are not available in artificial formulas, are responsible for this
- It is not enough for the nutrients to be present in the milk: they should be present in the right quantity and the right forms so that the baby can use them. This is called bio-availability. The bio-availability of nutrients in human milk is perfect for human babies
- The baby easily digests it because it contains the right kind of milk proteins
- Human milk is rich in antibodies and immunity-boosting factors. This helps the baby's ability to resist mild to severe infections. Babies, who are exclusively or almost exclusively breastfed, have significantly fewer gastrointestinal, respiratory, ear, and urinary infections. Antibodies in human milk directly protect against infection. Breast milk also appears to have properties that help boost a baby's own immune system. If the baby does develop an infection, then it will be milder if the baby has been breastfed
- It is at the perfect temperature
- Breast milk cannot get spoilt because it is available on demand and does not have to be stored
- Most importantly, breast milk is free!
- For the mother who breastfeeds, the risk of breast cancer is reduced

Why early breastfeeding?

Whether it was a vaginal or caesarean birth, nursing immediately after birth has advantages for a mother. Early breastfeeding:

- Intensifies the mother-child connection. The hormone oxytocin that is released when you breastfeed is also called the 'cuddle hormone' and promotes bonding. Oxytocin also helps the uterus contract
- Provides stimulation to help the milk start flowing
- Provides the baby with the immunological advantages of colostrum (the thin colourless fluid which is secreted in the first few days, before the actual milk starts flowing)

Neha asked: With my first baby, I did not get enough milk in the first 1 or 2 days. My mother and grandmother scared me that I was starving the baby and I started with milk supplements. I really want to give exclusive breastfeeds for the little one I am expecting. Will I have enough milk?

My answer: Be confident in your ability to feed your baby. Don't worry; remember that almost all mothers, even those who have had a caesarean section, will be able to produce enough milk for their babies. All it requires is patience and perseverance. It takes at least three to four days to establish proper flow of milk. A crying baby does not equate to a starving baby. In the first week, babies will lose weight and that is a normal phenomenon. A week to ten days after the delivery, the baby will start gaining weight and this is the best proof that you have enough milk.

Should you be giving anything other than breast milk?

It is absolutely important to give your baby breast milk exclusively for the first six months. Do not give sugar solutions or commercially available milk supplements unless there is an overwhelming reason and your paediatrician advises you to do that.

Even if you have had a caesarean, you can put the baby to breast in a few hours, with help. Do not let the nurses or other paramedical staff give the baby anything other than breast milk.

When does the milk start flowing?

For the first three days, you will produce only a thin, watery secretion that is called colostrum. This is vital for the baby because it is rich in antibodies and protects the baby against infection. Milk will start flowing on the third or fourth day after the baby is born. Once lactation is established, you may find that the milk may leak from your breasts even if you hear the baby cry. This is Nature's way of making sure your baby has milk when he needs it.

> The baby's cry and the baby suckling at your breast are both essential to send signals to your brain. The flow of breast milk is set off by these signals. The more the baby suckles, the better the production of milk.

How often should you feed?

When you first start breastfeeding, you can start feeding every one-and-a-half to two hours. As the milk starts flowing, you should continue to keep this interval. This way the baby will get hungry and suckle better. Some people recommend 'demand feeding' which means you feed the baby whenever she cries. This might be exhausting and feeding the baby at regular intervals might be easier. In a few weeks, the baby will settle into a pattern and will feed every two to three hours. At nights, if the baby is sleeping, you can wait without giving a feed for up to 3–4 hours.

The quality of milk varies within a given breastfeeding session. **Foremilk** is the milk first swallowed by the baby and has a lower fat content and is thin. **Hindmilk** is produced as the infant continues to breastfeed over the next several minutes. The fat content is higher, it is thicker, and this is what satisfies the baby.

How long should you feed?

In the beginning, you might find that the baby may feed for only 5–10 minutes at each breast. Within a few days, the baby will start suckling for 15–20 minutes at each breast. The more the baby suckles, the more the milk will flow. You can tell your baby has finished on a breast when the suckling slows down and the breast becomes soft. Then, offer the second breast to your baby. Change the breast you start with, each time you nurse. For example, if you started feeding with the right breast and then moved to the left, with your next nursing session start on the left breast.

What if your milk flow does not get established?

Occasionally, a mother might find that she has difficulty in establishing milk flow. You might be prescribed drugs called galactagogues, which stimulate your brain to produce prolactin, which is the hormone that helps you

Meghna asked: I am getting so many suggestions to increase the amount of milk I produce for the baby. My mother is suggesting fenugreek, my aunt wants me to eat lots of garlic and my mother-in-law wants me to drink three glasses of milk every day. What advice should I follow?

My answer: There is not a single mother who does not worry whether she will have enough milk. Have faith in Nature, which will ensure that you will produce enough milk to nourish your baby. All these traditional methods have been around for generations but scientific studies have not proved their efficacy. A very small study showed that babies seemed to suckle longer when mothers ate garlic. Garlic definitely flavours breast milk with its unique smell; however, there isn't much research to back up the ability of garlic to increase breast milk.

You need to drink milk as part of good nutrition but you need not go overboard. Two glasses of milk and 2 cups of curds will fulfill your dairy requirements.

produce milk. Two of the commonly used galactagogues are domperidone and metoclopramide (both these drugs are commonly used to treat nausea and heartburn). These medicines should be taken only with a prescription from your doctor.

Tips to help the milk flow

- Sit in a calm and quiet atmosphere
- If you can, use towels soaked in warm water (and squeezed half dry) on your breast for 5 minutes before you start
- Calm your baby by putting her on your shoulder and patting her—when she is screaming with hunger she will have a hard time finding your nipple (though some babies can be completely inconsolable!)
- Don't hesitate to get the help of a professional. If after you get home, you find that the baby is not taking to the breast, go back to the hospital and let a senior nurse help you learn the technique again. There are lactational specialists: see if you can find one near you
- Keep yourself well hydrated. Drink lots of fluids through the day

Sundar asked: I never thought we could get so stressed about this little baby! My wife and I constantly worry that he is not getting enough milk. How can we be sure that he is okay?

My answer: There are some ways to assess that your baby is getting enough milk.

- Your baby should get an average of 8–12 feeds in a day, with each feed lasting 10–15 minutes
- With adequate feeds, the baby will pass urine 4–6 times during the 3rd and 4th days, and this increases to 6–8 times on day 5 and after
- Meconium (black-green stools) will change to transitional stools (yellow-brown) within approximately 3 days of birth and the baby will have 3–4 stools per day after day 4
- Weight loss is normal and your baby will lose 5–7 per cent of his birth weight in the first few days. The weight loss usually stops in 5–7 days and then he will regain his birth weight by 2 weeks of age. With adequate feeds, a baby will gain 15–40 grams per day

Positions for breastfeeding

The breastfeeding pillow

Getting into a comfortable position is one of most the important things for successful breastfeeding. For a long time women have been using a regular pillow to raise the baby comfortably to the level of the breasts. You can use as many pillows you need to get into a comfortable feeding position. There are also breastfeeding support pillows being made specifically for this purpose.

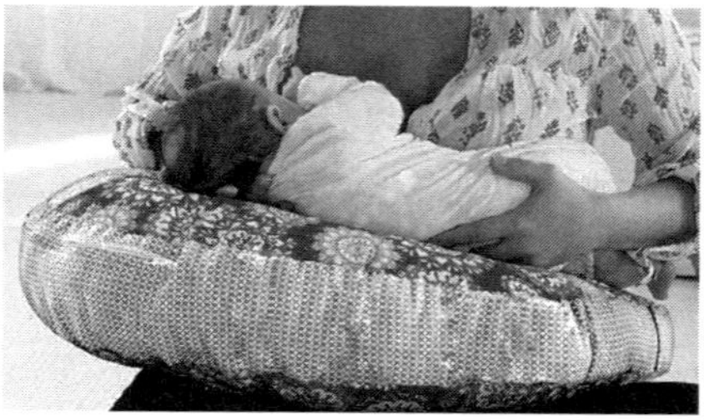

Breastfeeding pillows come in different shapes: 'C' shape, 'O' shape, and the crescent shape. The 'C' shape tends to be the most common shape and is generally easy to fit around your waist, at the same time providing a place to support your arm comfortably. Do remember that you will be using it only for a year or so and in your enthusiasm, don't go and buy the most expensive one!

Cradle hold

This position is a very natural one. If you are feeding on the left breast, you use your left arm. You cradle your baby with her head resting in the bend of your elbow. Her body lies on the forearm and your palm supports her sweet little bottom.

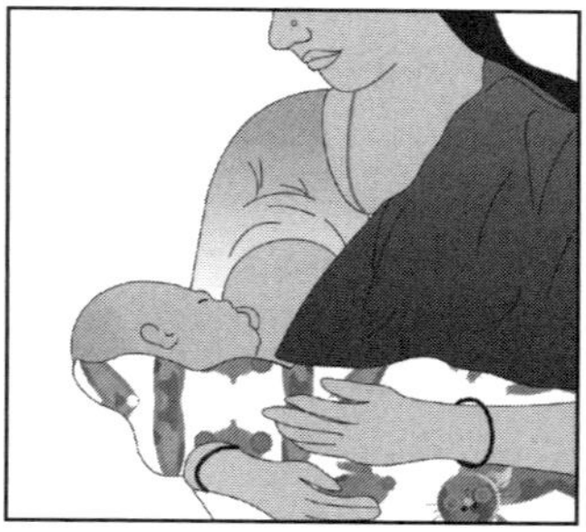

With the other hand, cup your breast, placing your thumb above your nipple and areola and the other four fingers below the nipple. Light compression with the fingers and thumb will make the nipple more prominent and easier to latch on to.

If the cradle hold is used, the baby can rest on a pillow. This is particularly useful after a caesarean section because the pillow will cover the tender incision. Many mothers find the cradle hold more comfortable after the first few days of recovery from surgery, but not in the first one or two days.

After a caesarean

It might a little difficult to find a completely comfortable position for breastfeeding immediately after a caesarean section. The nursing staff can be a great help in lifting and positioning the baby initially, so that there is no pressure on the incision. The movements of one of the arms may be restricted due to the placement of the IV fluids. Usually, the IV fluids will be removed after the first 24–48 hours and you will then find it easier to hold and manipulate your baby.

The side lying position

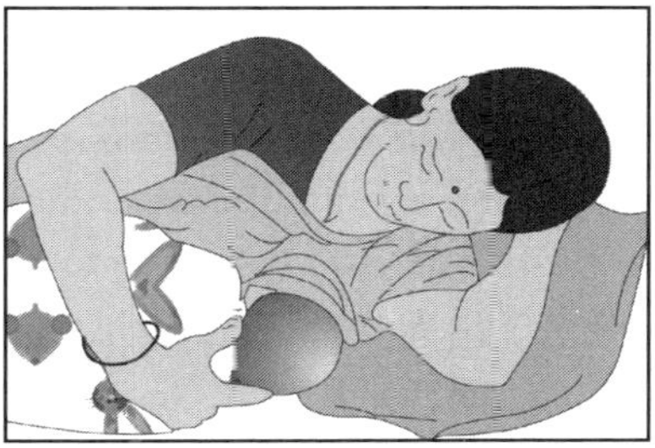

This position is great when you are feeding in the middle of the night and are too tired to sit up. The baby should be placed on her side, facing your body. Your elbow can be placed under her head to support it, and to turn her head towards the breast. She should always be directly facing the breast so that she won't have to turn her head to nurse. A rolled up towel placed behind the baby can help keep her from pulling off the breast as she relaxes during the feeding.

This is also the preferred position in the first few days of having had a caesarean section. You should turn slowly onto your side, and put a rolled up towel next to the incision in case the baby kicks.

Breastfeeding: 'latching on'

What is latching on?

The way the baby grasps the mother's breast with the mouth, to be able to suckle properly, is called latching on. With proper latching on, the baby

- Opens her mouth wide
- Grasps not just the nipple but also most of the areola (the dark area around the nipple)
- Her tongue will be well applied to the under surface of the nipple.

Latching on correctly is the key to successful and painless breastfeeding. If the baby does not latch on properly, you may develop cracked or sore nipples and the baby may not get enough milk.

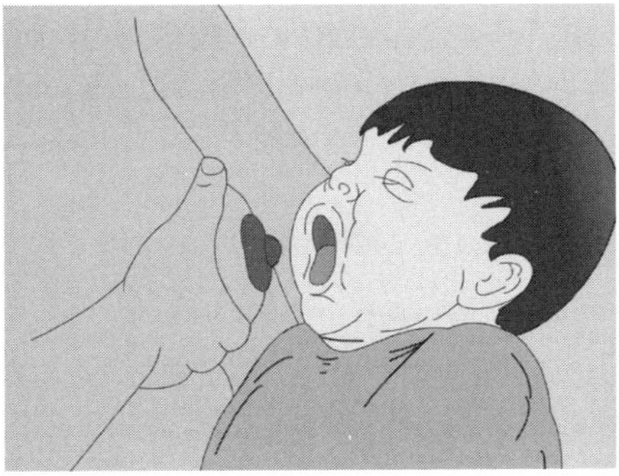

Baby opening her mouth wide

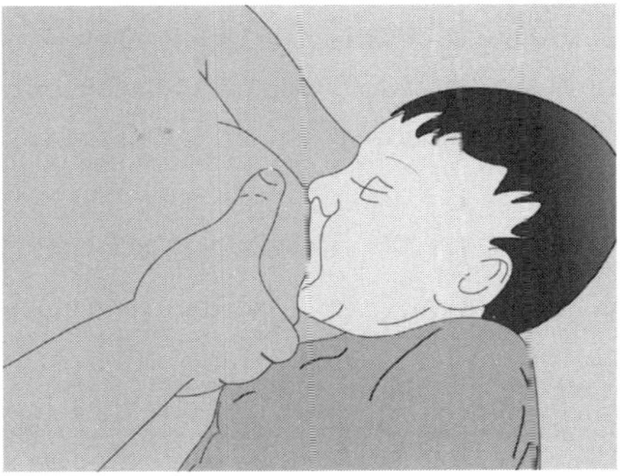

Baby correctly latched on

Tips for proper latching on

- Learn to recognize your baby's early signals for hunger. He will usually start smacking his lips and try to suck on his fingers. This is the best time to offer him the breast. Once he starts crying and screaming with hunger, he may become inconsolable and it may take longer to calm him down and have him latch on
- Cradle the baby's head on your elbow. Gently stroke the cheek facing you. This will stimulate the rooting reflex that will make the baby turn towards you. Support your breast with 4 fingers below and the thumb above. You can also spread your fingers to have your index finger above the nipple and the other three fingers below. Place your fingers far enough behind the areola (the dark area surrounding the nipple) so that the baby will have enough place to hold on to
- Now lightly rub the nipple across the baby's upper lip or nose. This will make her open her mouth wide. It might take one or two tries before your baby opens her mouth wide enough to latch on properly
- At this point, it will be tempting to stuff the breast into her mouth–don't! Pull her quickly towards your breast and she will latch on
- Make sure that her lower lip is not tucked in and that her mouth is covering both the nipple and areola. Her tongue should be well applied to the under surface of the nipple. When the baby's mouth is properly applied, the suctioning action of the mouth, tongue and lips will ease the milk out of the milk glands
- If the baby has not latched on properly, it may be painful. Release the baby's mouth and try again
- Once your little one is properly latched on, you can lightly depress the breast with your finger to prevent it from blocking the baby's nose. Elevating her head slightly may also provide a little breathing room. But as you manoeuvre her, be sure not to loosen the baby's grip on the areola

Releasing the breast from the baby's mouth

Do not pull the baby's mouth off the nipple. The suction from the baby's mouth will cause the nipple to become sore. Insert your little finger gently between the baby's gums, release the suction and then move your baby away from the breast.

Burping the baby after breastfeeding

As babies suckle on the breast, they swallow air. Babies burp to release air trapped in their stomach. Usually, breastfed babies tend to swallow less air when feeding, as compared to bottle-fed babies. However, it is a good idea to burp the baby when you switch from one breast to the other and also at the end of the breastfeeding session. Usually babies outgrow the need to be burped by 4–6 months old because they learn to suckle without swallowing too much air. Of course there are babies who will always need burping, without which they will spit-up and regurgitate milk.

Methods of burping

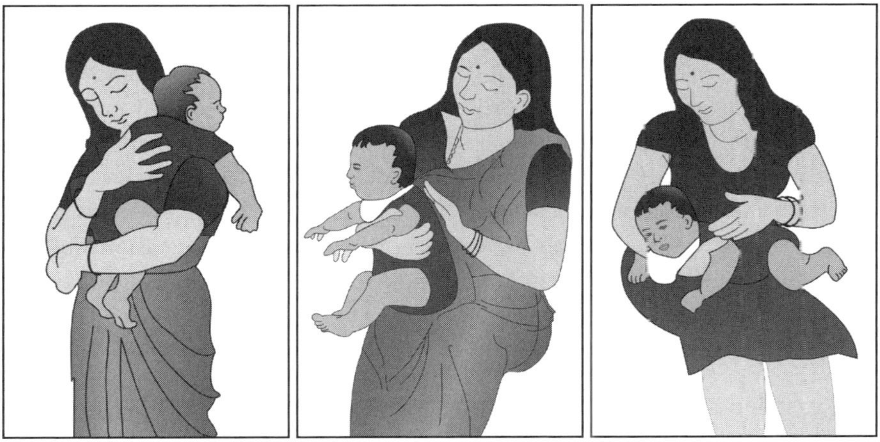

On your chest or shoulder

Hold your baby against your chest with her chin or cheek resting on your shoulder. Gently pat or rub her back. Don't forget to place a cloth over your shoulder to protect your clothes from spit-up.

Sitting on your lap

Sit your baby on your lap facing away from you. Lean him over your arm, while supporting his head. Gently pat or rub his back. Put a cloth bib on your baby and a cloth over your lap to catch any spit-up.

Face down across your lap

Lay your baby face down on your legs so he's lying across your knees. Support his head with one hand. Pat or rub his back with the other hand. Use a cloth to catch any spit-up milk.

Sometimes the baby just won't burp. If you don't get a burp after a few minutes, try a different position.

Manasa asked: As soon as he finishes feeding, my baby struggles to pass gas and also passes a little bit of motion. Is that normal?

My answer: Milk is the baby's only food and milk tends to generate gas—that is quite normal. To pass gas, the baby will grunt and strain. His face may turn quite red with the effort. He may also scream his head off if he has colic, which is again caused by the milk. When he does pass gas, he may also leak a little bit of stools with it. He may leak stools after every feed, in addition to his regular passage of stools 3–4 times a day. As long as it is only a small quantity and not large watery stools, it is not diarrhoea (learn more in **Chapter 47**, *Your new baby*).

Breastfeeding after a caesarean section

Having had a caesarean will not have an adverse effect on breastfeeding. Even the initiation of breastfeeding need not be delayed. Though there will be some discomfort because of the pain of the stitches, you will be encouraged to start breastfeeding as soon as possible. As soon as you are fully conscious and alert and able to hold the baby, you can begin breastfeeding. Mothers who have epidural or spinal rather than general anaesthesia will generally be able to hold the baby sooner and nurse her.

Pumping and storing your breast milk

There are times that you may not be able to breastfeed your baby directly. You may have delivered prematurely and the baby may be in the nursery, or you may be a working woman who has to be away from the baby for several hours during the day. To ensure that you continue to make enough milk, the breasts must be pumped at regular intervals. If you feed the baby 8 times a day, your body will make enough milk for it. If you feed only 2 times a day, the breasts will produce just enough milk for two times a day. That is why it is important to remove milk during the times your baby normally would feed.

Expressing milk with your hands can be painful and may lead to sore nipples. Use a manual or electric breast pump. Some companies rent out electric breast pumps.

Before you express breast milk, be sure to wash your hands with soap and water. The breast pump parts and bottles must be washed and kept clean. Breasts and nipples do not need to be washed before pumping.

The milk can be stored in feeding bottles in the fridge. You can warm the bottle in a water bath or microwave, before feeding the baby. Any milk that a baby does not finish must be thrown out.

Ensure that the baby is brought to you as soon as you are awake enough to be able to hold the baby. You will, of course, need assistance for the first few times. The earlier you start breastfeeding, the sooner you will master the art of holding and satisfying your baby.

Having the baby's father or another person staying with you in the hospital room can be a great help in lifting the baby, changing position, changing diapers, and so forth. You can be up and about soon after the caesarean, but for the first few days your ability to move around is restricted. Having a person in your room to assist you can help establish breastfeeding early.

Common problems during breastfeeding

Remember that the **size of the breast** does not relate to the amount of milk produced. Smaller breasts are no reason for anxiety and will produce enough milk to nourish the baby.

Retracted or inverted nipples

The nipple, instead of pointing outward, is retracted into the breast. Tell your doctor about this during the antenatal check-up. Drawing out the nipple daily during your bath, with lubricant applied to the fingers, is sufficient. If the inversion persists, the nipple can be pulled out with certain techniques that your doctor can instruct you about.

A breast pump may be used for a few minutes before a feed to help pull the nipple out. Some mothers use a nipple shield. After the baby has suckled for a few minutes, the nipple will protrude out. The shield can be removed and the baby can be put directly onto the breast.

Breast engorgement

It is common to have your breasts become heavy, hard and painful, especially soon after delivery. This is called engorgement and happens because of swelling of the breast tissue or excessive milk distending the breast.

You might get relief by feeding the baby more often. Pumping of milk may be required to soften the areola and allow better latch-on. Warm fomentation or ice packs are both effective in relieving the pain. A mild painkiller like ibuprofen and firm support with well-fitting underclothes are recommended.

Sore and cracked nipples

When you start breastfeeding for the first time, the nipples are still soft and there may be a certain amount of discomfort when the baby starts suckling.

If the baby's mouth is positioned properly, there should be no pain. If the baby does not latch on properly, the nipples can be very painful during feeds and can develop cracks. Placing a drop of milk on each nipple and allowing this to air dry after breastfeeding may help.

Nipple creams and a nipple shield can be used for temporary relief but learning the proper method of latching on is the best treatment.

Breast infection and abscess

Occasionally, bacteria from the baby's mouth can enter the breast and cause an infection. The breast can become painful and there may be a hard, red patch. In the early stages, this infection is called **mastitis**. You might develop severe tenderness of the breast and have a fever. Mastitis might resolve with antibiotics. When the infection gets worse, there may be a collection of pus in the breast called a **breast abscess**. The only treatment would be to remove the pus either by aspiration through a needle or by a surgical incision.

When you decide to stop breastfeeding

Once you have breastfed your baby for as long as you want and now want to stop, you may feel some discomfort for a few days due to engorgement. Do not try to pump out the milk because that will stimulate the breast to make more milk. You have to stop the feeds completely even if your baby isn't too happy with it. Wear a tight-fitting bra. Use ice packs for the discomfort. Paracetamol or ibuprofen will help with the pain. If the discomfort is too much, your doctor may prescribe a drug to suppress lactation (see section on Suppression of lactation, below).

If you do not want to stop breastfeeding abruptly, you can drop one feed at a time every 3–4 days till you reach a point where the breasts don't get engorged. This might take about a month. Your baby also may feel more comfortable being weaned off this way.

Breast care

To make sure that you reduce the problems encountered with breastfeeding, follow this routine:

- Clean your nipples with cotton soaked in water after every feed. Pat the breast dry and make sure the nipple is completely dry before putting the bra on again
- Wear a supportive bra. Nursing bras with a front opening flap are useful

- Change breastfeeding positions to encourage proper latching-on and lessen soreness
- If you apply a nipple cream for sore or cracked nipples, wash it off before you feed the baby
- Avoid deodorants and perfumes for a while

Extra nutritional requirements during breastfeeding

You need an additional 500–700 calories/day during breastfeeding. Make sure you get enough protein in the form of dals, milk, curds (yogurt), eggs and meat. Protein intake should be 25 g/day. Iron and calcium supplementation must be continued throughout the duration of breastfeeding. Vitamins and minerals should also be supplemented.

Does the food you eat affect the baby?

New mothers are often worried that the food they eat may affect the baby by passing through the milk. You need not worry. Make sure you eat a balanced diet. What you eat will not affect the baby but a healthy diet can improve the quality of milk.

Do the medications you are given affect the baby?

Many mothers are worried that the medications prescribed for them after delivery will adversely affect their babies. The medications used for pain relief are usually not a problem, and are routinely given to the mothers of newborns. If an antibiotic has been given at the time of the caesarean section, it too will not affect the baby. Although these medications do pass into the milk in very small amounts, the volume of colostrum or milk produced during the first few days of nursing is small, so the amount ingested by the baby is minimal.

If you are placed on any medication for an illness, do let your doctor know that you are breastfeeding.

Giving milk substitutes

Breastfeeding is no doubt the best option for babies. Unfortunately, in certain circumstances, the mother may not be able to feed the baby.

Neither cow's milk nor buffalo's milk are easily digested by babies so are not recommended. Commercially available milk formulas are manufactured under sterile conditions. They try to reproduce mother's milk using a complex combination of proteins, sugars, fats, and vitamins. The disadvantage of milk substitutes is that they do not contain the antibodies and immunity boosting properties of breast milk. They are also very expensive.

Sterilizing bottles and rubber nipples

Bottles and nipples need to be sterilized before the first use and then washed and sterilized again before every use. Bottles and nipples can transmit bacteria if they are not cleaned and sterilized properly.

Any milk that a baby does not finish must be thrown out. Bottles left out of the refrigerator longer than 1 hour should not be used.

Present day milk powders do not require very hot water for mixing. After pouring warm water into the bottle, add the milk powder and then shake the bottle. Do not mix the formula in a separate tumbler and then pour it into the bottle. This can lead to infection.

Suppression of lactation

Suppression of lactation may be required in certain situations:

- When you have fed your baby for as long as you want and now have decided to stop breastfeeding
- In the unfortunate event of a stillbirth
- If the mother has an infection that may be transmitted to the baby if breastfed, for example HIV, or active tuberculosis in the lungs

There are no scientific studies that have shown that jasmine flowers or cabbage leaves wrapped around the breast can cause the milk to dry up. It is an old wives' tale.

Cabergoline is the drug of choice as it is well tolerated. It can be given as a single dose of 1 mg or two doses of 0.5 mg.

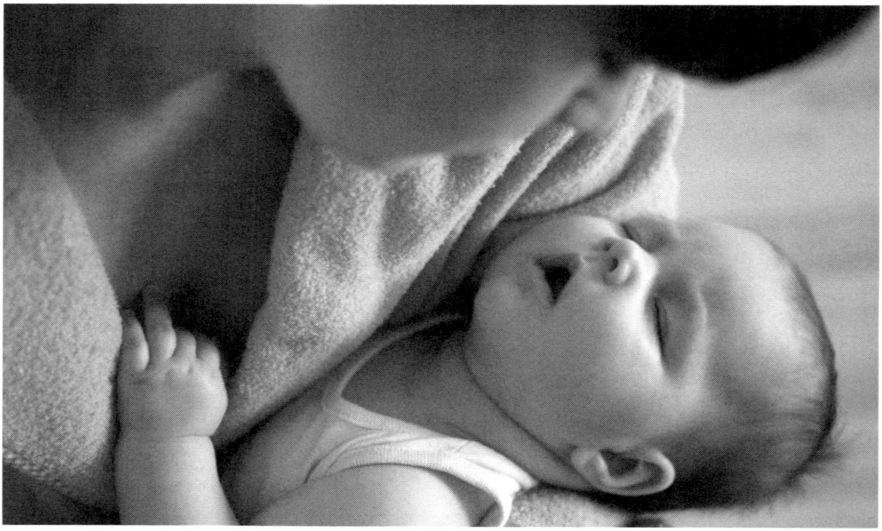

Old wives' tales

- Don't eat dal, channa, rajma, or potatoes because it will give the baby gas. **Not true!** These substances don't even enter breast milk and so have no effect on the baby.
- Avoid mangoes—it will cause the baby to have jaundice. **Not true!**
- Don't drink too much water because it will dilute the milk. **Not true!** You need to drink plenty of fluids to keep yourself hydrated and to help in milk production.
- If your hair is wet when you feed the baby he will catch a cold. **Not true!**
- You should not eat while you feed the baby as it will cause indigestion in the baby. **Not true!**
- If your baby doesn't feed from both breasts for a long duration she needs supplements. **Not true!**
- If your breasts aren't engorged and spurting milk you aren't producing enough milk. **Not true!** As long as your baby is passing urine and motion enough number of times and is showing a steady increase in weight, you have enough milk.
- Don't drink coffee or tea when you feed the baby as it dries up your supply. **Not true!**
- It is important to give your baby water because she will be thirsty otherwise. **Not true!** All the water the baby requires is obtained from her milk intake.
- Keep alternating breasts every 10 minutes. **Not true!** Feed on a breast till the baby stops sucking and your breast feels soft. The baby needs to suck for at least 15–20 minutes on each breast to get the fat-filled hind milk.

CHAPTER 28

Your diet after delivery

Shonal has just had a baby. Her family is after her to eat much more than she usually does. They tell her it is important because she is breastfeeding. Is this necessary? She is concerned about putting on weight. She also wants to regain her pre-pregnancy figure.

If Shonal eats a balanced, healthy diet and follows a strict exercise regimen, she can be fit, continue to breastfeed and nourish her baby, and not put on unwanted weight.

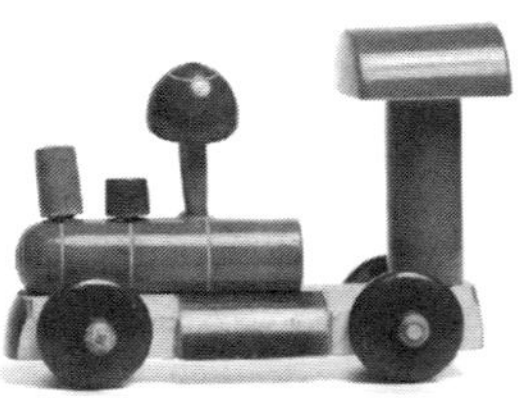

28

Your diet after delivery

So you have had your baby! Suddenly, all the necessary and unnecessary advice you got throughout your pregnancy from friends and relatives seems to have doubled. When you reach out for that piece of mango, your mother-in-law is horrified. 'You can't eat that', she says, pulling the fruit away. 'You have just delivered!' Your mother wants you to have a tablespoon of ghee with each meal. An aunt who has come to see the baby checks with your mother if you are getting a special mix of dried fruits and nuts.

Who should you listen to? Having just delivered, do you really need to have a special diet? Can you eat normal food or does everything have to be specially prepared for you? If you have had a caesarean section, will certain kinds of food affect the wound?

> Culturally, Indians tend to have many restrictions on diet for a woman after delivery. These may not always have a basis in science. Common sense and an emphasis on a balanced diet should dictate what you eat after a delivery.

A balanced diet along with plenty of fruits and vegetables is essential.

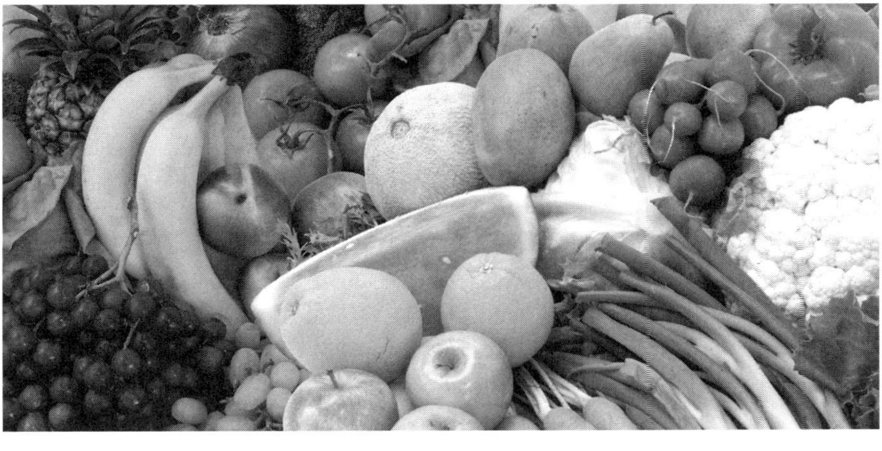

After the delivery, you will find that you have lost more than half of the weight that you had put on during pregnancy. Some of the weight that disappeared instantly after delivery includes:

- The baby (2.5–3.5 kg)
- The placenta and amniotic fluid (1 kg), and
- Retained water (2 kg)

You still have another 4.5–5.5 kg to lose, if you had put on the appropriate amount of weight in pregnancy (about 10 kg). That excess weight that you are still carrying is due to an increase in the fat stores in your body. These few kilos are what you still need to lose to regain your pre-pregnancy weight.

It is important to eat a balanced diet adequate for the increased caloric requirements for breastfeeding and at the same time, lose the excess fat that you have accumulated during pregnancy.

How much weight should you have gained in pregnancy?

The amount of weight you should gain in pregnancy depends on your pre-pregnancy body mass index (BMI). BMI is calculated as your weight in kilos divided by your height in metres^2.

> Obesity in women starts very often in pregnancy. If you don't lose all the excess weight after the delivery, you will put on even more in a subsequent pregnancy. This additional weight tends to accumulate each year.

If you have gained the ideal amount of weight in pregnancy, then you will find it easier to reach your pre-pregnancy weight. If you have gained more than you should have, then you will have to work harder to shed that weight.

BMI before pregnancy	Ideal weight gain in pregnancy
Less than 18 (underweight)	12–14 kilos
18–25 (normal weight)	10–12 kilos
25.1–29.9 (overweight)	8–10 kilos
30 or more (obese)	6–8 kilos

A balanced diet after delivery

You do not have to eat large quantities because you are breastfeeding. It is important to eat a balanced diet. There are no foods that will affect the baby. There are no foods that you should not eat after the delivery. There are many old wives' tales that restrict what a woman can eat after the birth of a baby but these have no scientific basis.

When you are breastfeeding, you should consume adequate dairy products (two glasses of milk and two cups of curds), proteins in the form of grains, nuts, pulses, eggs, meat, fish or poutry, a limited amount of carbohydrates to provide you energy, and plenty of fruits and vegetables.

Vitamin and mineral supplements

It is important to be on a combination supplement of iron, B-complex and folic acid for a few months after a delivery. A calcium supplement is essential throughout the time that you are breastfeeding.

Deena said: I'm always hungry after I breastfeed but I really want to lose the pregnancy fat. How can I diet?

My answer: Eating healthy does not mean you have to starve. Your body is burning up calories because you are breastfeeding. If you now balance this out with good, healthy food you not only will help with the nursing, you will lose weight too. You can also eat small, frequent meals so that your energy levels stay up.

The problem arises when you eat a diet high in carbohydrates. Cut the rice and chapatis to a minimum. You can fill up with greens cooked with dal, dishes made with whole lentils (like rajma and channa) lots of vegetable side dishes and salads. If you eat eggs, they are an excellent source of proteins. You can eat meat dishes as long as you don't eat large quantities of carbs along with them. Keep saturated fats to a minimum.

Old wives' tales

- Eat plenty of ghee. It will help the uterus heal. **Not true!** You will only put on unnecessary weight. Ghee is a saturated fat and should be taken in moderation.
- Avoid spicy food and hot or cold drinks because it will harm the baby. **Not true!**
- Eat lots of garlic: it will increase milk flow. **Not true!** Garlic by itself does not increase the flow of milk. It changes the smell of milk and that may tend to make the baby suckle more.
- Ajwain water helps digestion. **Not true!** There is no scientific evidence to support this.
- Avoid certain kinds of lentils (channa, rajma), root vegetables and certain fruits because it will cause the baby to be colicky. **Not true!** There is no food that you should particularly avoid. If you find that the baby gets colicky every time you eat a specific food, then you can avoid it.

CHAPTER 29

Getting fit after delivery

Samhita has always been careful about what she eats though she has never been a fitness freak. Her best friend had a baby two years ago and got back into shape within a year. Samhita is inspired and has promised herself that she will not let herself go after the delivery and will work hard to regain her pre-pregnancy figure.

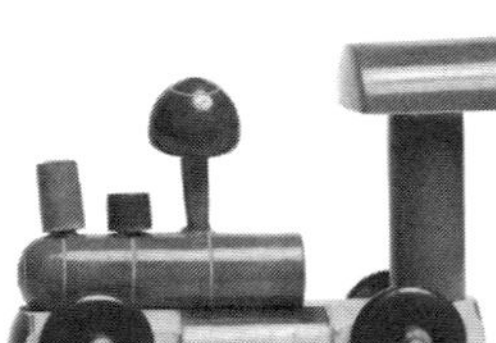

29

Getting fit after delivery

It has been a roller coaster ride through the pregnancy. You have come home with your little bundle of joy. After a few weeks, you have settled into somewhat of a routine and now your thoughts are turning to that wobbly post-pregnancy tummy. Will you get your figure back? Will you be able to lose weight? The two things that you have to contend with after a delivery are:

- Extra fat deposits (especially over the abdomen)
- Poor abdominal tone

This is why postnatal exercises are as important as antenatal exercises. To begin with, you can start slowly but within a month after a vaginal delivery, you should be able to push up your activity level comfortably.

Abdominal fat vs poor abdominal tone

It is normal for women to put on weight around the waist during pregnancy. However, the more difficult thing to handle is the loss of tone of the abdominal muscles. After the delivery, for a few weeks, you may find that your abdominal wall is flabby and tends to balloon out below the waist.

> It is absolutely important to start working on the abdominal muscle tone as soon as possible after delivery. Once the muscle tone is lost for a prolonged period of time, it is difficult to get it back.

The main muscle that lines the front of the abdomen is called the rectus abdominis. This is the muscle that body builders turn into a 'six-pack' with exercise. As the uterus grows, the rectus abdominis is stretched. The tone of this muscle can be damaged in various situations:

- Repeated stretching (in women who have had more than one child)
- Overstretching (in women who have had twins or a large baby)
- Women who have had poor intake of protein all their lives and have a thinner rectus abdominis to begin with (the damage to the abdominal wall can happen even with one pregnancy)

Lack of tone in the abdominal muscles not only changes your shape, it also leads to low back pain and bad posture because abdominal muscles play a big role in keeping your spine upright.

Remember that losing abdominal fat is possible with a sensible diet and exercise but regaining abdominal tone is only possible with abdominal exercises specifically aimed at restoring muscle tone. Getting back your abdominal tone will stand you in good stead all your life.

When should I start postnatal exercise after delivery?

Vaginal delivery

Remember that after a vaginal delivery, there is no reason that you cannot start walking around the house in a day or two. After a month, you can start a good fitness regimen.

Walking is a great form of exercise and should be resumed when you are comfortable and pain free. It is also a great way to get out of the house for a little 'me' time.

Caesarean section

If you have had a caesarean section, it would be normally recommended that you start light exercises a month after the surgery. Six weeks after the surgery, you should be able to start postnatal exercises, after having obtained a clearance from your obstetrician.

In the beginning, you can restrict the duration of exercise to 15 minutes but can gradually work your way up to 45–60 minutes a day.

Tips for healthy exercising

- Exercise twice a day
- Repeat each set of movements about ten times in every session, gradually increasing the number of repetitions
- Remember to keep your breathing slow and smooth
- Work up your stamina gradually
- Try and take a few classes with a physical trainer or watch a video and learn the exercises
- Keep yourself well hydrated

Why bother with postnatal exercises?

Postnatal exercises have many benefits. They help in:

- Strengthening the pelvic floor muscles which prevent leaking of urine

- Preventing lower back pain
- Restoring your body to a healthy shape - that flabby abdominal wall has to be worked on!
- Boosting energy levels

Abdominal diastasis or abdominal wall separation

After delivery, some women may find that when they raise their heads to get up, the abdomen bulges in the midline, starting from the top of the abdomen all the way to the pubic bone. If you put your fingers in that bulge, you may find that there is a gap between the rectus muscles of both sides. **Diastasis** or **abdominal wall separation** will have a gap of 2 cm or greater between the two sides of the rectus abdominis muscle. Sometimes the separation can be very prominent.

This condition will not cause any physical problem. If it is quite pronounced, your tummy will bulge out. Some women are extremely bothered by it. Routine abdominal crunches will actually worsen the condition. *Special exercises for diastasis are given later in the chapter.*

If the abdominal muscle separation is very prominent and is causing you to feel self-conscious, you doctor may suggest an *abdominoplasty* If the muscles of your abdomen are also very lax, the surgery may not be useful.

A sampler of exercises

Pelvic floor (Kegel's) exercises

Kegel's exercises are specifically focussed on the pelvic floor muscles that support the uterus, bladder and bowel. They are useful both for prevention and treatment. By keeping the pelvic floor muscles toned, the risk of urinary leakage with ageing can be reduced.

Kegel's exercises are recommended both during pregnancy and after delivery. Well-toned pelvic floor muscles make it less likely to develop prolapse of the uterus.

> **Achala asked:** I had my baby six weeks ago. I find that sometimes I'm not able to control my urine when I have to go to the bathroom. Is that going to be a problem?
>
> **My answer:** Loss of bladder tone happens commonly during pregnancy and may persist for a while after delivery. Most of the bladder tone will come back spontaneously. You should also help it along by doing Kegel's exercises.

To learn how to identify and contract the pelvic floor muscles, the best method is to try and stop the flow of urine as you are urinating. You may not succeed initially, but with practice, the basic move can be mastered. Stopping and starting the urine stream should only be used initially to learn the technique, and should not be done all the time—it may lead to bladder dysfunction. Another technique to initially identify the muscles is to insert two fingers inside the vagina and to attempt to squeeze the surrounding muscles. The vagina can be felt to tighten around the fingers and the pelvic floor will be felt to move upward. When the muscles are relaxed, the pelvic floor can be felt moving down to the starting position.

Once the pelvic floor muscles have been identified, the exercise can be done in a sitting or standing position. The exercises can be done while watching television, working on the computer or whenever there is some free time. The exercises should be done three times a day.

- Empty your bladder
- Contract the pelvic muscles for 10 seconds and then relax for 10 seconds
- Repeat this sequence a total of 20–30 times at each session.
- Care should be taken not to contract the muscles in the abdomen, thighs or buttocks
- Breathe freely while doing the pelvic floor exercises

Back and abdominal exercises

Hold each position for 10–20 seconds. Repeat each set at least 10 times. Use an exercise mat for greater comfort.

Exercise 1

Lie on your back and bend your knees with your feet slightly apart. Breathe out and tighten your abdomen, pulling your abdominal wall towards the spine. Press your pelvis downwards to flatten your low back against the floor.

> During these exercises, always pull your abdominal muscles towards your spine. Do not let your abdomen bulge out. Doing that not only will it not restore muscle tone, it can worsen abdominal diastasis (see alongside).

Exercise 2

Lie on your back. Bend your knees and keep them together. Tighten your abdomen, pulling your abdominal wall towards the spine, and flatten your low back against the floor. Bring both knees to the right side so as to let your right knee touch the floor as far as possible. Return to the starting position and rest. Repeat on the left side. Repeat for 10- 15 sets.

Exercise 3
Pelvic bridge
This is a great exercise after delivery since it works both on your abdominal and pelvic muscles.

Bend your knees and place your feet flat on the floor with your feet six to eight inches apart. Your palms should be flat on the floor alongside your body. Relax your upper body and back while drawing in your abdominals and squeezing your pelvic floor muscles. Press your hands and forearms into the floor and slowly push your pelvis up towards the ceiling. Hold the position for a slow count of three (you can increase it to a count of ten as you get more comfortable with this). Slowly lower your body back to the start position. Perform two to three sets of 12–15 repetitions, allowing 30–60 seconds rest between sets.

Exercise 4
Cat stretch
This is a great exercise to stretch and strengthen the muscles in your lower back. It helps in relieving low back pain that is common after childbirth. It also helps in preventing low back pain later in life.

Kneel on all fours, keeping both hands and the knees on the floor. Start by taking a deep breath. As you exhale, tighten your abdominal muscles towards your spine, and round your back, letting your head drop. Your back should be curved toward the ceiling. Hold this pose for a count of 10 before relaxing back into the original position.

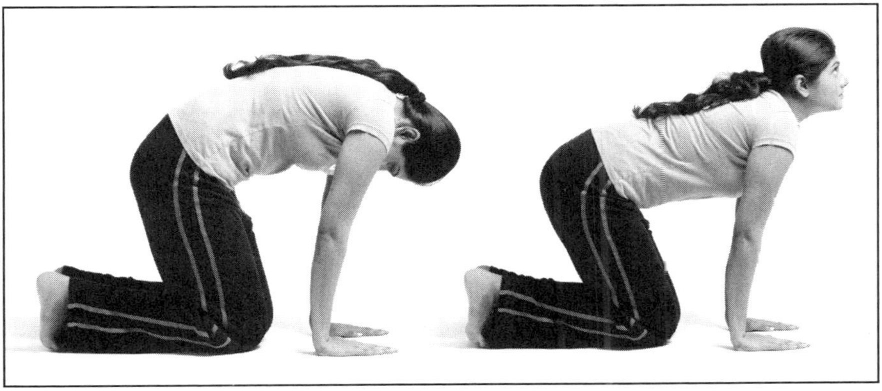

Cat stretch position 1 *Cat stretch position 2*

Exercise 5

Head and shoulder lift

Lie on your back and bend your knees, keeping your feet together and flat on the floor. Tighten your abdomen, and press your pelvis downwards to flatten your low back against the floor. Slowly lift the head, chin toward your chest, and contract you abdominal muscles toward the floor. Stretch both hands towards your knees, hold for 3–5 seconds, and lie down slowly. Complete 10 repetitions.

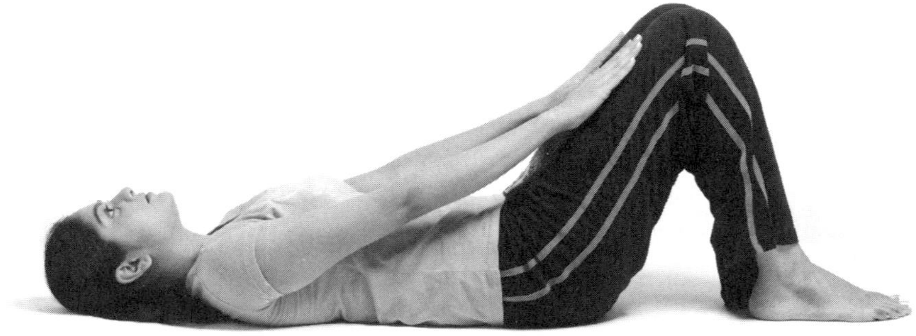

Head and shoulder lift position 1

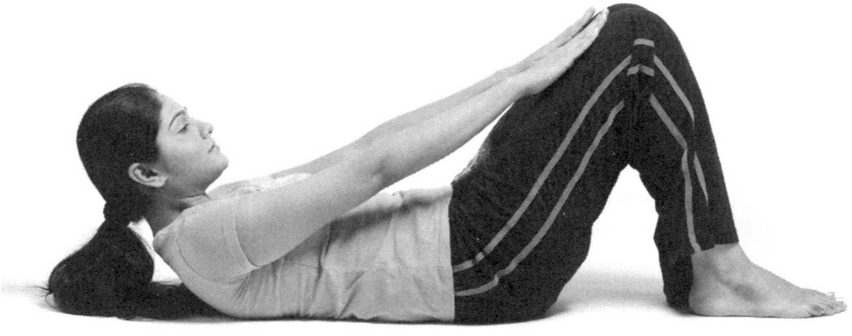

Head and shoulder lift position 2

Exercise 6

Abdominal crunch

Lie down with hands crossed over the chest or behind the head, feet on the floor, knees bent. Contract the abdominal muscles towards the spine and lift your head and shoulders off the floor, bringing the rib cage towards the lower belly. Lower slowly back to start and repeat 10 times.

Exercise 7

Oblique crossover crunches

Lie on your back and cross the right foot over the left knee. Place your left hand under your head. Lift the shoulder blades off the floor and twist to the right, bringing the left shoulder and elbow towards the right knee. Lower back down and repeat for 10–15 reps before switching sides.

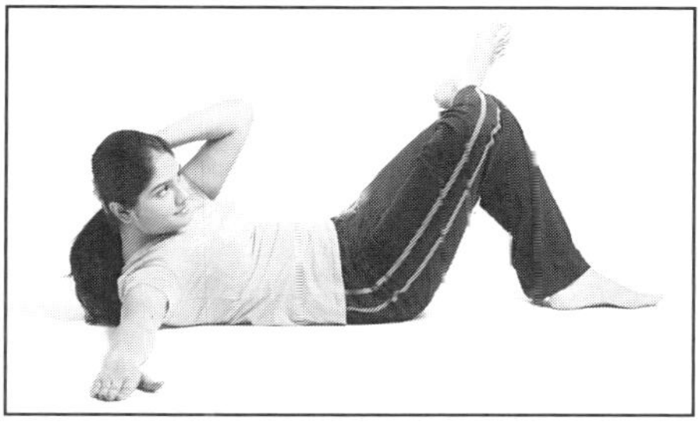

Oblique crossover crunch

These are just a few suggestions for exercising your abdominal muscles. You need to have determination and discipline to regain your pre-pregnancy shape. Exercise will help you keep fit and boost your energy levels.

Exercises for abdominal diastasis (abdominal wall separation)

The following exercises are recommended to help build abdominal strength, though they may not always reduce the size of the diastasis.

- **Core contraction:** In a seated position, place both hands on your abdominal muscles. Slowly contract the abdominal muscles, pulling them straight back towards the spine. Hold the contraction for 30 seconds, while maintaining the controlled breathing. Complete 10 repetitions.
- **Upright push-up:** With feet together arms-length away from wall, place hands flat against the wall, contract abdominal muscles toward spine, lean body towards wall, with elbows bent downward close to body, pull abdominal muscles in further, with controlled breathing. Release muscles as you push back to starting position. Complete 20 repetitions.
- **Squat against the wall:** Also known as a seated squat, stand with back against the wall, feet out in front of body, slowly lower body to a seated position so knees are bent at a 90° angle, contracting abs toward spine as you raise body back to standing position. Complete 20 repetitions.

Towards a flat abdomen

The disadvantage of Indian clothes is that they hide many body flaws! Do not hide behind loose clothes after the delivery. Always be aware of your abdominal muscles. Make it a point to keep pulling in your tummy muscles. Walk with a good posture, with your shoulders pulled back and your tummy tucked in. Encourage the return of a flatter abdomen by pulling in your deep abdominal muscles whenever you think about them, when walking, when cooking, when driving, when working and even when feeding your baby.

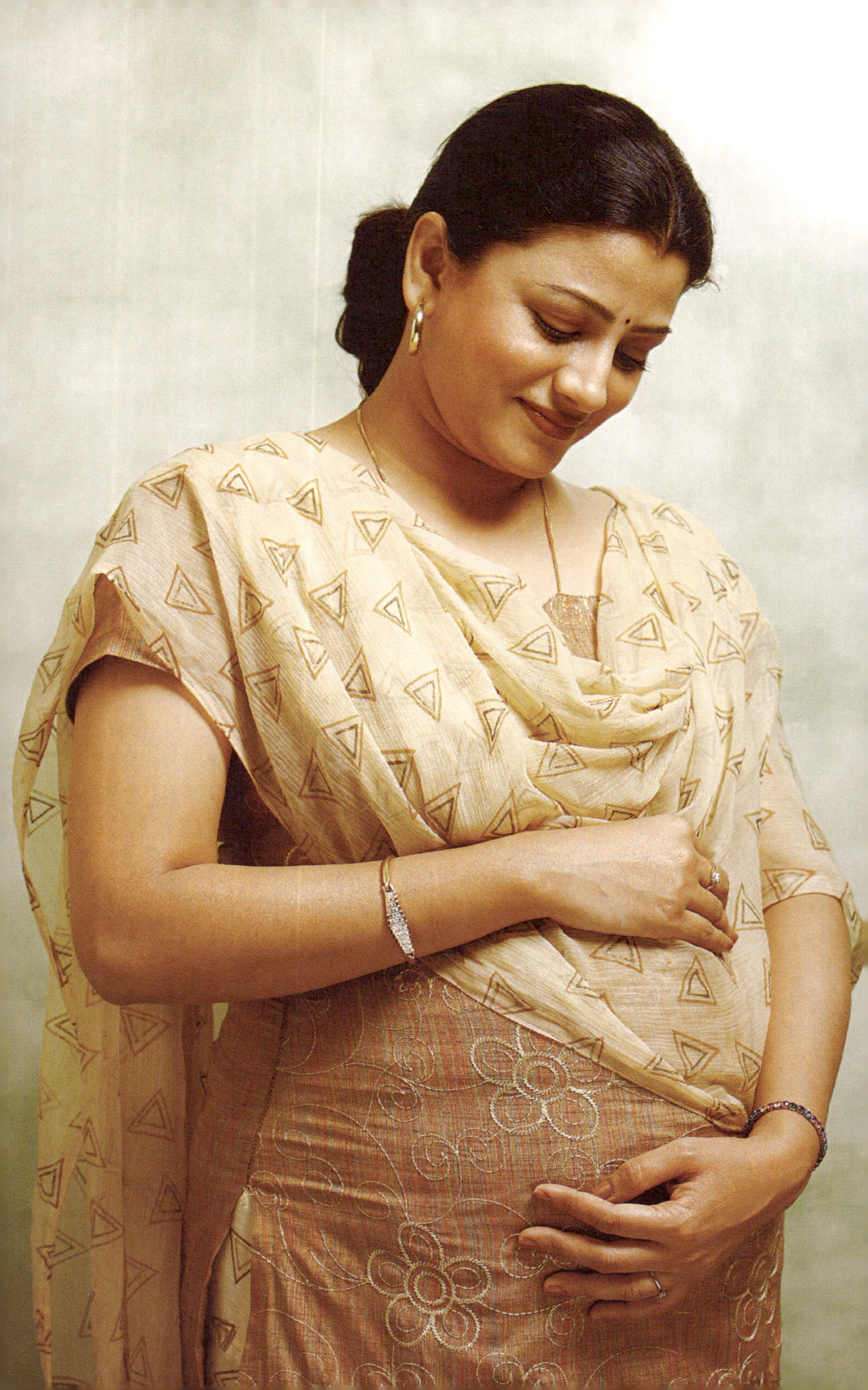

When things go wrong

CHAPTER 30

Miscarriage

Shantha is fighting back tears. She is holding on tightly to her husband's hand. He too, is looking stunned. At their routine third month check-up, their obstetrician has told them that the baby inside the uterus has not grown beyond two months. Shantha has had a missed miscarriage.

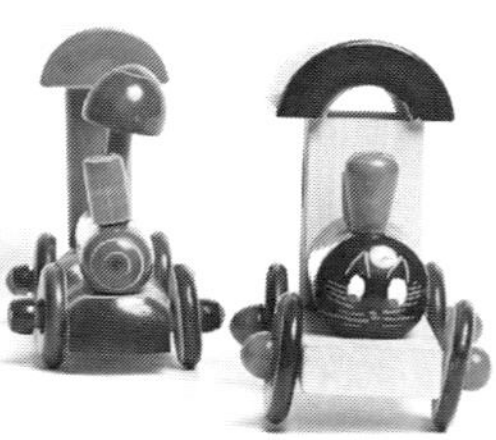

30

Miscarriage

Being told that you are undergoing a miscarriage is distressing. Even more disturbing is the lingering feeling that you may have in some way caused it. To compound this needless guilt, misinformed relatives and friends give you a list of things you may have done that places the blame of the miscarriage squarely on your shoulders.

It is important to realize that miscarriage is a natural process and cannot be caused by something you did or didn't do. About 15–20 per cent of women who conceive will lose their pregnancy in a miscarriage. There is no reason why you will not be able to have a baby the next time you try.

What is a miscarriage?

A miscarriage is the spontaneous ending of a pregnancy before the fifth month (20th week) of pregnancy. The medical term for miscarriage is spontaneous abortion.

Most miscarriages occur during the first 16 weeks of pregnancy. Many occur within the first 10 weeks. Some women miscarry even before they know they are pregnant.

Why does a miscarriage happen?

It is often difficult to pinpoint the exact cause of a miscarriage. However, most miscarriages are caused by problems that occur during fertilization, when the sperm and the egg fuse to form an embryo. The commonest cause of a miscarriage is an abnormal number of chromosomes—either too many or too few. Often, the foetus does not develop at all, or it may develop abnormally. **Miscarriage is the body's way of ending a pregnancy that is not developing normally.**

Chromosomal abnormality is the commonest cause of a miscarriage. The foetus may have an abnormal number of chromosomes—either too many or too few. Though this can happen at any age, women older than 35 have an increased risk of having a miscarriage because of this reason.

What are the symptoms of a miscarriage?

Possible symptoms include:

- Bleeding, which can range from a few drops of blood to a heavy flow. The bleeding may start with no warning or there may be a brownish discharge first
- Cramping pain in the lower abdomen
- A gush of fluid from the vagina without bleeding or pain. This may mean that the membranes have ruptured
- A clot-like whitish tissue may pass out of the vagina. Try to keep this material so the doctor can examine it

Sometimes, it happens that there is minimal or no bleeding and pain, but the foetus has died and symptoms of early pregnancy have disappeared. The diagnosis is made only when an ultrasound examination is done. This condition is called a **missed miscarriage** or **missed abortion**.

Jharna asked: I am pregnant for the second time. In my first pregnancy I miscarried in the third month. I had fallen once in the bathroom before the miscarriage. My mother-in-law told me I was careless and the fall caused the miscarriage. How do I prevent a miscarriage this time?

My answer: Please tell your mother-in-law to back off and not blame you for the miscarriage. A fall cannot cause a miscarriage. The baby is well protected within the uterus. It was just a coincidence that you fell a few days before the miscarriage. It is a human tendency to connect the dots and create a cause and effect phenomenon!

Travelling to work or working long hours also will not cause a miscarriage. Please do not give up your job (and your independence!). Sitting at home will only make you put on unnecessary weight (because of lack of activity and overeating) and bore you to tears.

Travelling by two-wheeler, auto, bus or car does not cause a miscarriage. Many husbands are worried that the potholes on the roads will cause a miscarriage. This is just a misconception.

In addition, there is no evidence that emotional stress, physical overactivity or sexual activity causes miscarriage in a normal pregnancy.

Another common myth is that eating papayas, mangoes or pineapples will cause a miscarriage. Absolutely untrue! Your grandmother may also forbid you to have sesame seeds but again, this is only a myth that it can cause a miscarriage.

Can a miscarriage be predicted?

When you see your doctor because of spotting or bleeding in early pregnancy, two tests that help in predicting a miscarriage are:

- Blood levels of the pregnancy hormone (hCG)
- Ultrasound imaging

Blood levels of hCG

If you have bleeding in the first trimester and your doctor suspects that you may have a miscarriage, she might order a blood level of hCG. In a normally growing pregnancy, the level of hCG will go up rapidly in the first three months. A miscarriage can be predicted if

- The hCG level is much lower than it should be for that period of pregnancy
- If the hCG level does not double in 48 hours

Ultrasound scan

Even if the baby's heartbeat is seen, the following ultrasound findings may predict a poor outcome:

- A gestational sac that is *abnormally small*
- The baby is *lying very low* in the uterus, almost ready to be expelled
- A *slow heartbeat*, less than 100 beats per minute at 6–8 weeks of pregnancy, predicts an increased chance of miscarriage. Your doctor will ask you to come back after a week to recheck the heartbeat
- *A blood clot (subchorionic haematoma)* between the baby and the uterine wall may occur spontaneously. Though a small blood clot is not associated with an increased chance of miscarriage, large blood clots can be. Blood clots will get absorbed by themselves though you may have bleeding on and off for a few days or weeks

How is a miscarriage diagnosed?

Most often, on a routine check-up your doctor may do a pelvic exam to check the size of the uterus and find that the size of the uterus does not correspond to the duration of pregnancy. Miscarriage may also be suspected if you have had bleeding accompanied by lower abdominal cramping.

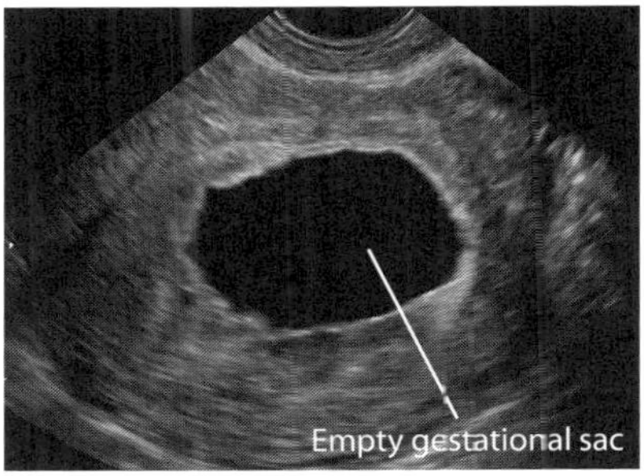

Missed miscarriage ('blighted ovum')

A missed miscarriage (see below) is diagnosed when the gestational sac is *empty*. This is also called a *blighted ovum*. If the foetus is seen, absence of the heartbeat confirms a missed miscarriage.

An ultrasound scan is also useful in confirming if the uterine cavity is completely empty after a miscarriage.

What are the types of miscarriage?

Threatened miscarriage

An ongoing (live) pregnancy associated with some bleeding is called a *threatened miscarriage*. The first symptoms are usually vaginal bleeding with or without mild period type pain. The amount of bleeding may vary, from just spotting, to a gush with clots.

Approximately 25 per cent of all pregnant women have some degree of vaginal bleeding during the first two trimesters. In a threatened miscarriage, the baby's heartbeat can be seen on ultrasound and there is a good chance that the pregnancy will continue to term.

Your obstetrician may advise rest in bed for 2–3 days. The bed rest may stop the bleeding and the pregnancy may continue normally. Special precautions such as stopping exercise, staying off your feet as much as possible and avoiding sex may be necessary for one or two weeks.

Hormonal therapy with progestogens has been used over the years to treat threatened miscarriage. However, medical research has failed to produce strong evidence to support the need for hormonal tablets or injections in case of a threatened miscarriage.

Inevitable miscarriage

Miscarriage becomes inevitable if the bleeding and cramping increase, and the cervix (mouth of the uterus) begins to open. An inevitable miscarriage means that nothing can be done to prevent the miscarriage.

Incomplete miscarriage

The miscarriage is incomplete if only a part of the contents of the uterus is expelled. There can be excessive bleeding because the uterus tries to flush out the remaining tissue. A dilatation and curettage (D&C) or suction procedure may be required to remove the remains of the foetus and placenta from the uterus. If the bleeding is not heavy, a medical evacuation may be done. For this, tablets of misoprostol may be inserted in the vagina or given orally to complete the miscarriage.

Complete miscarriage

When the uterus expels its contents entirely, it is called a complete miscarriage. The pain and bleeding will stop after you have passed a large clot-like whitish tissue out of the vagina.

Missed miscarriage

In a missed miscarriage the foetus has died but the body does not recognize the pregnancy loss. There is no bleeding or expulsion of the pregnancy tissue. Though many women may have a disappearance of pregnancy symptoms like nausea and vomiting, in some women the placenta may still continue to release hormones, so you may continue to experience signs of pregnancy.

If a missed miscarriage is diagnosed in early pregnancy (less than 6 weeks), misoprostol tablets are placed in the vagina or given orally to encourage expulsion of the tissue (medical evacuation). A D&C (surgical evacuation) may be required if the medical evacuation does not work. A D&C may also be done if you are more than 6 weeks pregnant, or have had a caesarean in a previous pregnancy, in which case misoprostol cannot be used.

Are you Rh negative?

In any pregnancy it is important to know your blood group and Rh type.
In the case of a miscarriage, if you are Rh negative your doctor will advise you on the need for an injection after the miscarriage to prevent future problems (see **Chapter 39**, *The Rh factor and your pregnancy*).

When can you try for another pregnancy?

Give yourself time to heal both physically and emotionally before you try for another pregnancy. Apart from the physical reasons to avoid a pregnancy, it is also important to wait until you have dealt emotionally with the loss. Your obstetrician may advise you to avoid sexual intercourse for 2–4 weeks after a miscarriage. Depending on your age, you can wait three to six months before trying for another pregnancy. Use some form of birth control till then. Your obstetrician will advise what is best for you.

Some women do have repeated miscarriages. A series of three or more consecutive miscarriages is called recurrent pregnancy loss (see section on Recurrent pregnancy loss below). These miscarriages may be caused by conditions that can be treated. If you have had two or more miscarriages, it is important to be tested to determine and treat the cause.

Pallavi asked: I had a miscarriage a year ago. We want to try for another pregnancy now. Should we have any tests before we go ahead? My doctor suggested a TORCH test.

My answer: If you have just had one miscarriage, no tests are needed before you try for another pregnancy. If you have had two or more miscarriages, you and your husband may need to be tested before attempting another pregnancy.

The TORCH panel is a blood test that checks for toxoplasmosis, Rubella, cytomegalovirus and herpes infection in the mother. Since these infections do not cause repeated miscarriage, **this test is absolutely unnecessary** and has long been abandoned in relation to miscarriage.

Do not blame yourself for the miscarriage

Most miscarriages are spontaneous and not precipitated by anything you did. Grief, anger and feelings of guilt are common and completely normal reactions to a miscarriage. Allow yourself to grieve over the loss of the baby. Seek support from relatives and friends. You may find it helpful to talk to others who have had miscarriages. You may be afraid that your miscarriage means that you won't ever be able to have a baby. Remember that for most women, the next pregnancy is normal.

Dos and don'ts after a miscarriage

Your recovery will take 4–6 weeks. You may have some spotting and discomfort for a few days.

- Restrict your activity for 2 weeks. This **does not** mean bed rest. You can carry on light housework
- Avoid intercourse for 2 weeks. Discuss birth control with your doctor before you resume intercourse
- Your doctor will see you for a review after 4–6 weeks
- Continue your iron supplements for 1–3 months, depending on your doctor's advice
- Low-impact exercises, such as walking or swimming, will not hurt you. You can start 2 weeks after the miscarriage. Gradually exercise more as you feel better

When should you call your doctor after a miscarriage?

If you are recovering from a miscarriage, call your obstetrician immediately if you have any of these symptoms:

- Heavy bleeding
- Severe abdominal pain
- Foul-smelling discharge from the vagina
- Fever with chills

These may indicate that you either have a piece of tissue left behind in the uterus or that you have developed an infection.

When you get pregnant again

It is natural to be anxious when you get pregnant again. However, since most miscarriages happen due to an abnormal number of chromosomes in that particular pregnancy, the chances of miscarrying again are very low. **After one miscarriage, your chance of carrying the next pregnancy to term is 80 per cent, the same as women who have never had a miscarriage.** If you have had two miscarriages one after the other, even then your chance of having a normal pregnancy is as high as 70 per cent.

Mahadevi asked: I had a miscarriage with my last pregnancy. Many of my friends say that it happened because I was too active. My mother and husband want me to quit my job because I have to travel 1 hour to work each way. They tell me that when I get pregnant again, I should stay at complete bed rest for the first three months. Is this true? Was it my fault that I miscarried?

My answer: Absolutely not. Miscarriage happens for many reasons and the most important one is that Nature does not allow an abnormal foetus to grow. A woman's activity does not precipitate a miscarriage. If the pregnancy is normal, nothing can dislodge it. **If the pregnancy is abnormal, even lying in bed without moving will not prevent a miscarriage.**

Just because you had a miscarriage the first time does not mean that you have to change your lifestyle. You can be as active as you normally would be.

Complete bed rest has its own problems. Complete bed rest is quite a punishment for young women who are used to being active. Not using muscles can cause joint pain and muscle aches. Prolonged bed rest can actually weaken leg muscles and can cause them to waste away. Bed rest can also increase the risk of dangerous blood clots in the veins of the legs.

Boredom and anxiety can cause mood swings. If you already have another child, he might feel frightened or confused, seeing you confined to bed. For a family that normally depends on two incomes, loss of your job can cause financial stress. Bed rest without decreasing dietary intake can lead to the piling on of unwanted kilos, which in itself can lead to complications.
In plain words, bed rest has nothing to recommend it!

RECURRENT PREGNANCY LOSS

When there have been 3 or more miscarriages, it is called recurrent pregnancy loss. Many experts suggest that investigations should be started if a woman has lost two pregnancies one after the other. Two to five per cent of couples attempting pregnancy will face this problem (which means that 95–98 per cent of you will be fine!).

The loss of a pregnancy, no matter how early or late, can cause feelings of intense grief and despair. Many women feel they are somehow defective and unable to have a baby. You may feel discouraged. You and your husband may be troubled and even overwhelmed by these feelings. Remember it is not your fault. Most women can expect to have a normal pregnancy even after having had more than one miscarriage.

Many factors can lead to recurrent miscarriage though the cause cannot be found in almost 50 per cent of repeated miscarriages.

If a woman loses her pregnancies repeatedly before the 10th week of pregnancy, it is called **recurrent early pregnancy loss**. If the pregnancy losses occur between the 10th and the 20th week (5th month) of pregnancy, it is called **recurrent late pregnancy loss**. It is important to differentiate between the two because the causes for the two may differ.

Known causes of recurrent pregnancy loss

Parental age

The risk of miscarriage is highest when the mother is 35 or older, and the father is 40 years or older.

Obesity

Recent studies have linked an increased risk of miscarriage with a BMI of 30 kg/m^2 or more. The best thing you can do for yourself is to get down to an optimal weight before you try for a pregnancy. Medical problems related to obesity, such as diabetes and polycystic ovaries, can also lead to repeated miscarriages.

Presence of the APA (or APLA) syndrome

This is the most important treatable cause of recurrent pregnancy loss. The mother has specific antibodies called antiphospholipid antibodies (APA) that can cause many problems in pregnancy, including miscarriage.

The APA syndrome is diagnosed by a blood test. It can be treated with blood thinners like low-dose aspirin tablets and heparin injections. Both these medications reverse the abnormal blood clotting caused by the APL antibodies and result in a live birth in 85 per cent of women treated.

Problems of the uterus

Septate uterus

A septate uterus is a defect present from birth that divides the uterine cavity into two by a wall of tissue called a septum. This may lead to repeated miscarriages. This is treated by surgically removing the septum.

Cervical incompetence (or cervical insufficiency)

Cervical incompetence is a condition in which the cervix opens painlessly, leading to preterm delivery. This condition occurs most frequently between 18 and 24 weeks of pregnancy and requires prompt medical attention.

Cervical incompetence

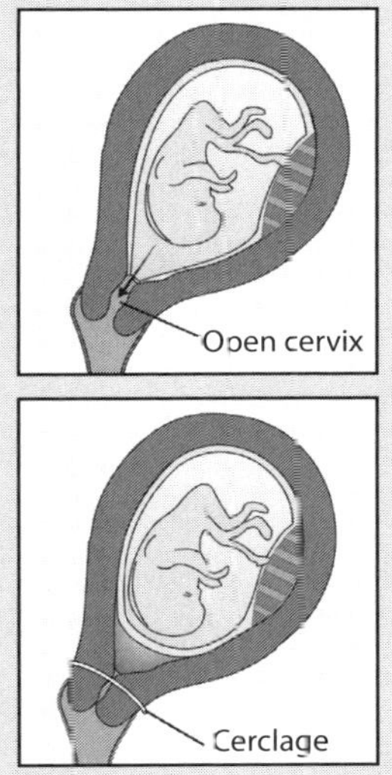

The cervix (mouth of the uterus) normally stays tightly closed till it is time for the baby to be born at term. In some women, the muscle fibres in the cervix are abnormal and will relax too early, usually between the 4th and 6th month of pregnancy. This happens painlessly and is usually heralded by light bleeding from the cervix, along with profuse white discharge and/or the rupture of membranes.

Take the instance of Menaka. She has been pregnant three times. The first two times she lost the pregnancy just at the beginning of the 5th month. She had no pains but started leaking water. By the time she got to the hospital the mouth of the uterus was completely open. She had definite cervical incompetence. With the third pregnancy, a stitch was placed on the mouth of the uterus in the 3rd month. This is called **cervical cerclage**. She carried the baby to term and is now the happy mother of a pretty baby girl.

Tests for recurrent pregnancy loss

The common tests done for couples that have had two miscarriages or more are:

- A blood test for the presence of antiphospholipid antibodies
- Evaluation to rule out an abnormality of the uterus: this involves a good quality ultrasound scan (including a 3D scan) or a hysteroscopy

(where a thin, lighted telescope-like instrument is introduced into the uterus) that will reveal abnormalities of the uterus that could lead to repeated pregnancy loss

- A chromosomal test for the couple: this is usually done if there have been three or more miscarriages. Sometimes one of the partners has a chromosomal abnormality that can get passed down to the foetus and cause a miscarriage. Even in this case, the couple has a 75 per cent chance of having a normal pregnancy

Can repeated miscarriage be treated?

APA syndrome

If it has been clearly established that there are antiphospholipid antibodies present in the blood stream, then this can be treated with blood thinners like low-dose aspirin tablets and heparin injections. Both these medications reverse the abnormal blood clotting caused by the antiphospholipid antibodies and result in a live birth in 85 per cent of women treated.

The low-dose aspirin tablets are started as soon as you start trying for a pregnancy or as soon as a pregnancy test comes positive. The heparin is started once the pregnancy is confirmed by early ultrasound and the heartbeat is identified.

Cervical incompetence (or cervical insufficiency)

The cervix (mouth of the uterus) is held shut by a stitch. This stitch is placed during a surgical procedure under anaesthesia. The suture is usually placed through the vagina. In some women, the procedure has to be done through a cut in the abdomen or even through a laparoscope. The suture is removed before delivery.

Septate uterus

The septum can be removed surgically to end with a single uterine cavity. Removing the septum results in a high chance of a pregnancy going to term.

Chromosomal abnormality in one parent

It is important to remember that even if there is a chromosomal abnormality in one parent, there is still a 75 per cent chance of a normal pregnancy. In some couples, the doctor might suggest going in for in-vitro fertilization (IVF). Once the embryos are formed, they can be tested and only the normal embryo is placed back in the uterus. This will ensure a normal, healthy and successful pregnancy.

Treatments of doubtful value

Bed rest

Prolonged bed rest for more than a few days has not been shown to be of any value in preventing miscarriage.

Hormonal therapy

It has been clearly proven that hormonal therapy with hCG injection or progesterone has no place in the management of repeated miscarriage. A recent, very large medical study called the PROMISE trial has proved categorically that progesterone does not result in any success in treating recurrent miscarriage.

Miscarriage: myths and misconceptions

Having a miscarriage is a sad event in any couple's life. It is almost impossible for you to believe that you did not do something that caused the miscarriage. To add to this, friends and relatives try to come up with some explanation for the miscarriage.

Remember that all the usual reasons given for causing a miscarriage are only myths and misconceptions.

The following are usually blamed but **do not cause a miscarriage:**

- Climbing stairs
- Strenuous activity
- Travelling by autorickshaw or in a bus
- Travelling on a bumpy road
- Travelling by air
- Having a fall
- Drinking something either hot or cold
- Eating fruits like papaya, pineapple and mango
- Eating sesame seeds
- Going out during a solar or lunar eclipse
- Having sexual intercourse
- Being emotionally upset

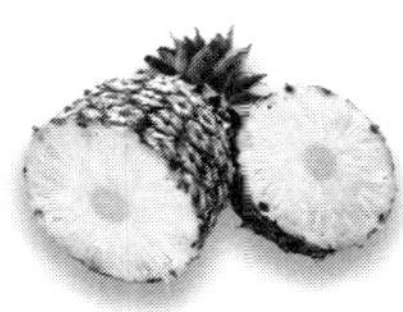

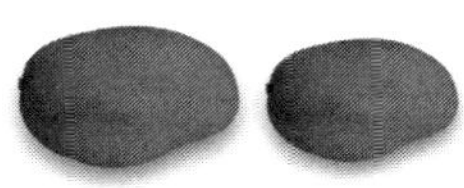

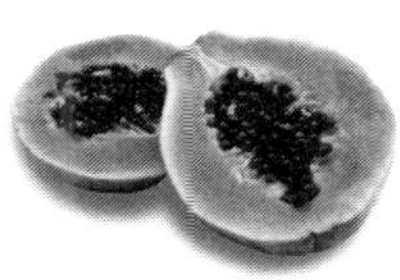

No, you don't have a 'weak' uterus

One of the commonest questions asked after a miscarriage is, 'Do I have a weak uterus?' There is nothing known as a 'weak' uterus. There is no medicine that 'strengthens' the uterus. Remember, miscarriages happen because the pregnancy is abnormal to begin with. A miscarriage is Nature's way of getting rid of an abnormal or defective foetus.

CHAPTER 31

Bleeding in pregnancy

Shanthi is frightened. She is two months pregnant. She woke up this morning to find a small amount of blood on her underclothes. She is extremely concerned.

Samhita is 28 weeks pregnant. She was working in her office when she had a feeling of wetness. On checking, she found she was bleeding. She rushed to her obstetrician.

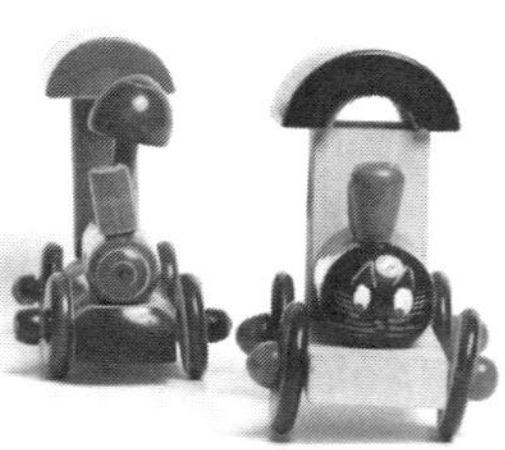

31

Bleeding in pregnancy

Did you know that 1 out of 4 pregnant women might experience light vaginal bleeding at some point during pregnancy, particularly during the first three months? Luckily, in the vast majority, the bleeding will have no impact on the pregnancy.

> Though you need not panic, it is important to seek medical help if you have bleeding anytime during pregnancy.

Vaginal bleeding is one of the more frightening experiences in pregnancy. It may vary from a small amount of spotting to heavy bleeding with clots and cramps. In pregnancy, even a small amount of vaginal bleeding can be alarming. Though bleeding may be a warning sign of an abnormality, it is not always a serious complication.

Vaginal bleeding in pregnancy has many causes. Bleeding can occur in any trimester. Slight bleeding may often stop on its own. Sometimes though, bleeding may be serious enough to be a risk to you or your baby. You should call your doctor or seek medical advice if bleeding occurs.

Bleeding in the first trimester (1–13 weeks)

Is it normal to bleed in the first trimester?

Though it is not normal to bleed early in pregnancy, it certainly is not an uncommon occurrence. Many women will experience spotting or bleeding in the first trimester of pregnancy. In most cases, women who experience slight bleeding in the first trimester go on to have a normal pregnancy. There are some signs and symptoms that may indicate that the bleeding is of serious concern.

Common causes of early pregnancy bleeding

Implantation bleeding: There might be a small amount of spotting or bleeding very early in pregnancy, about 10–14 days after fertilization. When the fertilized egg attaches to the lining of the uterus and starts burrowing

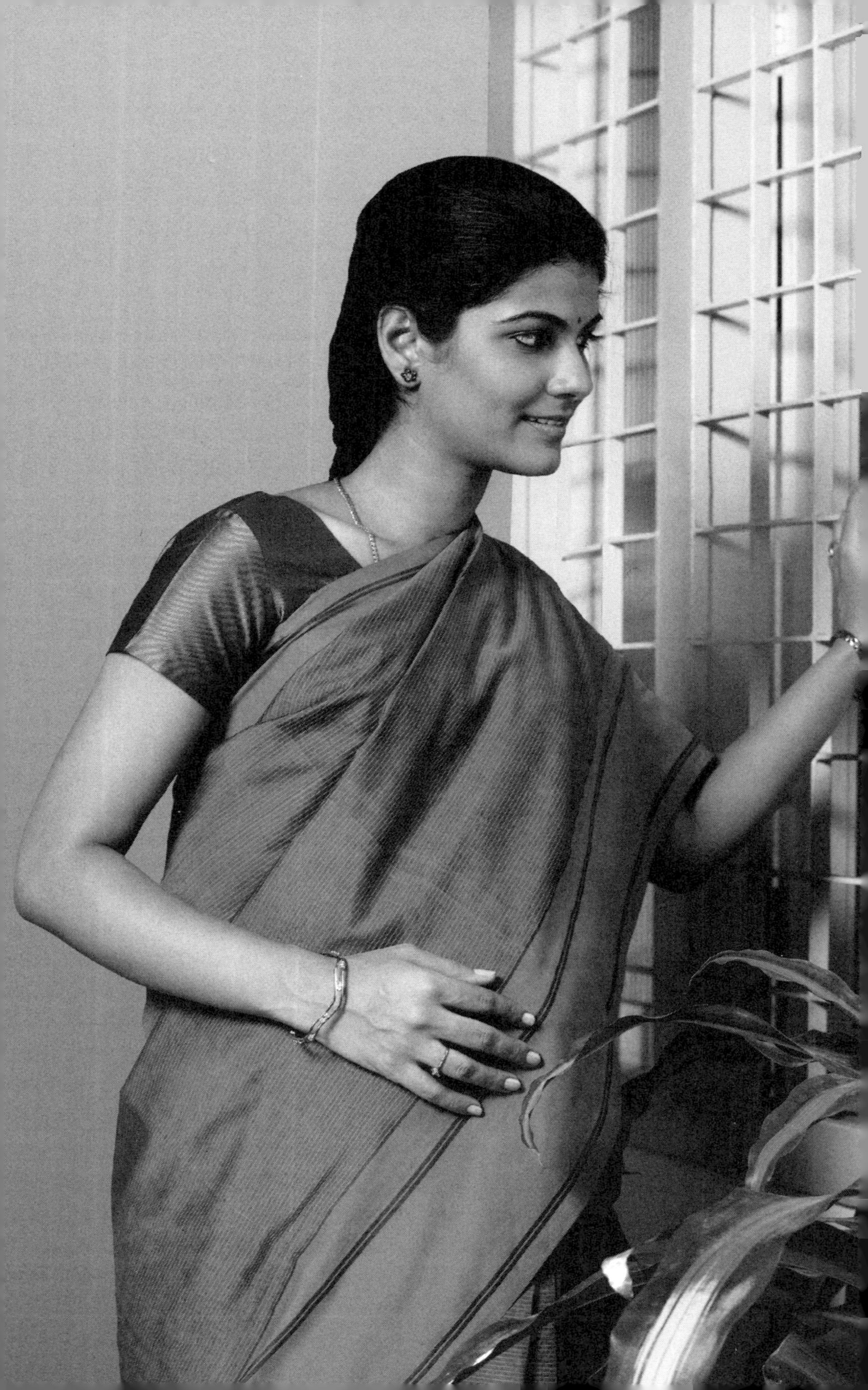

into the lining, there can be slight spotting. Some women actually mistake this light bleeding for a period and may not realize they are pregnant.

Mandy asked: I am three months pregnant. Once or twice after sex I noticed a little spot of bleeding on my panties. We are now really scared to have sex. Will it cause me to miscarry?

My answer: In pregnancy, the cervix (mouth of the uterus) becomes soft and congested. The cervix develops many more tiny blood vessels and some of these tiny vessels can bleed. There may be light spotting or bleeding after contact to this area, such as after intercourse or a pelvic exam. Occasionally, there might be a polyp on the cervix. A polyp is a non-cancerous growth that may bleed after intercourse.

This type of light bleeding in pregnancy is usually normal and will stop on its own. There is no reason to worry. Have a check-up and once your obstetrician gives you the go ahead, you can resume intercourse.

Miscarriage: Bleeding in the first trimester can be a sign of miscarriage. Miscarriage occurs in 15–20 per cent of pregnancies, most often during the first 12 weeks. Bleeding in the first trimester is always considered to indicate a possible miscarriage. It is called a *threatened abortion* Once you are examined and an ultrasound scan shows a good heartbeat in the baby, it indicates that the pregnancy will continue normally (see **Chapter 30**: *Miscarriage*).

Ectopic pregnancy: In some women, the pregnancy, instead of implanting inside the uterine cavity, will start growing in an abnormal place outside the uterus. This is called an ectopic pregnancy. A pregnancy inside the Fallopian tube (*tubal pregnancy*) is the commonest kind. A foetus implanted inside the tube can cause serious internal bleeding. Ectopic pregnancies must be treated immediately to save the life of the mother. Symptoms of ectopic pregnancy include vaginal spotting or bleeding, abdominal pain (which is usually worse on one side) and fainting.

Molar pregnancy (gestational trophoblastic disease): In this rare condition, the foetus does not form. Instead, the uterus is filled up with an abnormal mass made up of clusters of cysts. Bleeding is the most common symptom of a molar pregnancy. By itself, molar pregnancy is an uncommon cause of bleeding in the first trimester. A molar pregnancy may require treatment with suction curettage and drugs.

When should you seek immediate medical attention?

The vast majority of women who have some bleeding in early pregnancy go on to carry the pregnancy to term. It is urgent to call your obstetrician if the bleeding is:

- Heavier than a period
- Accompanied by severe cramps
- Accompanied by lower abdominal pain associated with fainting
- Associated with fever

Management of bleeding in the first trimester

Yes, it is scary. And yes, you will only think of the worst scenario. It is good to remind yourself that the majority of women with bleeding in early pregnancy will carry on to term.

Tests

When you have bleeding in the first trimester, your obstetrician will try to determine the cause of the bleeding. She will do a pelvic examination, may inspect the cervix and also may ask for an ultrasound examination. A blood test may be done to measure the pregnancy hormone (hCG). The blood test may be repeated after 48 hours because in a normally growing pregnancy, the hCG level will double in 48 hours (see **Chapter 30**, *Miscarriage*).

What can an ultrasound scan show?

An ultrasound scan can immediately rule out a miscarriage by identifying whether there is a foetal heartbeat or not. If there is a heartbeat, an ultrasound can also predict if the pregnancy will continue to grow or is destined for loss (see the Can a miscarriage be predicted? section in **Chapter 30**, *Miscarriage*).

An ultrasound can also identify an abnormal pregnancy like a molar or an ectopic pregnancy.

Bed rest

If the bleeding is slight, you may be advised bed rest for 2 or 3 days and limited activity at home. If the bleeding is moderate or heavy, you might be admitted to the hospital for a few days till the bleeding stops. You will be asked to gradually increase your level of activity and if there is no further bleeding for 1–2 weeks, you will be asked to resume your routine activity. It is best to avoid intercourse for two weeks following any vaginal bleeding.

Can hormones stop the bleeding?
Hormonal therapy with progestogens has been used over the years to treat threatened miscarriage. However, medical research has failed to produce strong evidence to support the need for hormonal tablets or injections in case of a threatened miscarriage.

Bleeding in the second trimester (14–27 weeks)

Bleeding in the second trimester is usually taken more seriously. It may be a signal for several conditions.

Miscarriage: Although miscarriage is less common in the second trimester than the first, a risk still exists.

Cervical incompetence or insufficiency: Occasionally, light bleeding from the cervix, along with profuse white discharge, may be a sign of cervical incompetence, a condition in which the cervix opens painlessly, leading to preterm delivery. This condition occurs most frequently between 18 and 24 weeks of pregnancy and requires prompt medical attention.

Preterm labour: Preterm labour can start off with vaginal bleeding and will then progress to cramping. If the obstetrician thinks that you are are at risk for preterm labour, she will advise bed rest and may also start you on tablets or injections which will arrest labour.

> Less worrisome causes of bleeding in the second trimester include a benign growth (**polyp**) on the cervix. The obstetrician can diagnose this when she inspects the cervix. Just as in the first trimester, bleeding may also follow intercourse since the cervix is soft and congested.

Management of bleeding in the second trimester
Your obstetrician will examine you to make sure there is no polyp causing the bleeding. She will also check the cervix to determine whether you are in labour or not. After that, she will ask for an ultrasound scan.

What can an ultrasound show (2nd trimester)?
An ultrasound in the 2nd trimester can help identify an incompetent cervix. It may also identify if there is any bleeding from the placenta. If there is any abnormality in the baby, it will be picked up.

Bed rest
If the bleeding is slight, you may be advised bed rest for a few days and limited activity at home. If the bleeding is moderate or heavy, you might be

admitted to the hospital for a few days till the bleeding stops. You will be asked to gradually increase your level of activity and if there is no further bleeding for 1–2 weeks, you will be asked to resume your routine activity. It is best to avoid intercourse for two weeks following any vaginal bleeding.

Cervical cerclage

If your doctor finds there is evidence of cervical incompetence (also called cervical insufficiency), an attempt will be made to suture the cervix shut (see **Chapter 30**: *Miscarriage*). The suture will be left in place till term and then it will be removed to allow for labour. Sometimes, the cervix may have dilated too much and the cerclage procedure may not be feasible.

Bleeding in the third trimester (28–40 weeks)

Bleeding late in pregnancy may threaten the health of the mother or the baby. Bleeding in the third trimester will usually require hospitalization.

Preterm labour: When there is mild bleeding associated with abdominal cramping or intermittent pain in late pregnancy **but before 37 weeks**, the first thing to suspect is preterm labour. A mucus 'plug' that covers the opening of the uterus during pregnancy is passed just before or at the start of labour. This results in a small amount of mucus and blood passing from the cervix. This is called bloody show. Preterm labour may also start with a gush of amniotic fluid (see **Chapter 32**, *When the baby comes too early: preterm labour and birth*).

Placental abruption: One of the emergencies that can occur before or during labour is placental abruption. This problem occurs only in 1 out of a 100 pregnancies. In this condition, the placenta separates or detaches from the uterine wall. This may cause vaginal bleeding. This can also be associated with severe abdominal pain. When the placenta becomes detached, the blood flow to the baby can get reduced or cut off. This endangers the oxygen supply to the baby and can jeopardize his health.

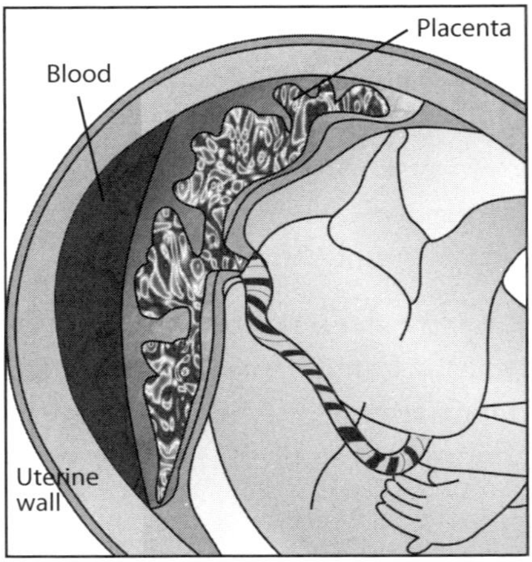

Placental abruption: the placenta has separated from the uterine wall

Who is at high risk for placental abruption?
Women who have had more than 1 pregnancy (the risk increases with each additional pregnancy), are over 35, have had an abruption before or who have high blood pressure in pregnancy, are at high risk for developing placental abruption.

Very rarely, severe blows (for example, during an accident) or other injuries to the abdomen can cause an abruption.

Placenta praevia: When the placenta lies low in the uterus, it is called placenta praevia. It may partly cover the cervix (partial placenta praevia) or completely cover the cervix (total placenta praevia). Placenta praevia occurs in 1 in 200 pregnant women.

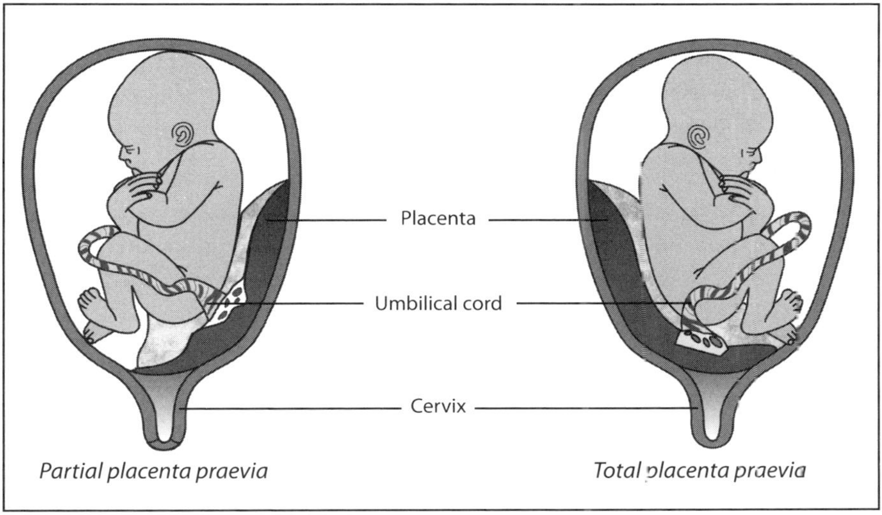

Placenta praevia can cause **painless** vaginal bleeding. Most of the time, this is managed conservatively. You might be admitted to the hospital for observation. If the bleeding stops, you might be allowed to go home. An elective caesarean section will be done when your baby is mature enough to be delivered. If the bleeding is profuse and uncontrollable, then an emergency caesarean section will be done, whatever the age of the baby.

Who is at high risk for placental praevia?
Placenta praevia is more common in women who have had more than one child, who have had a previous caesarean section, or who are carrying twins or triplets.

Management of bleeding in the third trimester

Bleeding in the third trimester requires immediate medical attention. You may need to be admitted to the hospital to find its cause. After labour has been ruled out, an ultrasound scan may be advised to determine the cause of the bleeding. If the bleeding stops and the health of the baby is not in jeopardy, you may be kept under observation for a few days or even weeks. If the bleeding has been profuse and a large amount of blood has been lost, a blood transfusion may be required.

Bleeding in late pregnancy can be a major health risk for both the mother and the baby. The problem might be serious enough to require early and immediate delivery of the baby, often by caesarean birth.

Samhita is 28 weeks pregnant. She was working in her office when she had a feeling of wetness. On checking, she found she was bleeding. She phoned her husband and told him to meet her at the obstetrician's clinic.

Samhita is rightfully worried. Bleeding in the second trimester is less common than in the first trimester.

Her obstetrician asked her whether she had had intercourse over the past 48 hours. Since the mouth of the uterus is very soft at this stage, sometimes there can be slight bleeding following intercourse. This is not harmful to the baby.

On examination, the mouth of the uterus was closed and showed no signs of premature labour. An ultrasound was done. The baby's heartbeat was normal. The placenta was lying a little low in the uterus. There was a small clot near the lower edge of the placenta.

Samhita was admitted to the hospital. Over the next two days, the bleeding changed from bright red to dark brown. Her obstetrician explained to her that this was a good sign. It meant that there was no fresh bleeding. She was discharged on the third day. She was advised to take it easy and avoid intercourse for the next two weeks.

Since she had no further bleeding, she went back to office after two weeks. She had two further episodes of slight brownish discharge. Her obstetrician explained that this was common. As the uterus enlarged, the placenta would keep moving away from the lower end of the uterus. The danger of bleeding would become less as the pregnancy progressed.

Samhita went into labour at 38 weeks and had a normal vaginal delivery.

Shanthi is frightened. She is two months pregnant. She woke up this morning to find a small amount of blood on her underclothes. She has no abdominal cramping or pain. She is extremely concerned.

Shanthi and her husband went to see her obstetrician. She had an internal examination. The mouth of the uterus was still closed. There was only slight bleeding present. Her doctor explained to them that this, along with the fact that she was not having any pains, was a good sign but only an ultrasound scan could confirm whether the pregnancy was healthy.

An ultrasound was done and she was delighted to see that the baby's heartbeat was seen clearly. Shanthi was having a 'threatened' miscarriage. Since there was very slight bleeding, Shanthi was asked to go home. She was advised to stay in bed for the next three days though she could get up to eat and to go to the bathroom. After three days, she had no further bleeding. She was asked to resume normal activity at home over the next week. She was also asked to avoid sexual intercourse for the next two weeks.

After a week at home, Shanthi had no bleeding. She resumed all her activities and started going out as usual. She had no further bleeding and had a normal delivery at term.

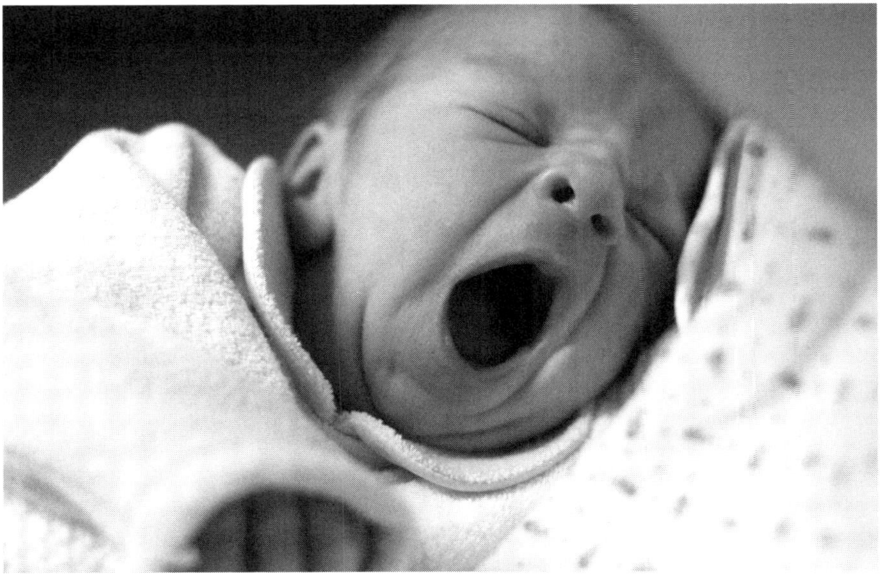

CHAPTER 32

When the baby comes too early

Susan is worried. Should she be hitting the panic button? She is only 8 months pregnant but since this morning, she has been having lower abdominal pain. In the beginning, it felt like menstrual cramping but now there is squeezing pain that comes every 10 minutes. Could Susan be in preterm labour?

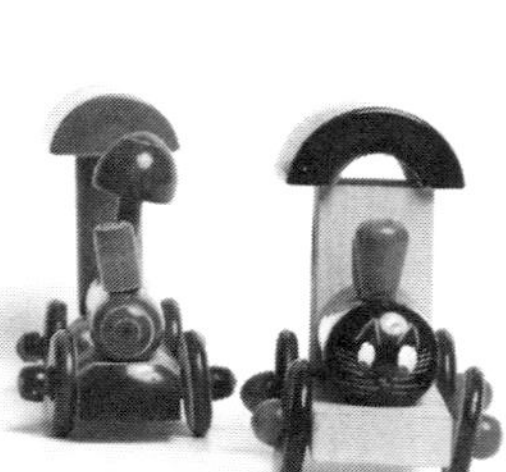

32

When the baby comes too early: preterm labour and birth

Your chances of delivering **at term** are very high. The majority of women will deliver at term—that means between 37 and 40 weeks. However some women could deliver a little earlier and a small percentage could deliver way too early. If your baby is born between 34 and 37 weeks, he could do very well, though he may require special care. Twenty per cent of Indian women deliver preterm, and India is the biggest contributor to the world's prematurity burden. **Before you get too worried, remember that your chances of having a full term baby are 80 per cent!**

What is preterm labour?

When labour begins after 20 weeks and before 37 weeks, it is considered preterm or premature. It is not known for certain what causes preterm labour to start, though certain pregnancies are prone to it.

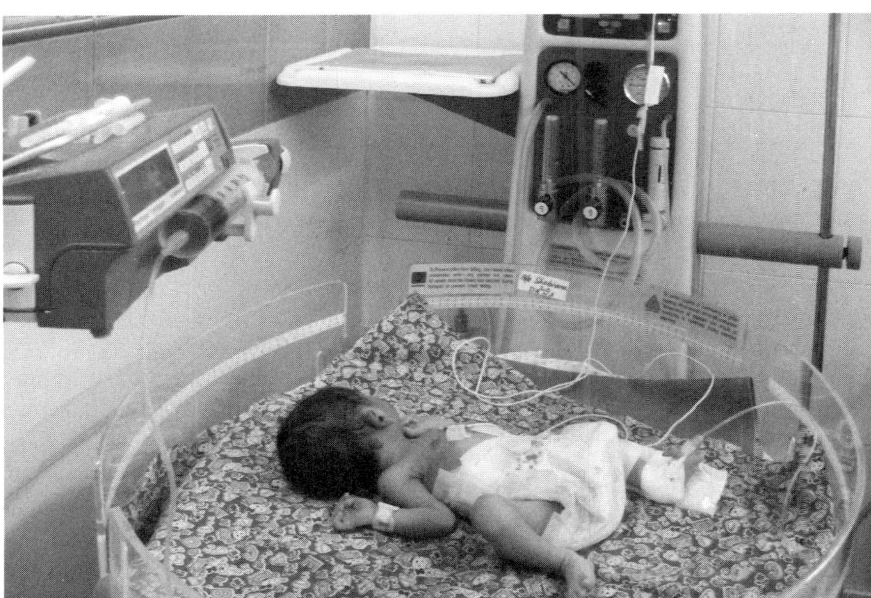

Luckily, even if labour pains start prematurely, in 30 per cent of women the pains may subside on their own without leading to preterm birth. Ten per cent of women with preterm labour pains may deliver within a week.

What can cause preterm labour?

Some pregnancies are at a greater risk for the occurrence of preterm labour.

- A previous pregnancy with preterm labour
- Previous miscarriages
- A mother who is very young (less than 17 years) or older than 35 years
- A mother who is underweight or overweight
- A uterus that is overstretched with twins (see **Chapter 36**, *Twins: double trouble?*), triplets, or excess amniotic fluid
- Urine infection (see **Chapter 44**, *Urinary tract infection in pregnancy*)
- Cervical incompetence (see **Chapter 30**, *Miscarriage*)
- A mother with high blood pressure or diabetes (see **Chapter 37**, *High blood pressure in pregnancy* and **Chapter 38**, *Diabetes in pregnancy*)
- A pregnancy following in-vitro fertilization (IVF)
- Prolonged or repeated bleeding in early pregnancy
- A growth restricted foetus (see **Chapter 34**, *Foetal growth problems: too small or too big*)
- A baby with physical or chromosomal abnormalities
- Smoking, stress and excessive physical activity

Can you do anything to prevent preterm labour?

Though many of the causes for preterm labour are not under your control, you can take some steps to help your baby reach term.

- Start your antenatal check-ups early and make sure you see your doctor for all the scheduled check-ups
- Try to space your babies adequately. Though 18 months is the shortest interval you should consider, an interval of three years between babies is ideal
- If you have any symptoms of a urine infection (see **Chapter 44**, *Urinary tract infection in pregnancy*), seek immediate medical treatment because it can trigger preterm labour
- Take care to avoid malaria (mosquito nets are very useful) because malaria is associated with preterm labour

- Keep your weight gain under strict control. Watch your diet and eat healthy. Excessive weight gain can lead to diabetes or worsen your diabetes. Excessive weight gain also makes you at risk for high blood pressure and preeclampsia
- If you have had a preterm birth before, your doctor may advise you to avoid intercourse in the third trimester because it may sometimes lead to contractions

Harini asked: I had preterm labour with my last pregnancy and delivered at 31 weeks. My daughter is doing well now but it was a very difficult time for the whole family. I am really anxious. How can I prevent another preterm birth in my next pregnancy?

My answer: Since you have had one preterm delivery, when you are pregnant again you will be given weekly progesterone injections starting from the 16th week of pregnancy, till 36 weeks. These injections will help prevent preterm labour and birth.

Treatments with **no proven benefit** include:

- Restriction of normal activity, or complete bed rest
- Having more frequent antenatal check-ups
- A stitch in the cervix if the length of the cervix is normal (more than 2.5 cm)
- A stitch in the cervix for someone who is pregnant with twins

What are the problems of preterm birth?

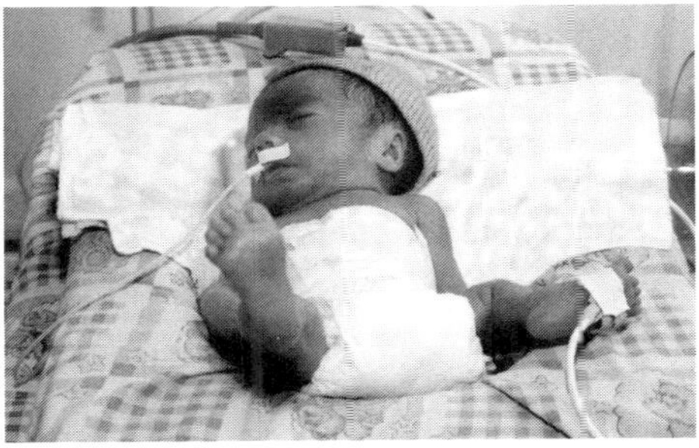

The earlier in pregnancy a baby is born, the greater the risk of serious problems for the baby. Many of the organs, especially the heart and lungs, are not fully-grown or mature. The biggest problem the preterm infant faces is called **respiratory distress syndrome** that results from being born before the lungs are mature enough to breathe air. Premature babies can also bleed into the brain, leading to potential brain damage. Preterm infants born after 32 weeks of pregnancy do better than those born earlier.

These babies require a specially equipped neonatal intensive care unit (NICU) to survive. Many hospitals in larger cities have well-equipped NICUs and the survival in these units can be very good.

Warning signs of preterm labour

If preterm labour is recognized early enough, delivery may be prevented or postponed in some cases. This will give the baby extra time to grow and mature. Even a few more days may mean a healthier baby. It is important to call your doctor or go to the hospital right away if you notice any of these symptoms:

- Watery, mucoid or bloody vaginal discharge
- Sudden increase in amount of vaginal discharge
- Pelvic or lower abdominal pressure
- Constant, dull, low backache that does not go away with rest
- Mild abdominal cramps like menstrual cramps
- Regular or frequent contractions or uterine tightening (sometimes painless), lasting beyond an hour
- A trickle or gush of fluid from the vagina

Am I in preterm labour?

Preterm labour can start with contractions (pains) or with rupture of membranes (a gush of amniotic fluid).

Contractions

You need immediate medical attention if your contractions

- Occur at least 4 times in a 20 minute period or if there have been eight contractions in an hour
- The contractions have been persisting for more than an hour

Rupture of membranes

There is a trickle or gush of fluid from the vagina. This indicates that the membranes have ruptured even though pains have not started. If it is just a little bit of leaking, how can you confirm that membranes have ruptured? Wear a sanitary pad and see if it continues to get wet. In any case, if you have doubts, it is best to go see your doctor who will confirm whether fluid is leaking.

Braxton-Hicks contractions

It is common to have Braxton-Hicks contractions after the 7th month. They will present as painless tightening of the abdomen in the last three months of pregnancy. They usually subside with rest and should not be mistaken for preterm labour.

How is preterm labour confirmed?

Are you having pains?

When you go to the hospital, your doctor will feel your abdomen to look for regular hardening of the uterus that will confirm contractions. You might also have an internal examination to assess the condition of the cervix. Preterm labour can be confirmed by finding out if thinning and dilatation of the cervix (mouth of the uterus) have occurred.

You might be monitored with a cardiotocograph (CTG) to see if you are having contractions.

Are you leaking fluid?
If you have ruptured membranes prematurely i.e., before pains have started, your doctor may do a speculum examination to see if there is fluid leaking from the cervix (mouth of the uterus). If there is leaking of fluid, an internal examination may be postponed till the obstetrician decides when and how the baby is going to be delivered.

Measurement of the length of the cervix

This ultrasound test is based on the fact that the risk of preterm labour increases if the cervix (mouth of the uterus) is short.

How is it done?
This scan is done with an internal (vaginal) probe. It is done between 16–24 weeks of pregnancy. In women with a previous preterm birth the cervix is considered short if it measures 2.5 cm or less. In women who have never had a preterm birth, it is considered short if it is 2.0 cm or less.

Who needs this test?
- Women who have had a previous preterm labour and birth
- Women with twins
- Women who have conceived after in-vitro fertilization (IVF)

It is not recommended routinely for women with no risk factors for preterm labour.

What if the cervix is short?
Your doctor will treat you with the hormone progesterone, or in some cases, might suggest a stitch to be placed in the cervix.

Treatment of preterm labour

Once preterm labour is suspected, your obstetrician will admit you to the hospital for observation. The objectives of treating premature labour are twofold:

- To try and stop labour, without jeopardizing the mother's health
- To ensure that if the baby is born in spite of preventive measures, then the lungs are mature enough for him to survive

Stopping preterm labour

Tocolytics are medicines that can stop contractions temporarily. The aim is to prevent delivery for at least 48 hours so that measures can be taken to help the baby's lungs mature. This also buys time to transfer the mother to a hospital that has a neonatal intensive care unit (NICU).

Helping the baby's lung mature

Steroids are administered if it appears that the chances are high of the baby being born before 34 weeks. Steroids cross the placenta and help the baby's lungs mature and also prevent bleeding into the brain. Steroids increase the baby's chance of survival. Steroids are most likely to help the baby when used between 24 and 34 weeks of pregnancy. Steroids are safe in pregnancy.

> **Steroids in pregnancy**
>
> Steroids are very safe in pregnancy. In addition to be being used to improve foetal lung maturity, steroids may be used in asthmatics in pregnancy and also to relieve the itching that occurs in the last few weeks of pregnancy (pruritic urticarial patches and plaques of pregnancy or PUPPP).

Protecting the baby's brain

Babies born before 32 weeks are at an increased risk for brain damage. In such cases the mother may be given magnesium sulphate to protect the baby's brain.

Delivery and care of a preterm baby

If your labour is progressing and your little one seems to be tolerating labour well, a vaginal delivery will be attempted.

If there is reason to believe that your little one may not be able to tolerate the stresses of labour, or if you have any complications, then a caesarean section may be advised.

Care of the preterm baby

Many preterm babies are very small and require special care. They are kept in an incubator to keep them warm.

Kangaroo Mother Care is an excellent method of treatment for very premature babies. The baby is held in skin-to-skin contact with the mother, for as long as possible each day. The mother's body warmth acts as an incubator. Babies undergoing Kangaroo Mother Care stay as warm as they would in an incubator. They bond better with their mothers, have fewer serious infections, go home sooner, and breastfeed better and longer.

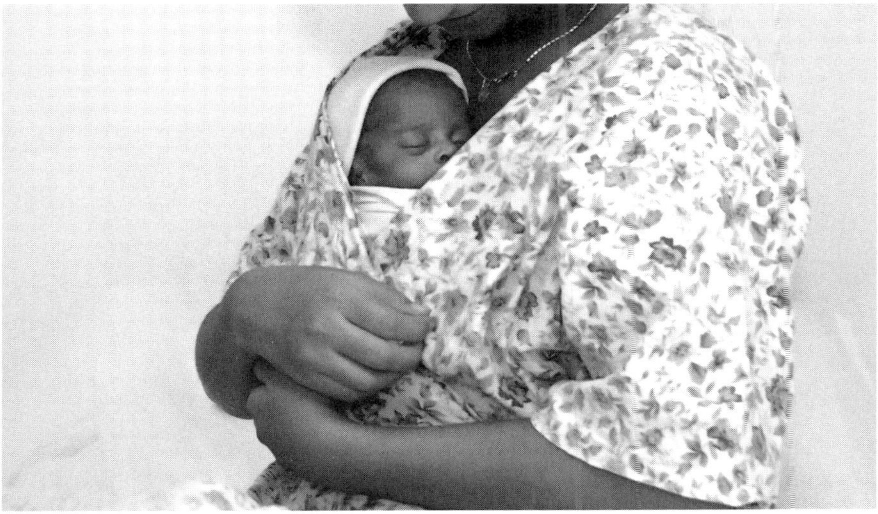

Kangaroo Mother Care for preterm babies *(Image courtesy: Fernandez Hospital, Hyderabad)*

The baby may also receive surfactant, a medication which, when administered, can prevent breathing difficulties in the baby and save the baby's life. You and your baby may be moved to a different hospital that can provide this type of care.

Today, with special care in a neonatal intensive care unit (NICU), even babies born between 28–30 weeks have a good chance of survival. Babies born between 32–36 weeks have an excellent chance of survival.

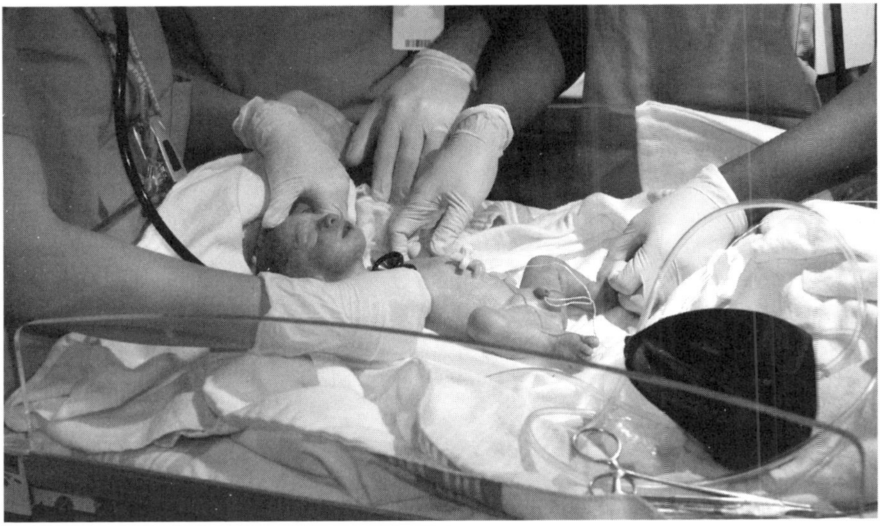

CHAPTER 33

When the baby is overdue: the postterm pregnancy

Seetha is getting impatient. Every day she gets calls from friends and relatives asking if she has delivered yet. The due date was three days ago and her baby seems to be quite comfortable inside the womb. The baby is showing no signs of wanting to come out! Seetha's husband is anxious and wants the obstetrician to deliver the baby immediately. Is this necessary?

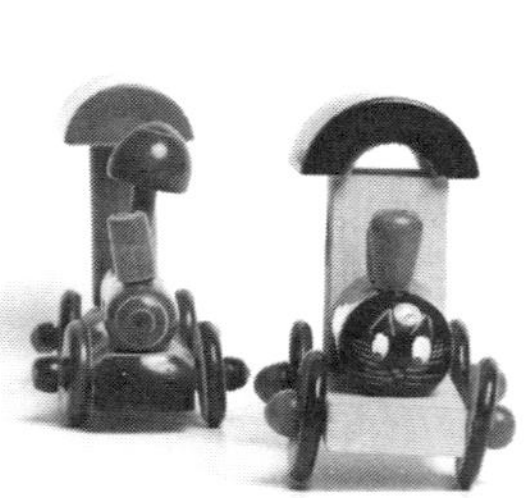

33

When the baby is overdue: the postterm pregnancy

Waiting for the birth of a child is an exciting and anxious time but when the baby does not arrive at the expected time, anxiety mounts, even when your doctor says everything is all right.

Why is my baby overdue?

Did you know that only 5 per cent of women deliver exactly on their calculated due date? Most will deliver just before or after the EDD. So you and your husband definitely need not get hung up on that date.

It's quite understandable that you are absolutely fed up of the pregnancy by now. Moving around is difficult, you can't sleep at night, your feet are swollen and you can't shake off this anxiety about why the baby refuses to come out.

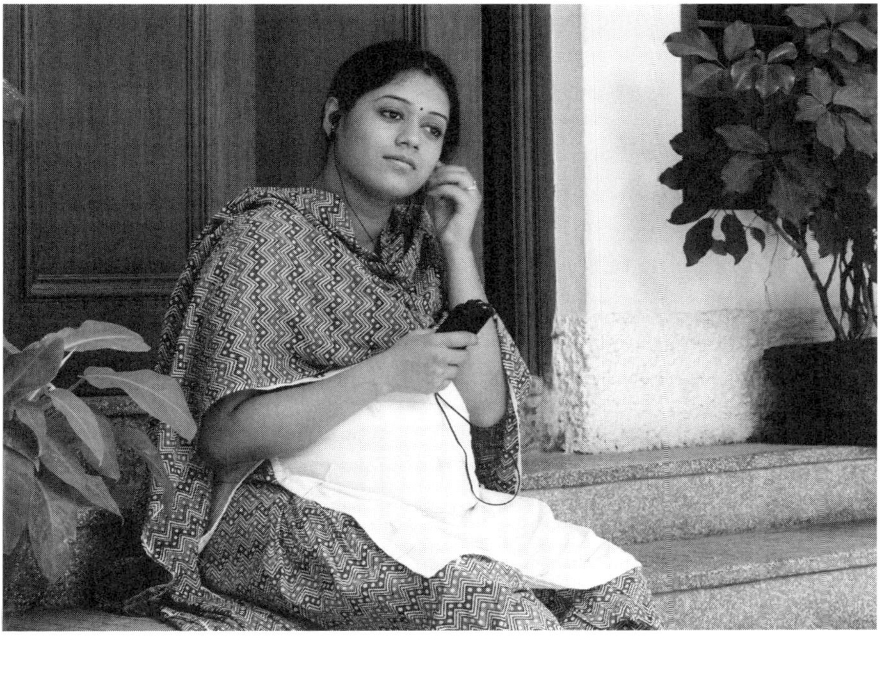

It doesn't help that the women you have been seeing at the doctor's clinic all seem to be delivering on time! Your family is also fretting and keeps nudging you to ask the doctor to get you delivered fast.

However hard it seems, don't lose sight of the fact that no pregnancy lasts forever (as it seems like this one is!) Labour could begin at any time. If it does not start spontaneously, measures will be taken to kick-start your labour.

What is postterm pregnancy?

Most women give birth between 37 weeks and 41 weeks of pregnancy. Very few babies are born exactly on their due date. It is quite normal to give birth as much as three weeks before or 7 days after the due date. It is important to remember that problems occur in only a small number of postterm pregnancies. Most women who give birth after the due date have no problems with the delivery and the newborn baby will do well.

By definition, a postterm (also called postdated) pregnancy is one that lasts 41 weeks or longer. Ten per cent of pregnant Indian women will deliver at or after 41 weeks.

> The due date (EDD) is just an indication about your expected time of delivery. It is calculated based on your last period but no one can know when you actually conceived. This means that the calculated due date is not perfect. Just remember that it is called *estimated* date of delivery or EDD, not *exact* date of delivery! Your sweet baby of course has no idea when she is supposed to be born—she just waits for hormonal signals to kick in and start off labour.

What are your chances of being overdue?

There are no specific causes that lead to a postterm pregnancy. However the chances of going beyond due date are higher if:

- You have had a previous postterm pregnancy
- Your mother had a postterm pregnancy
- This is your first pregnancy
- You are carrying a baby boy
- You are 35 or older
- The BMI is more than 30 kg/m^2 (obesity)

Are you really overdue?

This depends on how accurately your due date was calculated. A pregnancy may be incorrectly classified as postterm because of wrong dates.

If you have been having regular antenatal check-ups, an ultrasound scan would have been done in the third month or earlier that helps to calculate the most accurate due date (see **Chapter 13**, *Ultrasound scans in pregnancy*). If an accurate due date has been calculated, then your doctor can wait confidently for a week beyond that as long as the baby's health and yours, remain normal.

If your first ultrasound was done around the 5th month, the due date can be predicted within a range of 1 week: that means your date is +/- 1 week of the calculated due date.

Though not so common nowadays, some women may have their first scan later in pregnancy (after the 24th week, or 6th month). The later the ultrasound is done, the less accurate it is to fix a due date. If the due date has been calculated within a range of +/- 2 weeks, the pregnancy may falsely seem to be overdue.

Women with irregular periods

Women with irregular periods require an ultrasound in early pregnancy to establish an accurate due date. The due date should be confirmed as early in pregnancy as possible. Later, it becomes harder to set the due date accurately.

What are the risks of postterm pregnancy?

Apart from the physical aggravation of the pregnancy not coming to a happy ending when expected, an overdue pregnancy may have some unwanted effects on the baby.

The placenta is an astonishing organ that is created specifically to be the conduit between you and the baby, only for that one pregnancy. It carries oxygen and nutrition from you to the baby and removes unwanted waste products from the baby. However, it has an inbuilt, specific lifespan. Nature does not expect it to function well after 40 weeks of pregnancy.

As the pregnancy proceeds beyond 40 weeks, the placenta's function decreases and the baby receives less blood supply. This leads to certain complications that might jeopardize the baby.

- The amount of amniotic fluid around the baby decreases
- Less fluid may cause the umbilical cord to become compressed as the baby moves or as the uterus contracts

- Less oxygen reaches the baby, causing him to pass meconium (motion) into the amniotic fluid. This meconium can be aspirated into the lungs of the baby and can cause a problem called *meconium* aspiration syndrome. In this condition the baby has great difficulty in breathing when he is born
- In 15 per cent of pregnancies, less nutrition reaches the baby and the baby may lose some weight (see **Chapter 34**, *Foetal growth problems: too small or too big*)

How do we know the baby is healthy?

To confidently wait beyond the due date, your doctor has to ensure that the baby is handling the pregnancy well and is not facing any problems. A few tests will help in assessing the baby's health (see **Chapter 16**, *Tests of foetal well-being: is the baby tolerating pregnancy well?*).

Daily kick count

When the baby is healthy, he will move regularly inside the uterus. When he starts receiving less oxygen, he will move less. That is why your obstetrician will ask you to keep a count of how many times your baby moves inside, particularly when a baby is not born by the due date. You must contact your obstetrician if you feel the movements have become less. Instructions for doing the daily kick count are given in **Chapter 16**, *Tests of foetal well-being: is the baby tolerating pregnancy well?*

Non-stress test (NST)

A cardiotocograph (CTG) is used to record the baby's heartbeat. Looking at the recording, the obstetrician will be able to predict the baby's health. A healthy baby shows a specific pattern called a **reactive pattern** (see **Chapter 16**, *Tests of foetal well-being: is the baby tolerating pregnancy well?).*

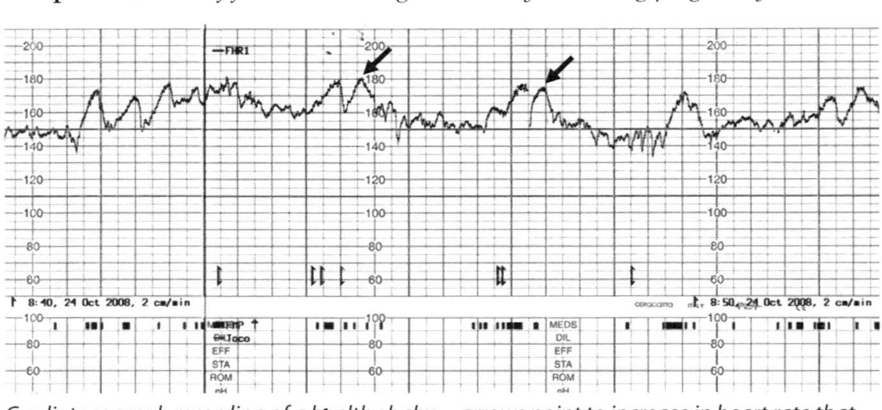

Cardiotocograph recording of a healthy baby—arrows point to increase in heart rate that indicates that the baby is getting adequate oxygen from the placenta

Amniotic fluid volume

The amount of amniotic fluid around the baby reflects the function of the baby's kidneys. If the fluid level remains normal, it is reassuring.

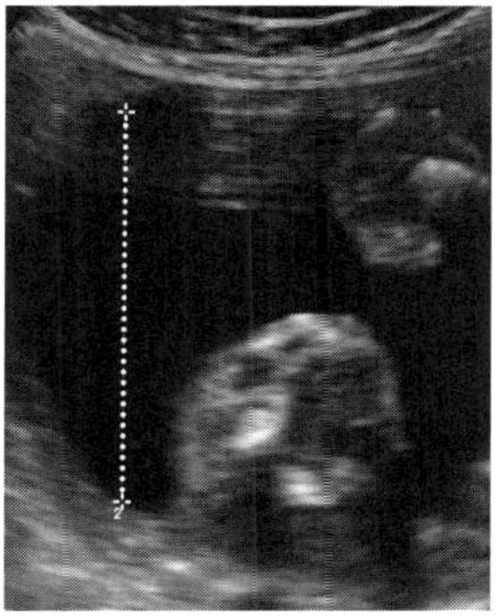

Measurement of amniotic fluid

When the oxygen supply to the baby decreases, the blood is shunted to the brain as a protective step. This diverts the blood away from the kidneys, resulting in a decreased production of urine. The amniotic fluid volume will start dropping. Decreasing amniotic fluid is an indicator of decreased placental function (see **Chapter 16**, *Tests of foetal well-being: is the baby tolerating pregnancy well?*).

Kick-starting labour

Stripping or sweeping of the membranes

This procedure, if done at around 40 weeks of pregnancy, has been shown to definitely reduce the number of women who go past 41 weeks. It can be done only if your cervix (mouth of the uterus) has started opening up a little.

This is a procedure where the obstetrician inserts the examining finger through the opening of the cervix and gently sweeps the finger around the inside edge, thereby detaching the membrane of the amniotic sac from the

Can you kick-start labour 'naturally'?

As you go past your due date, you will be flooded by any number of suggestions from your friends and family!

- 'Have sex!' says your best friend. Theoretically, having sex should make you go into labour because semen contains prostaglandins, the same hormone that makes your uterus contract. However, **there is no scientific evidence that this works.** Moreover, it may be quite uncomfortable to have intercourse at this stage of pregnancy
- 'Sweep and mop the house', says your mother. Sadly, you might end up with a clean house but no nearer labour. **This too will not help**
- Your grandmother wants you to have castor oil as a surefire method of inducing labour naturally. I will warn you right away: castor oil tastes and smells vile and can cause uncontrollable diarrhoea that may dehydrate you. Again, **no scientific evidence that this works**. It is just an old wives' tale

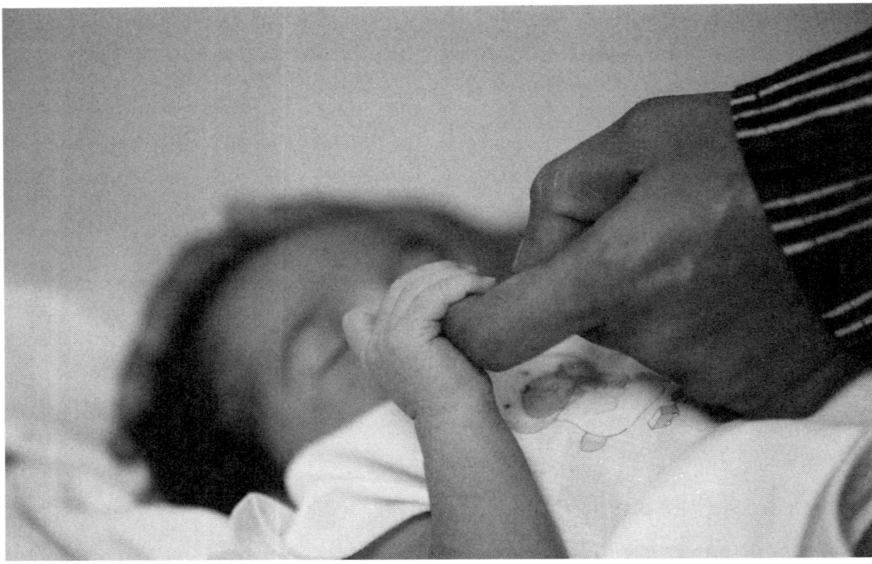

wall of the uterus. This may help start the process of ripening. This is done in the doctor's clinic. You go home and wait for pains to start. It works more effectively in women who have had a baby before.

How and when will you be delivered?

The decision about **how** you will be delivered will depend on

- Your medical health
- How ready your cervix is for induction of labour

The decision about **when** you will be delivered will depend on how the baby is tolerating pregnancy. Generally your doctor will wait till 41 weeks as long as the baby is doing well.

Assessing your readiness for induction

Obstetricians generally do weekly internal examinations after 38 weeks to assess if the cervix is thinning out (effacing) and opening up (dilating).

At 40 weeks

There are two options at 40 weeks.

- If you have not gone into labour by 40 weeks, a membrane sweeping will be done (see above)
- If the cervix is thinned out and opened up to 3–4 cm, and all other factors are favourable, the doctor will proceed with an induction to deliver you (see **Chapter 20**, *Augmentation and induction of labour*)

At 41 weeks

Induction of labour

If the cervix was not favourable at 40 weeks, or membrane sweeping was not successful, your doctor will definitely proceed with induction of labour. The labour pains will be monitored carefully and the baby's heartbeat will also be monitored throughout the process.

Caesarean section

A caesarean section will be done if the water around the baby is low or the non-stress test is not satisfactory. A caesarean will also be done if the induction does not work.

The postterm baby

At birth, approximately 15 out of a 100 postterm babies will show signs of *placental insufficiency*. This means that the baby did not get enough nutrition because the placenta was not functioning efficiently after the due date. The baby will be small and thin. The skin can be dry and peeling. These babies will do well after birth, once they start on their mother's feeds.

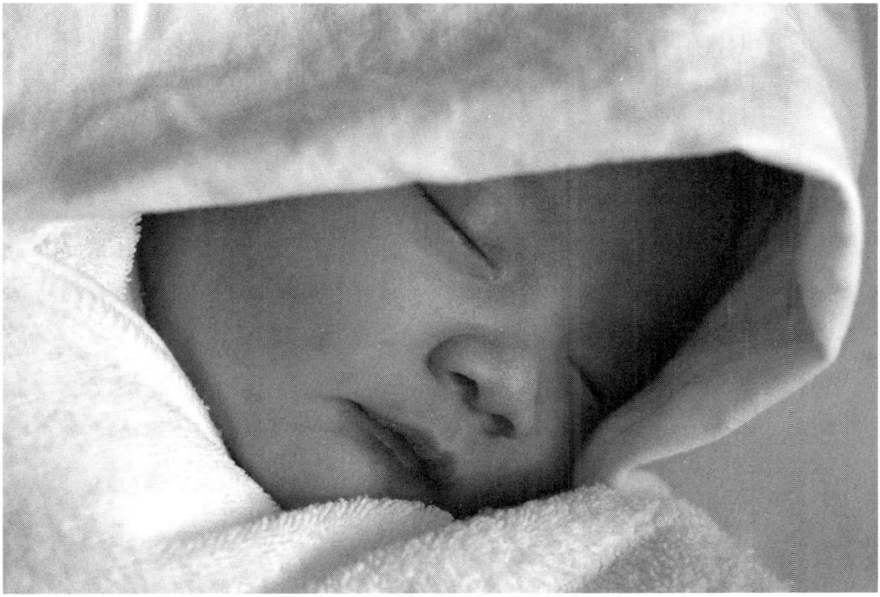

CHAPTER 34

Foetal growth problems: too small or too big

Supriya is 34 and has high blood pressure. During her routine check-up at 32 weeks, her doctor looked worried because the uterus looked smaller than it should. An ultrasound confirmed that the baby was not growing as well as he should have been. The baby has foetal growth restriction (also known as intrauterine growth restriction).

Shobana weighs 98 kg, and is in her 36th week. She has developed diabetes in this pregnancy. The ultrasound scan done this week estimates the baby's weight as 3.9 kg. This is a very large baby and has macrosomia.

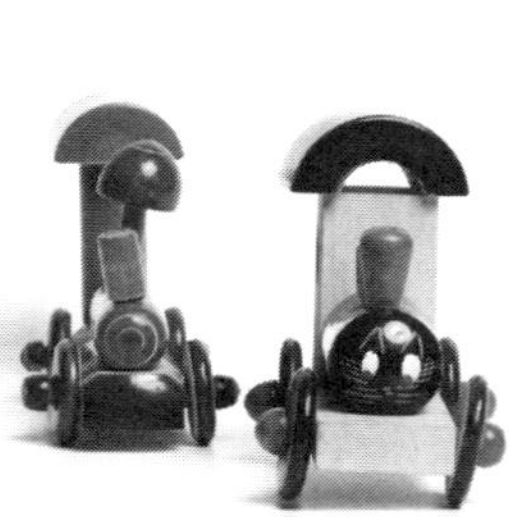

34

Foetal growth problems: too small or too big

When parents imagine the little one growing inside the womb, they only think of a chubby baby. Babies inside the womb are very much like children after birth: they grow according to the amount of nutrition they receive.

What growth problems can the baby have?

Foetal growth restriction and **macrosomia** are the two extremes of foetal growth disorders. In growth restriction, due to various reasons, the baby is smaller than it should be because he is not growing at a normal rate inside the womb. In other words, he is not able to reach his full growth potential. Macrosomia is just the opposite: the baby puts on excessive weight, especially having a disproportionate deposition of fat.

FOETAL GROWTH RESTRICTION (FGR or IUGR)

Every time you go for your antenatal check-up, your doctor checks the size of the uterus. This is probably one of the most important parts of the

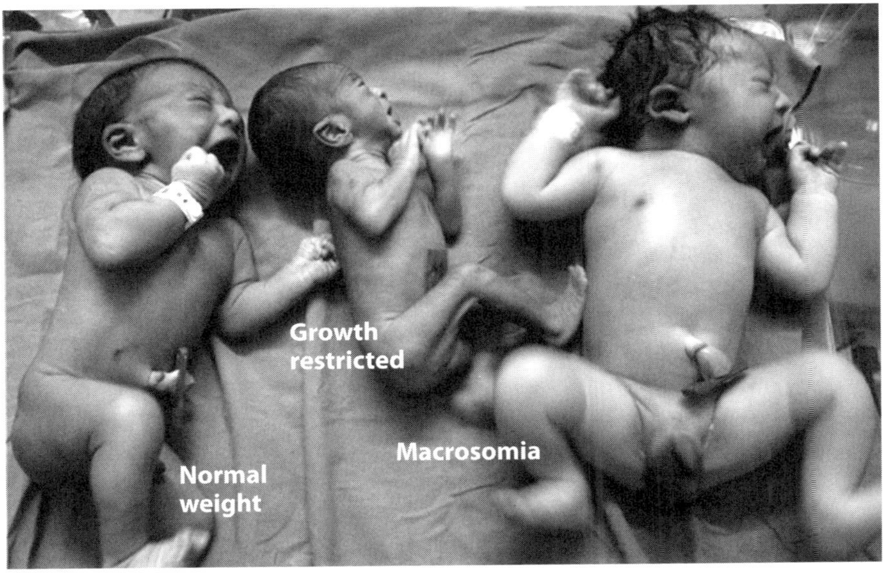

examination. You know why? At every check-up, the baby should have grown a little more and reached a certain size. If the baby does not show the expected rate of growth, your doctor may be concerned because that may indicate that the baby has **foetal growth restriction** (FGR), also called **intrauterine growth restriction** (IUGR).

FGR is usually diagnosed after the 28th week (in the third trimester) because this is the time that the baby puts on the maximum weight. If the baby does not put on the right amount of weight at this time, it is easier to suspect FGR.

Growth restriction and low birth weight are a major health issue in India because of the large number of babies born to ill-nourished women. One out of 5 babies born in India has a low birth weight. Though it is less common in middle-class women, it is still an issue.

What is foetal growth restriction?

The medical definition for FGR (or IUGR) is that the baby has an estimated weight below the 10th percentile for gestational age. Weight-wise, the World Health Organization defines FGR to be a baby weighing less than 2.5 kg. Neither definition is entirely accurate. Sometimes, the baby may appear small during the pregnancy but may be born at a normal weight and completely healthy.

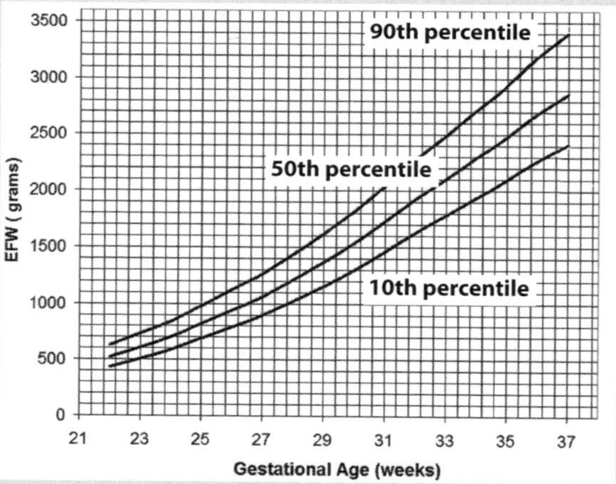

A baby's estimated weight is plotted on a graph to make it easier to visualize her growth. These growth charts are specific to a particular population (for example, Indian babies). The graph has three curving lines: the lowest is the 10th percentile (small baby), the middle one is the 50th percentile (average baby weight) and the 90th percentile (large baby). A growth restricted baby will have a weight below the 10th percentile and the macrosomic baby will be at or above the 90th percentile.

Are all small babies growth restricted?

When the doctor suspects that the baby is small, 50–70 per cent of those babies are actually **'constitutionally small'** and are perfectly healthy. It's important to remember that small parents have small babies. Indian mothers on an average, have smaller babies than Western mothers.

Only 20 per cent of small babies have **growth restriction**. These babies face problems inside the womb and after birth. Factors act on them inside the womb that prevent them from reaching their potential weight.

What are the risk factors for foetal growth restriction?

The basic problem in a growth restricted baby is the poor transfer of nutrition and oxygen from the placenta to the baby. Some of the conditions that affect placental function are:

Problems in the mother

- High blood pressure
- Diabetes
- Severe anaemia
- Being underweight
- Poor weight gain in pregnancy
- Short interval between one pregnancy and the next

Problems due to the placenta

- Placental abnormalities leading to poor function

Problems in the baby

- Chromosomal abnormalities
- Birth defects
- Twin or triplet pregnancy
- Infections like Rubella

How is growth restriction diagnosed?

During the usual antenatal check-up, if your doctor suspects that the baby is not growing the way he should be, an ultrasound scan will be ordered. A scan is the best tool to accurately diagnose FGR. Not only can an ultrasound measure the baby's growth, it may also identify a birth defect or infection that is causing the growth restriction.

Can growth restriction be treated?

Beneficial interventions

There are very few interventions that can actually be of benefit. Some of these are:

- Improving your dietary protein may help if you have a poor intake of protein in the first place. For vegetarians, this means increasing intake of dals (including rajma, channa), and dairy products. Eggs are an excellent source of protein. Non-vegetarians can add meat protein
- Increasing blood flow to the baby by lying on your side whenever you take a nap, for example, for an hour after breakfast and an hour after lunch. At night, try to sleep on your side as much as possible
- Low-dose aspirin started before the 16th week helps in women who have high blood pressure
- Stopping smoking helps

Interventions with no benefit

The following have **not** been shown to be of any benefit:

- Complete bed rest
- Protein powders and other so-called food supplements (such a waste of money!)
- Intravenous fluids
- Supplementation with l-arginine, zinc, calcium
- Oxygen therapy for the mother

Nirupama asked: I am 34 weeks and my doctor has told me that my baby is small. An ultrasound confirmed that my baby is growth restricted. My mother immediately bought me protein powder and I am having two teaspoons daily. Will that help?

My answer: There is absolutely no reason to waste money on 'protein powders'. The recommended serving size by the manufacturers is generally 10 g (containing 8 g of protein and providing 36 calories). A single serving therefore costs approximately a whopping Rs 40! The protein in these powders is usually provided by soy and milk protein. Compare this to the cost of 1 cup of yogurt (11.9 g protein and 144 calories), 1 large hard boiled egg, white only (6 g of protein, 30 calories) or ½ cup cooked rajma beans (7.6 g protein, 112 calories). So eat healthy and eat smart!

Is the baby safe?

When there is FGR, we know that the environment inside the uterus is not favourable for the baby. However, if the baby is delivered too early, the outside environment can be unsafe for a preterm baby.

To decide on the best time to deliver the baby, with the least risk, certain tests are done that will let your doctor know if the baby is safe.

You will be instructed on the daily kick count. The baby will be monitored with non-stress tests and ultrasound scans. Ultrasound is used to measure the baby's growth, assess the amniotic fluid volume and perform Doppler blood flow tests (see **Chapter 16**, *Tests of foetal well-being: is the baby tolerating pregnancy well?*).

When will the baby be delivered?

When the baby is very preterm, every day inside the womb improves the chance of the baby surviving after delivery. Your doctor will try to make the decision based on the balance between the baby's prematurity and how she is tolerating pregnancy. If the pregnancy has crossed 34 weeks, the chances of the baby doing well are very good.

How will the baby be delivered?

If the growth restriction is significant, the baby will not tolerate labour well. A caesarean birth might be the safest option.

Problems for the baby after birth

Growth restricted babies require a neonatologist for careful management of their health. They tend to have the following problems:

- Inability to maintain a normal body temperature
- Sudden drop in blood sugar levels
- Low blood calcium levels
- Problems with blood clotting

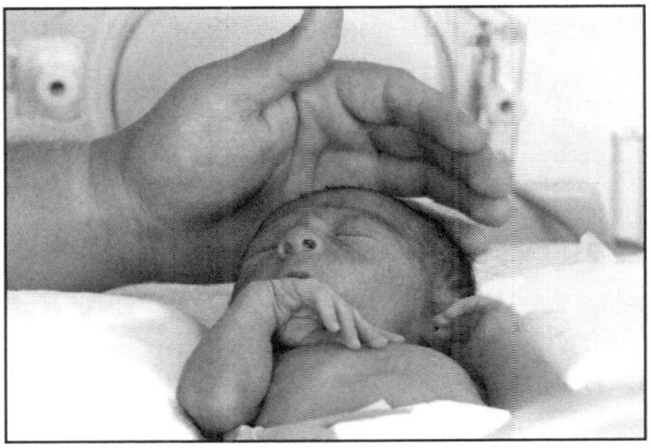

Once they start receiving proper nutrition, the majority of moderately growth restricted babies will do well. Babies with severe growth restriction can be a challenge for the neonataologist and the parents.

MACROSOMIA

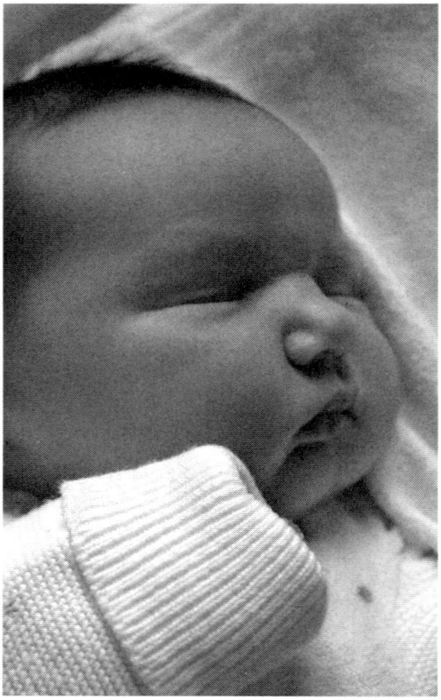

A macrosomic or large baby will have a weight at or above the 90th percentile for that particular week of pregnancy. This definition is country specific. For example, in the United States a baby is large if she weighs 4.5 kg or more at birth. However, in India a baby weighing 3.5 kg or more at term will be at the 90th percentile and so considered large.

As the double problems of obesity and diabetes are on a rise in India, more and more large babies are being born.

What's the problem?

Who doesn't want to have a chubby baby? Why is it a problem? Unfortunately, large babies can cause problems during delivery. Indian women are generally small-made and delivering a large baby can be a major predicament. The mother may have a difficult delivery with damage to the birth canal. The chances of a caesarean section are also very high.

Large babies themselves face problems. They may have a tough time navigating the birth canal and may lead to a major complication called shoulder dystocia. In this, the head gets delivered but the large shoulders get stuck in the birth canal. This can not only put the baby's life at risk, it can also cause nerve damage.

Who is at risk for having a large baby?

- Women who are obese (BMI more than 30 kg/m^2)
- Women with diabetes before pregnancy
- Women with diabetes that first developed in pregnancy but with poor control of sugar levels
- Excessive weight gain in pregnancy

Can macrosomia be prevented?

Though big women will have big babies, it is possible to decrease the chances of a large (macrosomic) baby. You don't need to be big to begin with—you may put on too much weight with indiscriminate eating and have a large baby.

Babies of diabetic mothers

Babies of mothers with longstanding diabetes, or poor control of blood sugar levels are not just large, they have a very specific distribution of fat. The chest is very large and wide and the neck is short. Their shoulders are definitely broad. That is why large babies of diabetic mothers are at high risk for shoulder dystocia and may cause difficult deliveries.

- Keep weight gain in pregnancy under tight control, especially if you are starting out with a high BMI (see **Chapter 10**, *Eating healthy in pregnancy*)
- If you are a diabetic, you should manage your sugar levels strictly by eating healthy and taking the prescribed medications properly. Your doctor will place you under the care of a nutritionist

How is macrosomia diagnosed?

During a routine antenatal check-up near term, your doctor might suspect that the baby is large. An ultrasound will be done to get the estimated foetal weight. Unfortunately, ultrasound diagnosis of macrosomia is not very accurate unless the baby is larger than 4.0 kg.

How will the baby be delivered?

Every mother with a large baby need not be delivered by caesarean section. If you have delivered a large baby vaginally in your previous pregnancy, your doctor will allow you to attempt a vaginal delivery with this pregnancy too.

A caesarean section will be suggested if the baby does not seem to fit into the pelvis. In a diabetic pregnancy with a large baby, a caesarean may be prudent because large diabetic babies have a body shape that makes it difficult for them to navigate the birth canal.

CHAPTER 35

Breech delivery

Suvarna has just visited her obstetrician. She still has three weeks to go before her due date. Her obstetrician has told her that the baby is in breech position. Suvarna is a little concerned. Is being in the breech position harmful for the baby? What kind of delivery will she have?

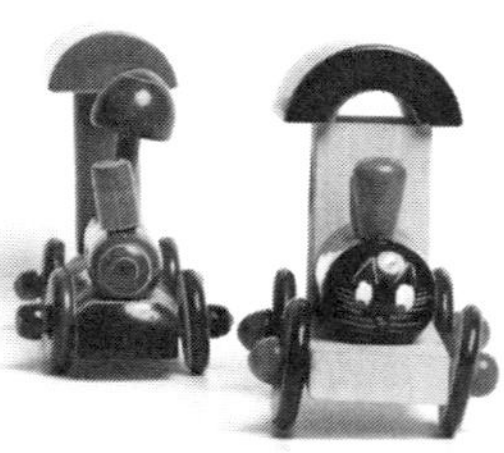

35

Breech delivery

In the early months of pregnancy, your baby is performing gymnastics inside the womb. In the span of a few minutes, the baby can be head-down, bottom-down or lying sideways. This is because there is plenty of space for her to move around.

The upside-down or breech baby

By the time you are 3–4 weeks from your due date, the baby is in more cramped quarters. She will still move around but won't be changing her position too much. She would have found her way into the ready-for-delivery position: head-down, close to your birth canal and with her bottom under your ribs. Once she has reached a stable position in the womb by 36–37 weeks, she will usually not move into a different position after that.

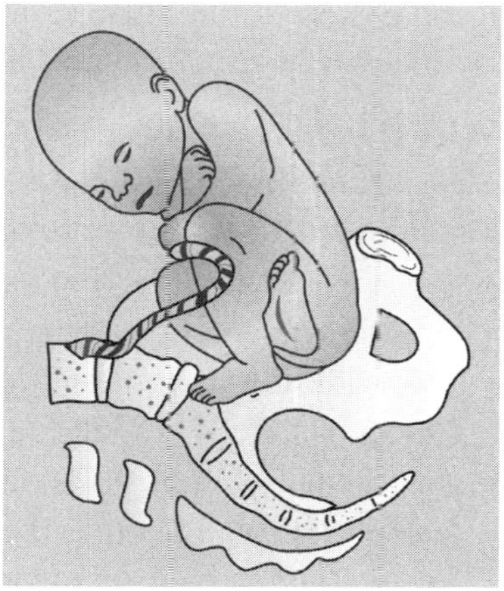

Baby in breech position

There are babies, however, who do not manage to get into the usual head-down position. Three to four per cent of all pregnancies will reach term with the baby still upside-down: the bottom and feet near the birth canal and with the head tucked under your ribs. This position is called breech presentation.

Types of breech presentation

There can be three types of breech presentations: complete, incomplete and frank.

A **frank breech** is the commonest type of breech presentation. With a frank breech the baby's legs are pointing straight up so that her feet are up by the head. The frank breech presentation is the safest position for a baby to be in if a vaginal delivery is to be attempted.

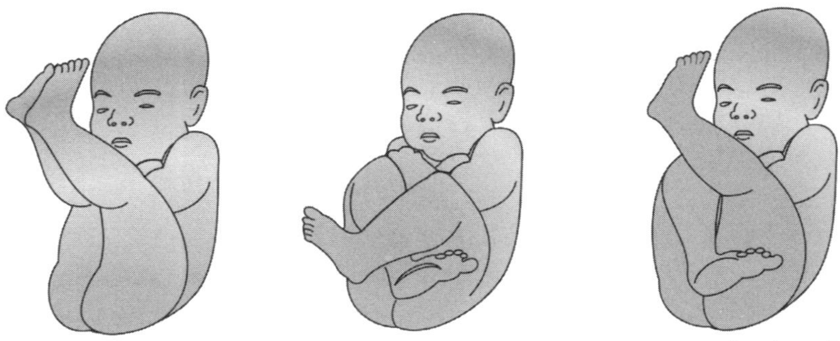

Frank breech Complete breech Incomplete breech

With a **complete breech** presentation, the buttocks are down, with the legs folded at the knees and the feet near the buttocks.

If the baby is in the **incomplete breech** position one or both hips are not flexed and the feet are often below the buttocks.

Why does breech occur?

Most of the time, there is no specific reason why the baby is in a breech position. However it is more common in certain pregnancies:

- *Prematurity* is the most common cause for a breech presentation. This is because there is more amniotic fluid around the baby and the baby is quite literally swimming in all that fluid. That means that it is very often in a breech presentation
- *Polyhydramnios* is a condition where there is excessive amniotic fluid. This too gives the baby too much space to swim around in and so she keeps flipping back into the breech position
- *Oligohydramnios* is a condition where there is too little amniotic fluid. This makes it difficult for the baby to move around and get into position
- *Twin* or *triplet* pregnancy
- Placenta lying very low or in front of the baby (*placenta praevia*)
- A baby with certain *birth defects*
- *Uterine abnormalities* that do not allow the baby to move around well (septate uterus or bicornuate uterus)

How is breech diagnosed?

In the last month of pregnancy, at every check-up your doctor will try to identify which part of the baby is in the lower portion of the uterus. If your baby is head-down, his hard, round head can be felt in the lower part of your abdomen. If he is in a breech position, his head will be felt closer to your ribs. If a breech is suspected, an ultrasound exam may be done to confirm the position.

The baby's position can keep flipping till the end of pregnancy, especially if it is your second or third pregnancy. It is not uncommon for the baby to get into the normal head-down position just before labour starts. In first pregnancies, the chances of the position changing after the 37th or 38th week are less. Sometimes, the baby can surprise the doctor, and the breech presentation is diagnosed during a pelvic exam when you are already in labour.

Changing the baby's position

If the baby is breech, your doctor may suggest **external version**, which is a procedure to manipulate the baby's position into the normal head-down position. This increases the chance of having a vaginal birth and therefore, is highly recommended. Version is not tried until 36–37 weeks of pregnancy. If it is done before then, the baby may still go back to being a breech.

Chitra asked: I am 37 weeks pregnant. My doctor told me my baby is in a breech position and wants to try and turn the baby into the proper position. Is this safe?

My answer: Your doctor has suggested an **external version**. If she can turn your baby into a head-down position, your chances are really good for a vaginal delivery and you can avoid a caesarean section. External version succeeds in more than half the cases. It will not be attempted if the amniotic fluid volume is low, if you have had a previous caesarean section or if there is a uterine abnormality.

You will be given a medication half an hour before the procedure to help relax your uterine muscles. The baby's heartbeat is recorded using a foetal monitor. Your doctor will do an ultrasound to see how the baby is lying in your womb. The position of the placenta and the amount of fluid around the baby are also checked. Scanning is done throughout the procedure to follow the position of the baby as the procedure is being done.

You will be asked to lie down on the examination table and keep your knees flexed (bent) to help relax the abdominal muscles. She will then place her hands on your abdomen, feeling the baby's parts, and gently manipulate the baby's body into the right position. The procedure is uncomfortable but not painful. If any problems arise with you or the baby, version will be stopped right away. After the version, the baby's heart rate is recorded again on a foetal monitor.

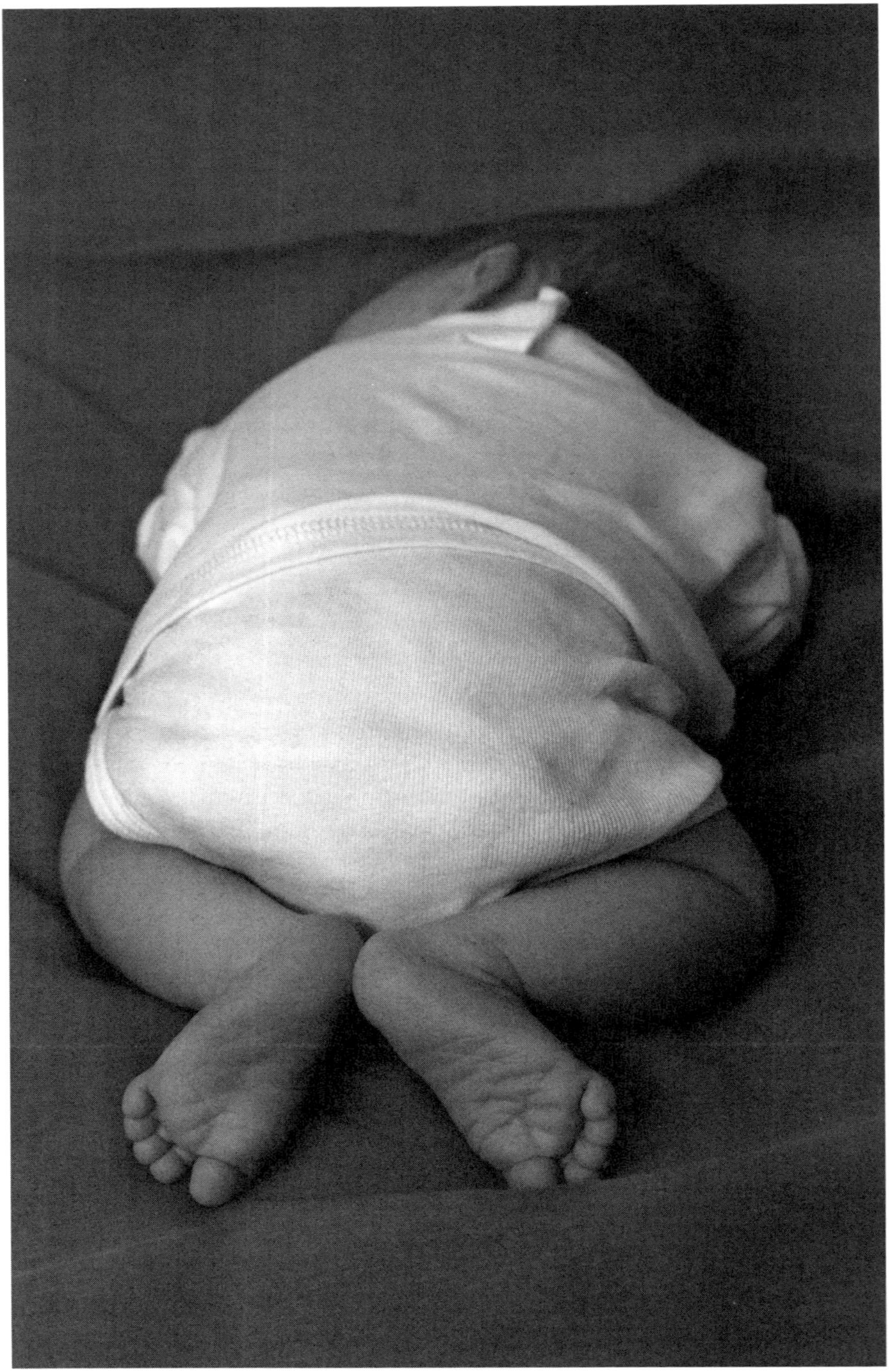

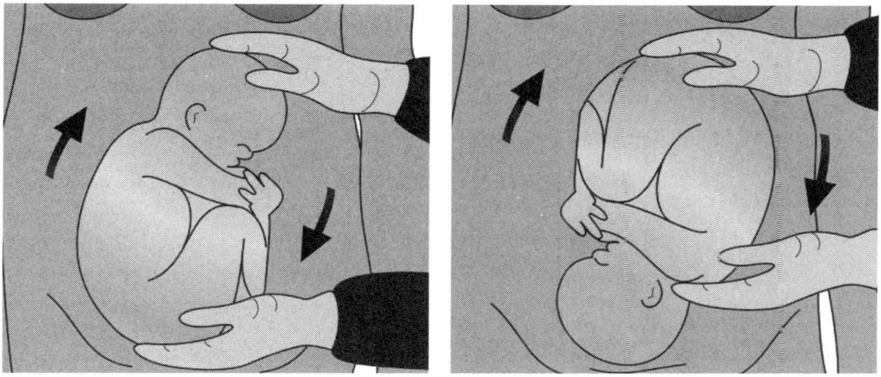

External version: turning the baby from breech to head-down position. The doctor will place her hands on your abdomen, feeling the baby's parts, and gently manipulate the baby's body into the right position.

Delivery of breech

The chances of vaginal delivery for a breech delivery have dropped dramatically in the past two decades after a medical study showed that the breech baby does much better with a caesarean section. Globally, 85–90 per cent of breech babies are born by caesarean section.

Vaginal delivery

If external version has not been successful and the baby is still in breech position at term, and you are particular about a vaginal delivery, you can discuss this with your doctor. If you have had a previous vaginal delivery, if the baby is in frank breech position, and if the baby is less than 3.5 kg, your obstetrician might try to deliver you vaginally.

Caesarean section

If it is known that the baby is in a breech position and a version has failed, an elective caesarean section may be planned. A caesarean section might be the better option especially in first pregnancies. If the breech presentation is discovered during labour, a decision for caesarean may depend on how far labour has progressed.

CHAPTER 36

Twins: double trouble?

Sunanda is exhilarated and at the same time nervous. She has had an ultrasound scan and discovered she is having twins! When she saw the two little babies inside her, her heart skipped a beat and then started racing. Her husband too is thrilled at this unexpected bonus!

Sheela and her husband have been trying for a pregnancy for a few years. They had undergone treatment with medications and have now conceived after a fertility procedure. She had her pregnancy confirmed with an ultrasound scan. She too is having twins.

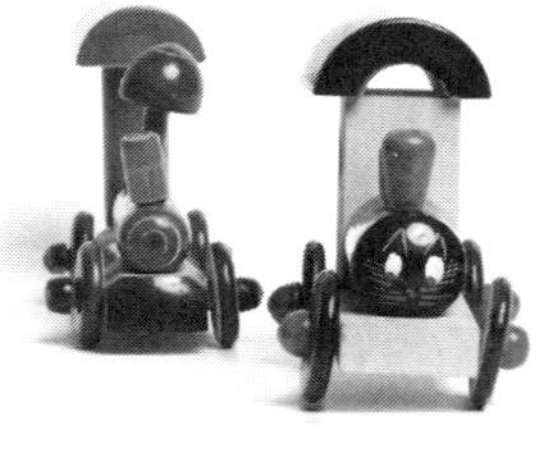

36

Twins: double trouble?

Some parents get very excited when they are told they are having twins. 'It's a double reward for a single pregnancy', they say. They are happy they can reach their goal of two kids with just one pregnancy! Soon, however, reality sinks in and they worry if a twin pregnancy is hard to go through. And what happens after birth? 'How do we manage two little ones at the same time?' they ask.

It is normal to have mixed reactions to the news of twins. You have to deal with the physical challenges of a twin pregnancy. You also worry about providing nutrition for the two babies in the womb, instead of just one. Though a twin pregnancy has its own set of complications, the majority of twin pregnancies will end with a double dose of happiness.

Different types of twins

Identical twins

Identical twins are formed when a single egg gets fertilized by a single sperm. The resulting zygote splits into two and forms two babies. Since

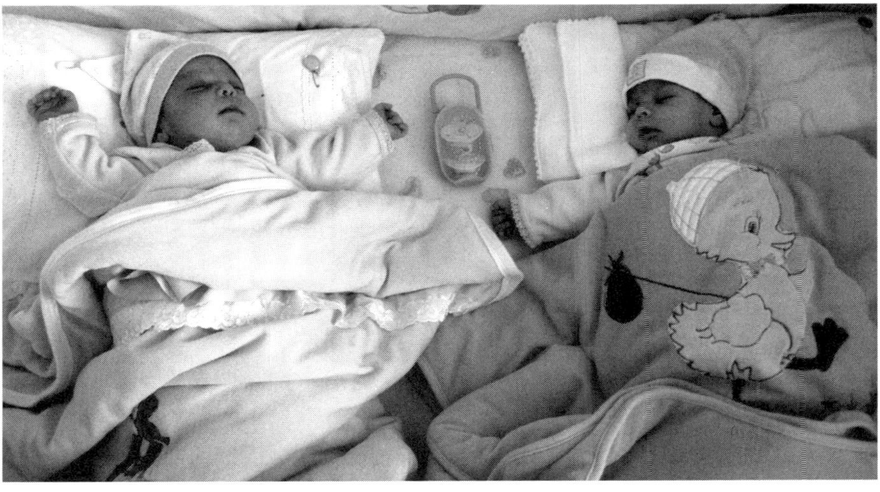

they are of the same genetic origin, they will share the same characteristics including being of the same sex and having the same blood group. Typically they are very similar in appearance.

> Did you know that identical twins are extremely similar but their fingerprints are not identical?

Identical twins may share a placenta, but each baby usually has its own amniotic sac.

Rarely, identical twins fail to completely separate into two individuals. These babies are known as *conjoined twins*.

Non-identical twins or fraternal twins

Non-identical twins or fraternal twins are formed from two different eggs (released during the same menstrual cycle) fertilized by two different sperms. They are like normal brothers and sisters, sharing some but not identical genetic material. They can be of different sexes and may have different blood groups. They can look similar or very different from each other.

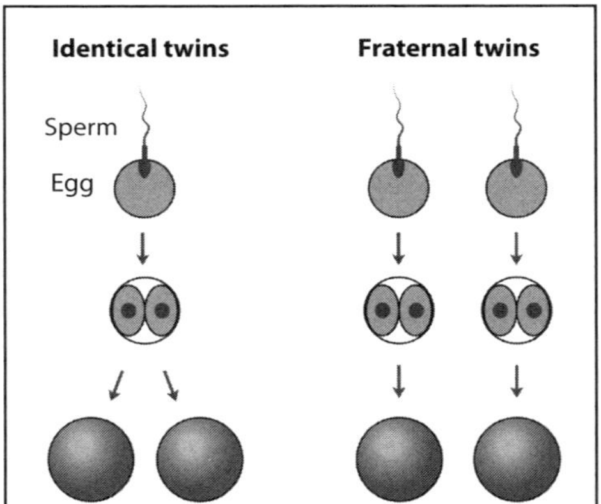

Separate amniotic sacs, shared placenta
Separate amniotic sacs, separate placentas

Fraternal twins each have their own placenta and amniotic sac.

> If a woman has triplets or more babies, they can be identical, fraternal or a combination of both.

How common is a twin pregnancy?

The chance of having **identical twins** has remained fairly constant throughout the world. The likelihood of having identical twins is uniformly **4 in 1000**. Only one-third of all twins in the world are identical.

The chance of having fraternal twins varies in different countries. In India the likelihood of having a fraternal twin is **9 in 1000**. Two-thirds of all twins in the world are fraternal.

Increased chance of having a fraternal twin

The chance of having a fraternal twin pregnancy increases if:

- You are one of fraternal twins
- You have a strong family history of fraternal twins. Your husband's family history of twins doesn't count
- You are 35 or older
- The BMI is more than 30 kg/m^2
- You have used fertility drugs to conceive. They can trigger the release of two or more eggs
- You have conceived through IVF (in-vitro fertilization or 'test tube baby'). This procedure typically involves implanting more than one embryo in the uterus and, therefore, is more likely to result in twins, triplets, quadruplets or more

Diagnosing a twin pregnancy

It is difficult for you to know early in pregnancy if you are carrying twins. One of the hints you might get is excessive vomiting. Since the double pregnancy is producing double the amount of hormones, the nausea and vomiting may be more than if you are carrying a single baby.

Physical examination

Usually your doctor may not be able to diagnose twins in very early pregnancy just from a physical examination. As the pregnancy grows, your obstetrician might suspect a twin pregnancy if your uterus is larger than expected.

Ultrasonography in twin pregnancy

Ultrasonography is an essential tool in the diagnosis and management of twin pregnancy (see **Chapter 13**, *Ultrasound scans in pregnancy*).

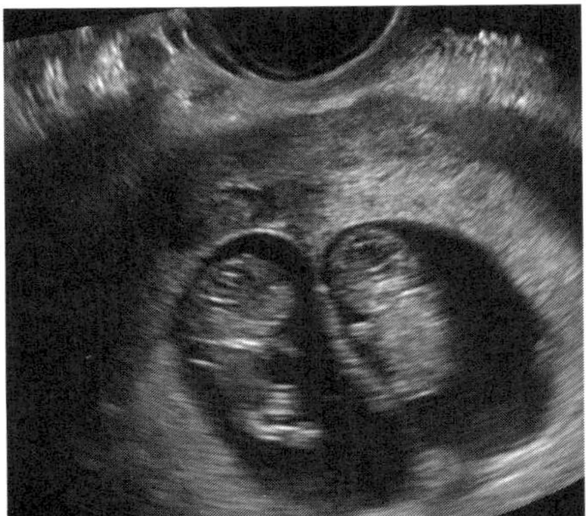

Twins at 8 weeks

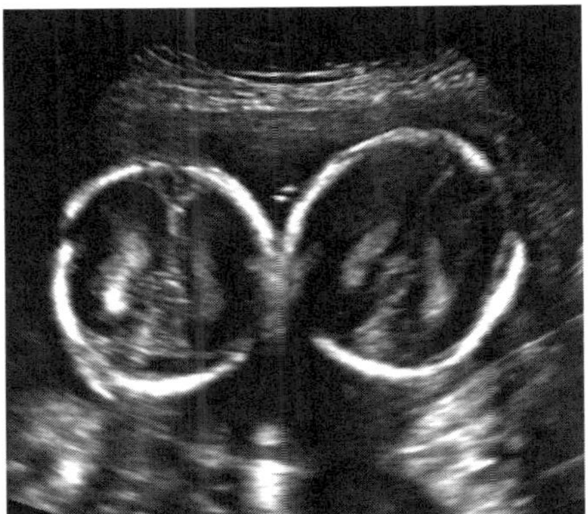

Twin heads seen at 20 weeks

A twin pregnancy can be identified as early as the 5th week of pregnancy. Your obstetrician may tell you that it is usually prudent to wait for one or two more weeks to confirm that it is actually a twin pregnancy because of the phenomenon known as the 'vanishing twin'.

The 'vanishing twin'

Sometimes, when an early ultrasound examination has shown the presence of twins, a repeat ultrasound done a little later in pregnancy may reveal that there is only one baby left in the uterus. You might or might not have experienced bleeding in early pregnancy. There is no known explanation for why one of the twins did not grow but certainly it is not because of anything you did or did not do. The remaining baby grows well and will not have any problem because of this.

Ultrasound imaging also helps in

- Tracking the growth of the babies
- Identifying any birth defects
- Evaluating how the babies are tolerating the pregnancy
- Identifying whether the baby closest to the birth canal is head-down or bottom-down (breech). This is important close to the due date to decide how your babies are going to be delivered

What to expect with a twin pregnancy

Having twins means that you need to take good care of yourself, thus ensuring that your babies grow well and are born with the least amount of complications. Having more than one baby also means that you may have more of everything!

- **More side effects:** Due to the increased amount of hormones produced, a twin pregnancy may result in an increase in the usual pregnancy complaints, such as nausea, vomiting, heartburn, sleeplessness and tiredness. As the babies grow, the physical discomfort due to the large abdomen may result in abdominal pain, shortness of breath and pressure on the bladder. As the pregnancy progresses, you might find it more and more difficult to find a comfortable position to sleep in.

Two babies, two heartbeats

Your doctor will listen for two heartbeats at each check-up. The heartbeats are heard at a distance from each other to make sure that both heartbeats are being located. If there is a doubt, the doctor will use an ultrasound to confirm both heartbeats.

- **More frequent check-ups:** Your obstetrician may schedule more frequent check-ups after the seventh month of pregnancy. This is to monitor the growth and development of the babies, monitor your health and watch out for signs of preterm labour (see **Chapter 32**, *When the baby comes too early: preterm labour and birth*).
- **More frequent ultrasound examinations:** Repeat scans may be advised to monitor the growth of the babies. Some twins may have a problem with growth and in some twin pregnancies one baby may grow more than the other. There are some complications that can occur specifically in twin pregnancies and these need to be carefully looked for.
- **More nutrition:** It is important for you to gain the optimal amount of weight. Eating a nutritious diet will ensure that the twins gain the right weight and are healthy at birth. When pregnant with twins, you will need to eat more than if you were carrying one baby. In addition to nurturing the babies, your diet must provide enough calories to meet your own energy needs.

  Concentrate on getting enough proteins because they are the building blocks of your babies' bodies. You too need enough proteins to keep up your energy (see **Chapter 10**, *Eating healthy in pregnancy*).
- **More rest:** Your doctor might recommend that you have more rest, particularly from the seventh month of pregnancy and beyond. Due to the increased volume of the uterus, you might find it uncomfortable to move around. It is nevertheless important to keep up a gentle exercise regimen. You might be asked to exert yourself less as you reach the last two months of pregnancy to decrease the chances of preterm labour.

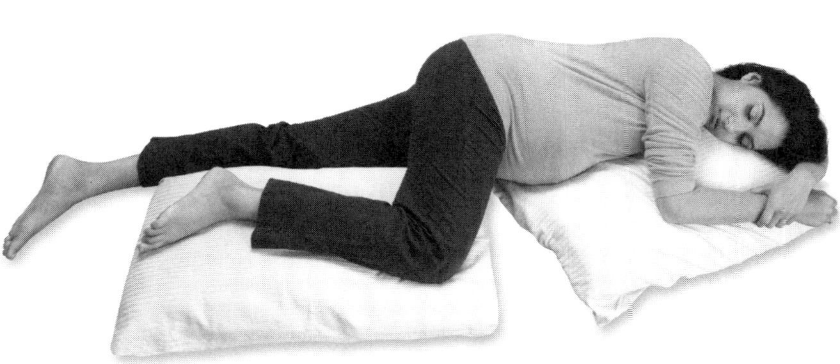

- **More iron:** Anaemia (a low red blood cell count) is more common in women who are pregnant with twins, so it is especially important to take your prenatal vitamins and iron as prescribed. Folic acid also is important for twins. It is hard to get all the folic acid you need just from your diet, so you need to take a prenatal vitamin that contains folic acid.

Iron and vitamin supplements

Your iron supplement should contain at least 60 mg of elemental iron. Most combined prenatal vitamins contain iron, vitamin B12 and folic acid and all three are required to avoid anaemia.

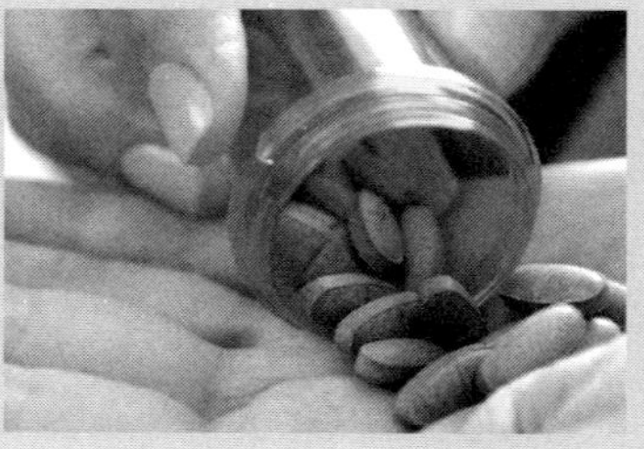

Urmila asked: I am 31 years old. I am pregnant for the first time and I just found out that I have twins. I was very excited but my husband wants me to quit my job and my mother-in-law says I should be at complete bed rest for the next three months because I have twins. Please tell me what to do.

My answer: It is always exciting to know that one is carrying twins. I am afraid I disagree with your husband. You definitely do not have to quit your job. You can certainly go to work and carry on all your responsibilities. Your mother-in-law is misinformed. There is absolutely no need for you to be at bed rest just because you are carrying twins.

Closer to the due date, your obstetrician may recommend slowing down, to prevent preterm labour. As the babies grow, there is an increased chance of going into labour, earlier than a woman carrying a single baby. You may find that after the 8th month, you get fatigued sooner. Nowadays, when many women can work from home, you might choose to stop going to the office and, if possible, work from home. Even if you have to take leave earlier than a woman who is carrying a single baby, it does not mean that you have to be at bed rest. You can continue to do light housework and go for your daily walks.

Double trouble: problems with twin pregnancy

Though most twin pregnancies will progress smoothly, the challenges for both you and your little ones are greater. This is the reason your doctor will see you more often after the 28th week.

What problems can you expect?

Overdistended uterus: As the two babies fight for space in your womb, you might suffer discomfort and pressure symptoms. Carrying all that extra weight will cause vague aches and pains. The other symptoms you will face are:

- Low backache due to the increased arching of your back
- Swollen feet: keep your feet up on a stool whenever you can and sleep with your feet propped on pillows
- Heartburn: small meals taken at frequent intervals will help. Ask you doctor for antacids. Don't lie down for at least two hours immediately after a meal
- Inability to eat because your stomach feels full with even a small quantity because the expanding uterus is pushing against your stomach. Eat several smaller meals a day (small portions will be easy to manage and will provide enough calories if taken at frequent intervals)
- Difficulty in breathing since the distended uterus is displacing your diaphragm upward

Preterm or premature labour: Preterm labour refers to contractions that cause the cervix to open before the 37th week of pregnancy (see **Chapter 32**, *When the baby comes too early: preterm labour and birth*). Labour generally begins at 37 to 41 weeks in most pregnancies with a single baby.

In a twin pregnancy, it is not unusual to go into labour between 36 and 38 weeks. The uterus is overdistended with the babies and this can trigger labour earlier than in a pregnancy with a single baby. You might be asked to be at rest and decrease excessive exertion from the 36th week of pregnancy.

Though much less common, labour may begin before 34 weeks. In that case you might be given steroid injections that help the babies' lungs mature faster so that they have an easier time breathing after birth.

Preterm birth: If preterm labour cannot be prevented or stopped once it has started, the babies may be born too early. Preterm birth is one of the commonest risks for twins. Twins born too early may face the same problems that any premature baby will face.

High blood pressure: When you are carrying twins, you have a greater risk of developing high blood pressure or preeclampsia. Preeclampsia is a condition in pregnancy in which there is high blood pressure along with protein (albumin) in the urine. Preeclampsia is 3–4 times more common

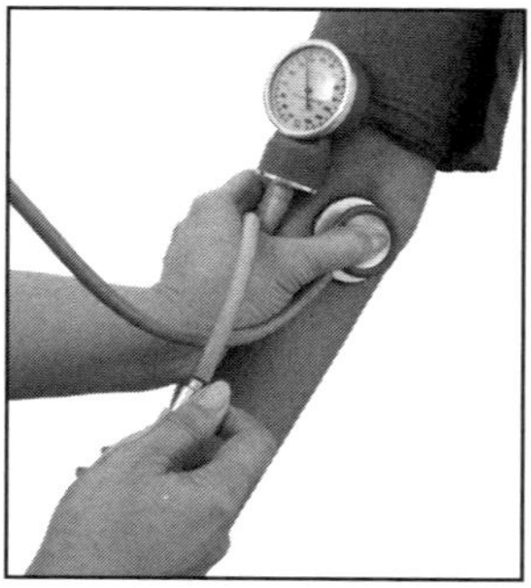

with twins (see **Chapter 37**, *High blood pressure in pregnancy*). Preeclampsia complicating pregnancy can have harmful effects on the babies. The blood flow to the babies is reduced and this results in less oxygen and nutrients reaching the babies, leading to foetal growth restriction (see **Chapter 34**, *Foetal growth problems: too small or too big*). The babies may need to be delivered early if the blood pressure becomes too high.

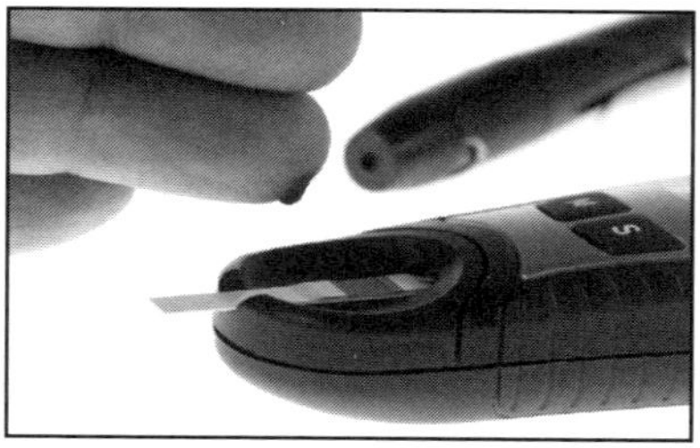

Gestational diabetes: Mothers of twins are more likely to develop gestational diabetes, a type of diabetes occurring in pregnancy (see **Chapter 38**, *Diabetes in pregnancy*).

Growth problems: Twins are more likely to be smaller than average. Ultrasound scans are done more often in a twin pregnancy, mainly to monitor the growth of the babies. The amount of amniotic fluid surrounding each baby also needs to be monitored.

Twins are said to have **discordant growth** if one is much smaller than the other. Discordant twins are more likely to have problems during pregnancy and after birth. Twins may be discordant because of poor functioning of the placenta.

Kick count in twins

Just as in a singleton pregnancy, it is always a good idea to keep track of how the babies are moving. Some mothers may actually be able to make out which baby is moving—that is because some twins are lying back-to-back and their little hands and feet are on opposite sides. However, most mothers will only feel a jumble of movements. Since the space gets cramped fairly early for twins, you will usually feel less sharp kicks and jabs after 32 weeks. You won't be able to keep a kick count for each baby but keep a general kick count (see **Chapter 16**, *Tests of foetal well-being: is the baby tolerating pregnancy well?*). If you think the movements are less even after one hour of observation, contact your doctor immediately.

Twin-to-twin transfusion: This is a rare complication and occurs only in identical twins. In this condition, a blood vessel in the placenta connects the circulatory system of one baby to the other. This causes one baby to receive too much blood and the other, too little.

Loss of one twin in early pregnancy: In some twin pregnancies, one of the babies dies in early pregnancy. You may have some spotting or bleeding from your vagina. This does not harm you or the other baby.

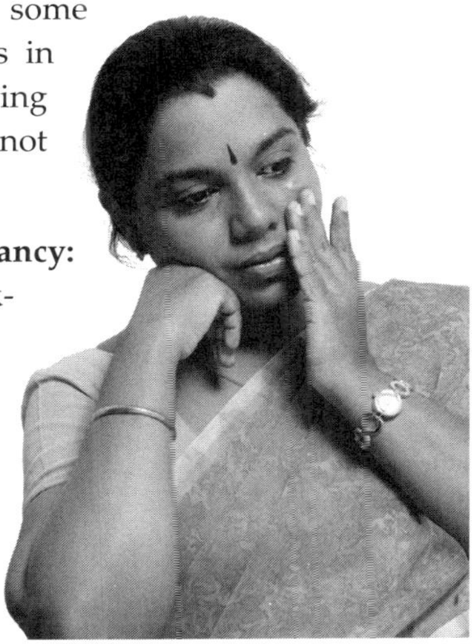

Losing one of the babies later in pregnancy: This situation is rare. At one of the check-ups, it might be found that one of the twins does not have a heartbeat. Though this is a more serious situation, with careful monitoring, you can often still have one healthy child. The support of your obstetrician and your family can help you go through this and deliver one live child, without any danger to your health.

An abnormal twin: In some twin pregnancies, an ultrasound scan may reveal that one of the twins is abnormal. You may still choose to carry the pregnancy to term, knowing that you can expect one normal baby. Your obstetrician will be able to guide you and counsel you about the pregnancy.

Delivery of twins

Most twins can be delivered vaginally, if the baby closest to the birth canal is coming down head-first. A vaginal birth may be possible even when the second twin is not in the head-down position, as long as the lower twin is in the head-down position. Once the first twin is born, the other twin can sometimes be turned, or delivered with feet or buttocks first. When the first twin is not in the head-down position, both twins are delivered by caesarean birth.

Your obstetrician will make the decision about the type of delivery depending on the position of each baby, the weight and health of the babies. The decision will also depend on whether you are having any complications such as preeclampsia or gestational diabetes. Rarely, complications after the vaginal delivery of the first twin may require a caesarean section for the second twin.

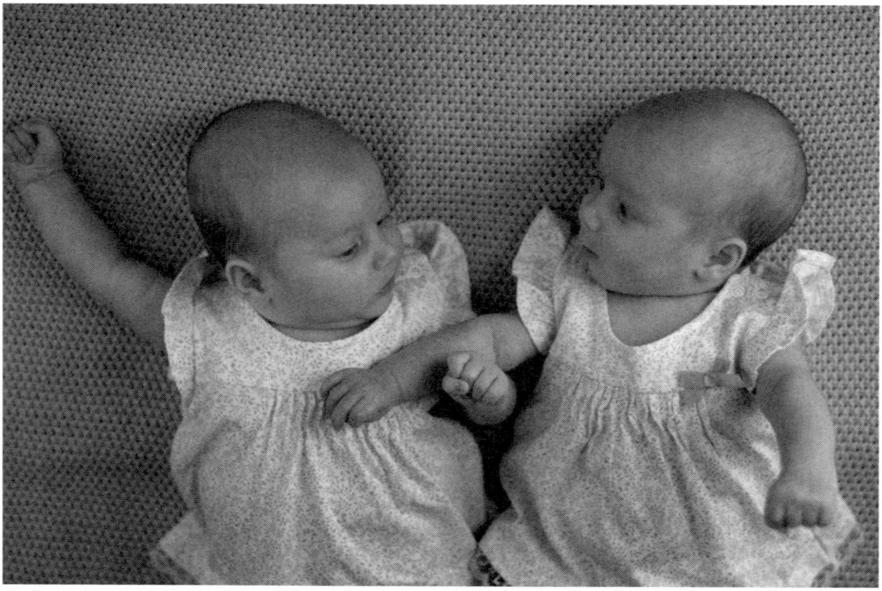

Labour, especially the pushing stage, can last longer with twins. Babies usually are born several minutes apart in a vaginal delivery, but it can take longer.

Caring for newborn twins

Delivering twins is the easy part! Once you take them home, you may feel a little overwhelmed by the constant demands of two infants. You may feel exhausted and sleep deprived. Make sure you have family members to help you in the first few weeks. Get as much rest as possible. Sleep when the babies are sleeping. Also take turns with family members to handle and care for the babies.

Most twins do well at birth and can be cared for like any other healthy babies. If the babies are born prematurely, they may be kept in the nursery in the hospital after birth. Some twins may need admission to a neonatal intensive care unit (NICU).

Breastfeeding twins

Breastfeeding twins can be a challenge. You may be concerned that you may not be able to breastfeed more than one baby. Remember that mother's milk is the best food for any infant. It has the right amount of all the nutrients the baby needs (see **Chapter 27**, *Breastfeeding*). When you breastfeed, your milk supply will increase to meet the amount needed by your babies. You will need to eat healthy foods and drink plenty of liquids. If you are exhausted and feel that you are not be able to breastfeed both babies despite your best efforts, your paediatrician may prescribe a milk supplement so that you can alternate between breastfeeding and supplement.

Names for twins

If you are having twins, use your imagination and name the babies with something unique! Some parents choose to name the twins with rhyming or interlinked names.

Some examples for a boy and girl combination are Maya and Mayank, Michael and Michelle, Neel and Neelanjana.

Two girls could be called Archita and Rachita, Manasa and Madhuri, or Devyani and Devanshi. Two boys could be called Vinay and Vijay, Tarun and Varun or Manav and Pranav.

What a great opportunity to come up with something appealing and attention-grabbing!

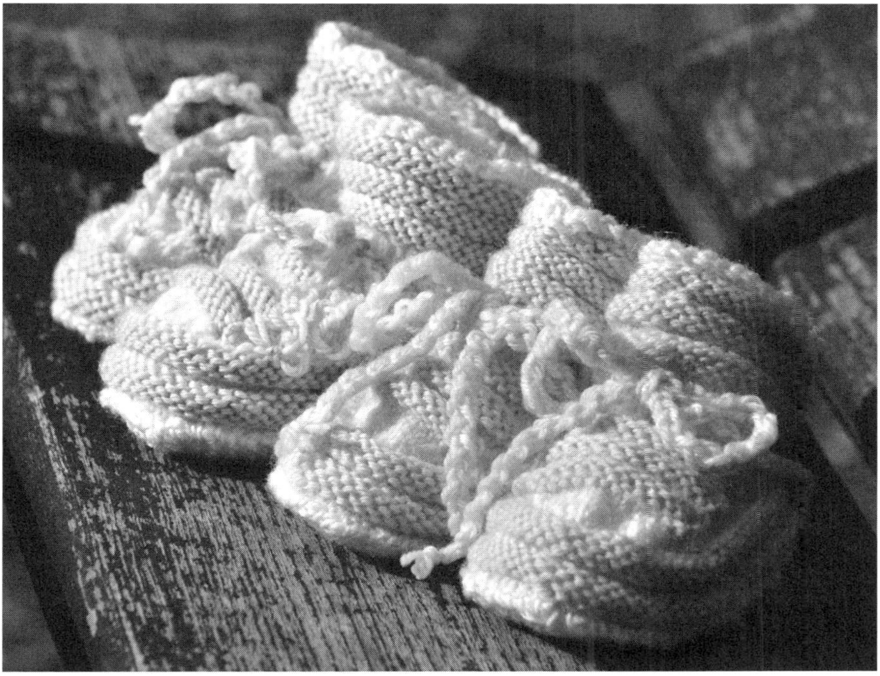

CHAPTER 37

High blood pressure in pregnancy

Sabrina has just come back from a check-up with her doctor. She is 34 weeks pregnant and her blood pressure was 140/90 at the check-up. Her doctor has told her to rest and come back after two days to check her blood pressure again. Sabrina is naturally concerned. How will the high blood pressure affect her and her baby?

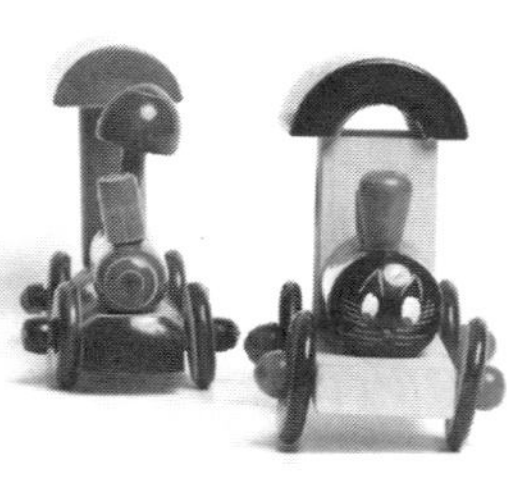

37

High blood pressure in pregnancy

Have you wondered why your doctor records your blood pressure at every antenatal check-up? Having a normal blood pressure is an important component of good health at any stage of life. In pregnancy too, a normal blood pressure through the course of the pregnancy will ensure good health for you and the baby. At each antenatal visit, a urine sample is also tested for the presence of albumin (protein). These two tests help in catching the earliest signs of hypertensive disease in pregnancy.

An elevation of your blood pressure isn't necessarily a signal to panic. High blood pressure in pregnancy is not uncommon. In fact, 10 out of a 100 pregnant Indian women will develop high blood pressure in pregnancy. About 70 per cent will occur in women pregnant for the first time. Though high blood pressure can cause problems for both the mother and the baby if not treated, the majority of women will still deliver a completely healthy baby.

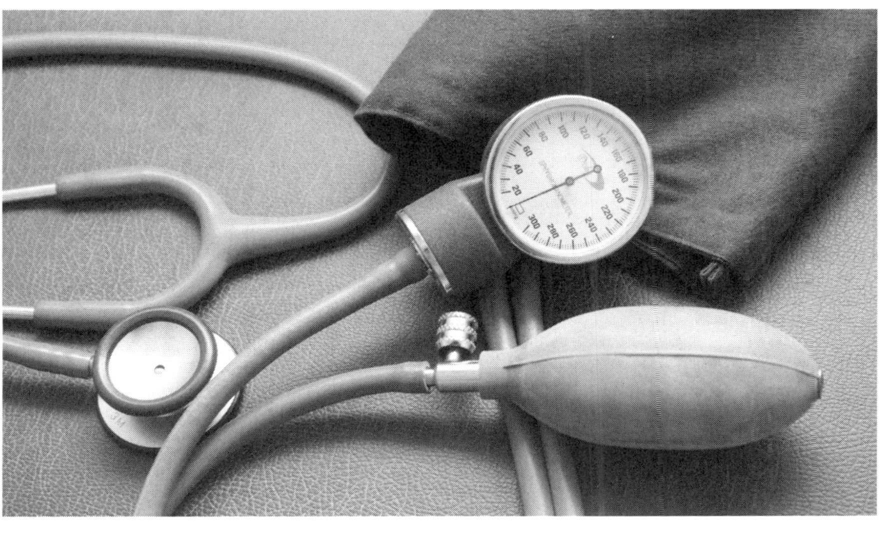

What is high blood pressure?

When the pressure in your arteries goes beyond a set limit, it is called *hypertension* or high blood pressure.

Blood pressure varies from person to person. It may even change with the time of day. It can increase if you are excited or if you exercise. It decreases when you are resting. These short-term changes in blood pressure are normal.

Blood pressure

Arteries are blood vessels that carry oxygen-rich blood from the heart to all parts of the body.

Blood pressure is the force of the blood pushing against the walls of arteries.

When your blood pressure stays persistently high, even after being checked two or three times, you are said to have high blood pressure or hypertension.

A blood pressure reading has two numbers, separated by a slash: for example, 110/80 (referred to as '110 by 80'.) The first number is the pressure in the arteries when the heart contracts. This is called the **systolic pressure.** The second number is the pressure in the arteries when the heart relaxes between contractions. This is the **diastolic pressure.** Though both systolic and diastolic rise in high blood pressure, a high diastolic reading is more problematic. Blood pressure is expressed as *millimetres of mercury (mm Hg).*

110	Systolic	Pressure in arteries when heart contracts
80	Diastolic	Pressure in arteries when heart relaxes

High blood pressure in pregnancy

In most pregnant women, readings of 120/80 or less are normal. If you are pregnant and your blood pressure is 140/90 or higher on two or more readings, you are considered to have high blood pressure.

If you have one high reading, don't panic. Did you know that many people get what is known as *'white coat hypertension'*? Just seeing the doctor in the hospital can send your blood pressure soaring for a short while. That is why another reading will be taken at least 4 hours later.

'Low' blood pressure?

It is very common for young Indian women to have a blood pressure of 90/60 or 100/70. This is absolutely normal. Unlike high blood pressure, there is no disease known as 'low blood pressure' in a healthy woman who is otherwise normal.

If your diastolic blood pressure is persistently over 90, then you will be considered to have hypertension in pregnancy.

Though high blood pressure in pregnancy can cause complications for mother and baby, serious problems can generally be prevented with proper prenatal care.

How does high blood pressure affect pregnancy?

When the mother has a normal blood pressure, there is good blood flow through the placenta. This enables the growing baby to get all the necessary nutrients and oxygen from the mother.

When high blood pressure occurs in pregnancy, the placenta is often abnormal and the blood flow through the placenta is affected. This effectively means that the baby is receiving less nutrients and oxygen.

High blood pressure in pregnancy can lead to:

Foetal growth restriction (intrauterine growth restriction): Decreased blood flow from the placenta causes growth restriction in the baby, resulting in low birth weight (see **Chapter 34**, *Foetal growth problems: too small or too big*).

> Growth restriction can be more marked in women who develop high blood pressure before 34 weeks of pregnancy or those who have uncontrolled chronic hypertension.

Preterm or premature delivery: When you have high blood pressure, there is an increased chance of delivering the baby before 37 weeks of pregnancy. This usually happens when the baby shows signs of receiving less nutrition or oxygen and the doctor will choose to deliver the baby rather than leaving him in the womb. Delivering the baby (even if he is premature) may also be the only way of treating high blood pressure that is worsening.

Types of high blood pressure in pregnancy

Chronic hypertension

Chronic hypertension is high blood pressure that has been present before pregnancy or that is diagnosed before the 20th week of pregnancy. It is also called **essential hypertension**. This form of hypertension will persist even after the delivery. The causes of chronic hypertension are not clearly understood, although heredity, obesity, diet and lifestyle may play a role.

During pregnancy, chronic hypertension may affect the growth of the baby. Most women with chronic hypertension have healthy pregnancies.

However, about 25 per cent develop a form of gestational hypertension called preeclampsia, which poses special risks (see below).

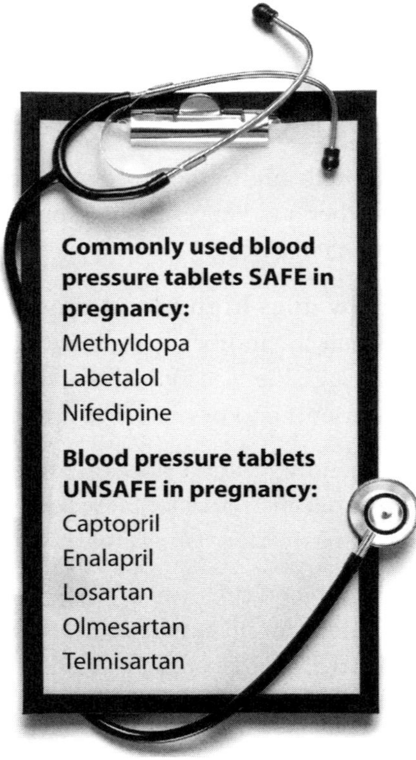

Preparing for pregnancy: If you have been taking medications before pregnancy to control your blood pressure, it is important for you to see your physician before attempting to conceive. This will ensure that the blood pressure is well under control before the pregnancy and therefore, will have the least amount of negative impact on your little one. This also will allow your doctor to switch you to a drug that is safe in pregnancy.

Gestational hypertension or pregnancy induced hypertension (PIH)

When high blood pressure is first detected after the 20th week of pregnancy, it is known as gestational hypertension. Your blood pressure usually returns to normal once the baby is born.

Once high blood pressure is detected in pregnancy, you will be required to see your doctor more often to monitor the blood pressure. Gestational hypertension may lead to preeclampsia and can jeopardize the health of the mother and the baby.

Preeclampsia

To this day, it is not clear why some women develop preeclampsia. Preeclampsia can occur anytime after the 20th week of pregnancy and up to six weeks after the baby is born.

When gestational hypertension is associated with one or more of the following signs, then the condition is called preeclampsia:

- Protein (albumin) in the urine
- Persistent headache
- Visual problems like blurring, double vision
- Rapid weight gain due to excessive water retention
- Swelling (oedema) of the hands and face

Who is at risk for developing preeclampsia?

Women are at risk of developing preeclampsia if they:

- Are pregnant for the first time
- Have had preeclampsia in a previous pregnancy
- Have a history of chronic hypertension
- Have twins or triplets
- Are 35 years or older
- Are diabetic
- Have kidney disease
- Are overweight

Eclampsia

When preeclampsia is associated with seizures (fits), it is called eclampsia. **Eclampsia is rare in women who receive regular antenatal care.**

This is a severe and dangerous situation for both the mother and the baby. Immediate delivery is sometimes the only way of saving the mother.

Management of high blood pressure in pregnancy

Limited activity

If there is only a mild increase in blood pressure, and you are not close to your due date, you might be advised rest. The best is to lie on your side for an hour after breakfast, two hours after lunch and to lie mostly on your sides in the night. Of course, this may not be possible if you are a working woman, so you might need to take a week or two off.

Durga asked: I am 34 weeks pregnant. Last week my doctor found that I have developed high blood pressure and he placed me on tablets. My mother-in-law has cut down my salt drastically. Why can't I have salt?

My answer: You need not change your diet for high blood pressure that appeared for the first time in pregnancy. You need not cut down on your salt, though I would suggest avoiding very salty food like pickles and chips, not because of the high blood pressure but because the high salt content is generally not good for you. Salt restriction is only advised for women with chronic hypertension. They should take less salt in their food.

Blood pressure medications

If the blood pressure does not get under control with these measures, you might be prescribed blood pressure medications. Methyldopa, labetalol and nifedipine are the most commonly used medications that are safe for both you and your baby. If the blood pressure does not come down to normal levels within a week in spite of drugs, you might be admitted to the hospital for a few days for adjusting the dosage of your medications.

You might also be admitted to the hospital if the blood pressure is abnormally high, and your medications will be monitored till the optimal dose is reached. If the blood pressure does not increase to very high levels, and if you do not develop preeclampsia, pregnancy may be allowed to continue until labour begins naturally.

HELLP syndrome

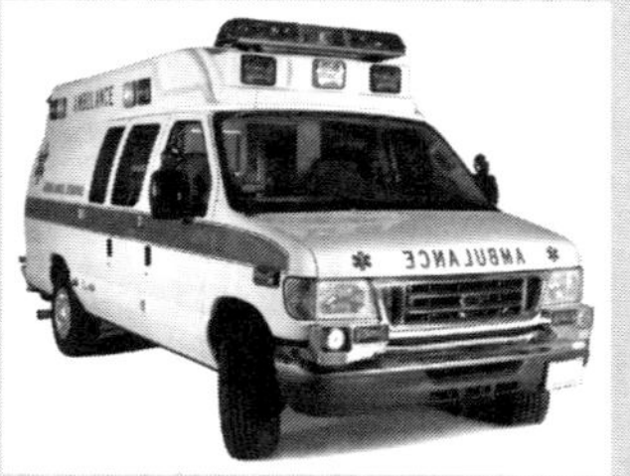

About 10 per cent of women with severe preeclampsia also develop a disorder called HELLP (Haemolysis, Elevated Liver enzymes, and Low Platelet count) syndrome, which is characterized by blood and liver abnormalities. Symptoms may include nausea and vomiting, headache, upper abdominal pain and general malaise. HELLP syndrome is a life-threatening condition. Women who develop HELLP syndrome during pregnancy require intensive monitoring. They almost always require immediate delivery to prevent serious complications.

Is the baby doing well?

Your baby's well-being will be closely monitored with non-stress tests and monitoring of the amniotic fluid volume (see **Chapter 16**, *Tests of foetal well-being: is the baby tolerating pregnancy well?*).

When will you be delivered?

Delivery will be considered if:

- There is persistent protein (albumin) in the urine
- The high blood pressure is having a harmful effect on your health
- The baby is not tolerating pregnancy

Delivering the baby is the only effective cure for severe high blood pressure, severe preeclampsia or eclampsia.

The decision is easier if you are closer to term because the baby will do well when delivered. If you are still preterm, your doctor will have to make a balanced decision based on your health and the baby's condition. The risk of prematurity is outweighed by the risk of progression to eclampsia. Eclampsia is a life threatening condition and is best avoided.

Either labour will be induced or a caesarean section will be done (if the conditions are not favourable or the baby cannot tolerate labour).

Preventing gestational hypertension and preeclampsia

Since nobody really knows why high blood pressure occurs in pregnancy, currently there is no way to prevent gestational hypertension or pre-eclampsia *in a first pregnancy*. However, the complications arising from high blood pressure in pregnancy can be minimized with regular antenatal check-ups and appropriate intervention.

Low-dose aspirin is given to prevent the recurrence of preeclampsia in some women (see box below).

Preventing high blood pressure and preeclampsia in the next pregnancy

Low dose aspirin (75 mg per day) may be started in the first trimester to prevent recurrence of high blood pressure in the present pregnancy in:

- Women who had developed high blood pressure before 34 weeks of pregnancy in an earlier pregnancy
- Women who already have high blood pressure before they become pregnant. It decreases the chances of developing preeclampsia

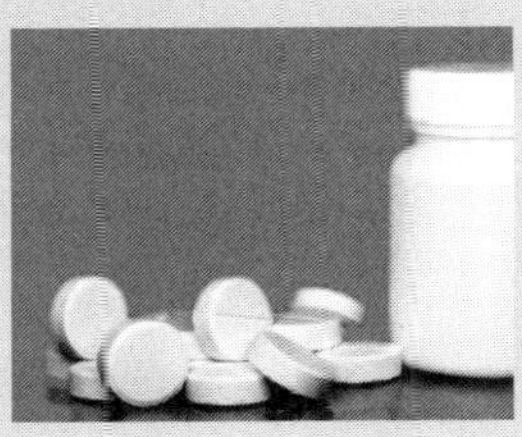

Is preeclampsia likely to recur in another pregnancy?

If you developed preeclampsia after the 37th week of pregnancy, you have a 20 per cent chance of getting it again with the next pregnancy.

However, if the preeclampsia occurred before the 32nd week of pregnancy, the risk of recurrence may be as high as 65 per cent in the next pregnancy.

CHAPTER 38

Diabetes in pregnancy

Sunanda is in her 28th week of pregnancy and has just been told that she has developed diabetes in pregnancy. Diabetes that develops or is first detected in pregnancy is known as gestational diabetes.

Sunetra, on the other hand, has been a diabetic for the past three years. She is 29 and pregnant for the first time.

Both have an excellent chance of delivering a healthy baby if they keep their sugar levels under good control. Their doctors will give them instructions and treatment that they must follow.

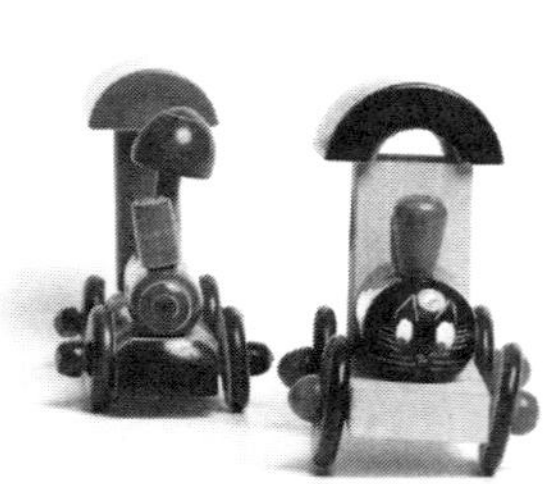

38

Diabetes in pregnancy

You went for a routine check-up in the 28th week of pregnancy. Your doctor asked you to undergo a routine blood test for sugar levels. The next thing you know, you are being told you have diabetes in pregnancy. When you are first diagnosed as having diabetes in pregnancy, the foremost thought that runs through your head is, 'Will my baby be fine?' You may also start stressing out about all the instructions you receive about diet, exercise and medications. Remember that you are not alone in this. The number of women developing diabetes in pregnancy has gone up almost 4 times in the past three decades.

Why is diabetes in pregnancy becoming so common?

In India, diabetes is now an epidemic. With changing lifestyles that involve access to too much food and an alarming absence of exercise, urban Indians particularly are facing the constant risk of diabetes. This

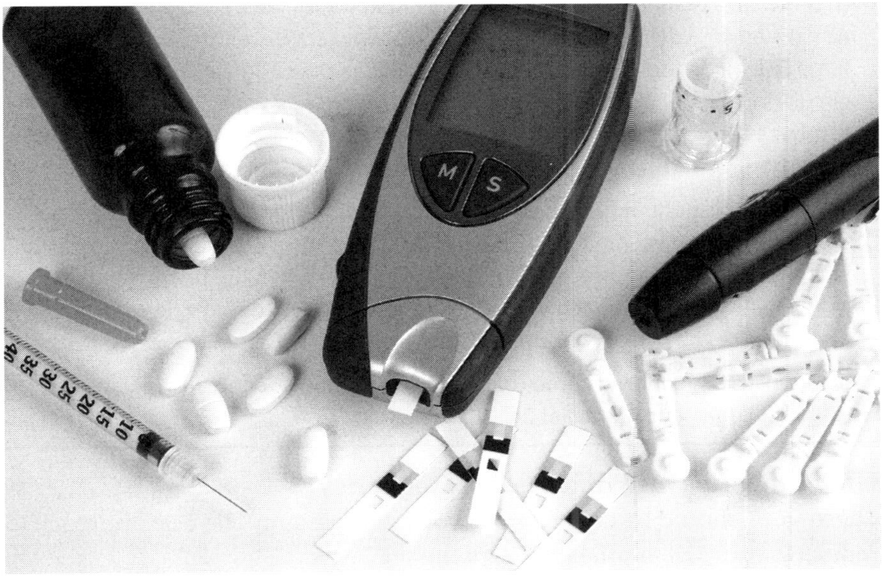

reflects too in the occurrence of diabetes in pregnancy. Three decades ago, 3 per cent of pregnant women developed diabetes. Today the rate in urban India is reported as 12 per cent, with some places reporting rates as high as 15 per cent.

Are you at risk for developing diabetes in pregnancy?

Sadly, just being an Indian increases your risk of developing diabetes in pregnancy. The risk of developing gestational diabetes increases with

- Age over 25
- Being overweight prior to pregnancy
- A strong family history of diabetes
- A history of diabetes in a previous pregnancy
- A baby weighing 4.0 kg or more in a previous pregnancy
- Having lost a baby late in pregnancy (stillbirth)
- High blood pressure, with or without high cholesterol levels
- Polycystic ovarian syndrome

Ameena asked: I am 29 years old and pregnant for the second time. I have completed 8 weeks. My first baby weighed 4.1 kilos at birth. My doctor tells me I am at high risk for developing diabetes and has scheduled me for a blood sugar test. Should I be worried?

My answer: Delivering a baby weighing 4.0 kilos or more is a red flag that you may develop diabetes in a subsequent pregnancy (or later on in life). Though all women who deliver large babies may not have (or develop) diabetes, a large baby is an indication that there might have been high levels of sugar circulating in your body. When the baby gets high levels of sugar from the mother's blood stream, he starts producing high levels of insulin to deal with the sugars. Unfortunately high insulin levels make the baby put on weight.

Your doctor is right in testing you early in pregnancy for the presence of diabetes. If you have high blood sugars early in pregnancy, there is a chance that the baby may be affected. The baby's organs form in the first 3 months of pregnancy and high sugar levels at this time may cause deformities and may also increase the risk of miscarriage.

If your blood sugar level comes back as normal, then your obstetrician will test your sugar levels again at 24–28 weeks.

How can you avoid diabetes in pregnancy?

These steps should be taken **before** you get pregnant. The best approach to reducing your risk of diabetes in pregnancy is:

- Optimize your pre-pregnancy weight. The closer you are to the optimum BMI for your height before you get pregnant, the lesser the chances of developing diabetes in pregnancy
- Build-in a regular exercise regimen to fit your lifestyle. There is strong evidence that brisk walking for at least 45 minutes, 5 days a week, can postpone the onset of diabetes for some years
- Reduce your waist measurement. There is definite correlation between abdominal fat and developing diabetes, at any age
- If one or both your parents have diabetes, or you have a sibling with diabetes, seek advice from your physician before you plan a pregnancy. Have your blood sugar levels tested. If your test shows that you don't have diabetes but have a tendency for diabetes (impaired glucose tolerance), get nutritional advice for a healthy diet and incorporate exercise into your daily routine

What are the types of diabetes in pregnancy?

The two types of diabetes in pregnancy are:

Gestational diabetes: This type of diabetes occurs first in pregnancy as a result of the changes that pregnancy hormones bring about. **It is diagnosed after the 20th week of pregnancy**

> Why do we need to know this? It is important to differentiate the two types because gestational diabetes has less of an adverse impact on the baby's health as compared to pregestational diabetes.

Pregestational diabetes: This type of diabetes is already present prior to pregnancy or **is diagnosed before the 20th weeks of pregnancy**. Even if you didn't know you had diabetes before you became pregnant, the fact that diabetes is diagnosed before the 20th week means you already had high levels of sugar when you conceived

Gestational diabetes

Diabetes caused by pregnancy is known as gestational diabetes. Gestational diabetes can develop in a woman who has not previously had the condition. It begins in the second half of pregnancy and is often diagnosed between the 24th and 28th weeks. The blood sugar levels, as a rule, return to normal after the baby is born.

Insulin is the hormone that normally controls blood sugars. It enables the body to break down sugar (glucose) to be used as energy. During pregnancy, the placenta produces certain hormones that prevent insulin from working efficiently and result in insulin resistance. When insulin becomes ineffective, the level of sugar in the blood rises, leading to diabetes in pregnancy. This effect is generally seen after the 24th week of pregnancy.

Developing gestational diabetes is a warning that you might develop diabetes later in life. It is important not to take this lightly. If you stick to a healthy diet, walk daily and maintain the appropriate weight for your height, you can postpone the development of diabetes.

Pregestational diabetes (diabetes diagnosed before pregnancy or in the first half of pregnancy)

If you have diabetes before pregnancy, you must be particularly careful about keeping your blood sugar levels well under control before you try for a pregnancy. Despite medical advances, babies born to women with diabetes, especially women with poor control of diabetes, are still at greater risk for birth defects.

Mahima asked: I am a diabetic. My husband and I want another child. How do I make sure that my baby will be healthy?

My answer: Your baby is particularly vulnerable in the first few weeks of pregnancy, when his organs are forming. Since you may not know that you are pregnant until the baby has been growing for two to four weeks, high blood sugars at this stage can be harmful to the baby. For this reason, good blood sugar control before you get pregnant is very important. To protect your baby from the very moment of conception:

- Keep you sugar levels strictly controlled
- Keep your HbA1C level below 6.5%
- Optimize your weight to be as close as possible to the ideal weight for your height
- Switch to a diabetic drug that is safe in pregnancy or to insulin shots with advice from your doctor
- Start folic acid supplements

Will you know if you develop gestational diabetes?

Unfortunately, in most women, gestational diabetes causes no symptoms. It is a silent disease and is usually discovered only following a blood test. That is why all women should be tested for diabetes in pregnancy.

How is diabetes diagnosed in pregnancy?

At the first visit

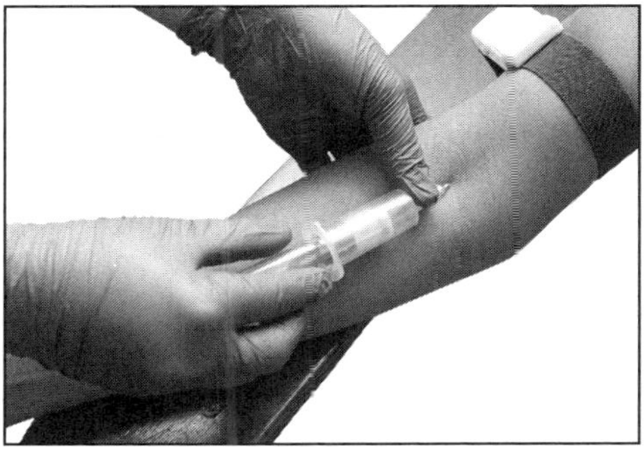

If you are not a known diabetic, you will be asked to undergo one of the following tests:

- Fasting blood glucose level
- 75 g oral glucose tolerance test (see below)

If the fasting blood sugar (or the 75 g 2-hour GTT) is normal, you will be tested next at 24–28 weeks.

In pregnancy, the fasting blood sugar tends to be lower than normal. If the fasting blood sugar (or the 75 g 2-hour GTT) is high, then it means you have pregestational diabetes and treatment will be started.

> When you are having nausea and vomiting in the early months, drinking a very sweet glucose drink may make you vomit. That is why many doctors prefer a fasting blood sugar test over a GTT.

Between 24 and 28 weeks of pregnancy

If the blood sugar levels were normal at the first visit, you will be advised an oral glucose tolerance test between 24–28 weeks of pregnancy.

Oral glucose tolerance test

The standard test recommended to diagnose diabetes in pregnancy is a **75 g 2-hour oral glucose tolerance test (GTT).**

How is the 75 g GTT done?

- It is done in the morning (preferably at or before 8 am)
- Do not to eat or drink anything except water for 12 hours prior to the test (for example, from 8 pm to 8 am)
- A fasting blood sample is first taken
- 75 g of glucose is given in 150 ml of water (adding lemon juice makes it easier to drink)
- Blood is drawn 1 hour and 2 hours after the drink
- If two or more of the glucose levels are higher than the normal values, a diagnosis of gestational diabetes is made

GTT explained

When you eat, your body immediately recognizes the input of calories. The food gets converted to sugar and the blood sugar level surges. Insulin is released to help absorb the sugar load and within an hour or two your blood sugar level comes back to normal. If your body does not produce enough insulin, or you have insulin resistance (when available insulin cannot be utilized) the blood sugar level stays high.

A GTT is a test where a 75 g load of glucose is given and the response of the body is measured. Diabetes is diagnosed when the fasting blood sugar level is high or the levels at the 1-hour mark or 2-hour mark (or both) are high.

Earlier, GTT in pregnancy used to be done over 3 hours with 100 g oral glucose load. However, that practice has been mostly replaced with the 2 hour 75 g GTT.

Why is diabetes in pregnancy a problem?

The good news is that gestational diabetes (that develops in the second half of pregnancy) may have minimal effects on the mother and the baby, if kept well under control. Unfortunately, poorly controlled diabetes in pregnancy is a double-edged sword that can affect both the mother and the baby. Pregestational diabetes is more of a problem but strict control of blood sugar levels can reduce the bad effects dramatically.

How does your diabetes affect the baby?

The following problems are less common with gestational diabetes and more common with pregestational diabetes.

- **Macrosomia:** When the mother's blood sugars are high, the baby's weight and growth may be excessive, leading to an overweight baby. With strict control of blood sugar levels, this problem can be avoided.

  How do high blood sugar levels cause problems? The baby produces insulin to combat the high sugar levels. The combination of high sugar levels and high insulin levels can make the baby excessively big (macrosomic). This in turn may cause complications during labour. The chances of caesarean section increase because the baby may be too big to be born through the

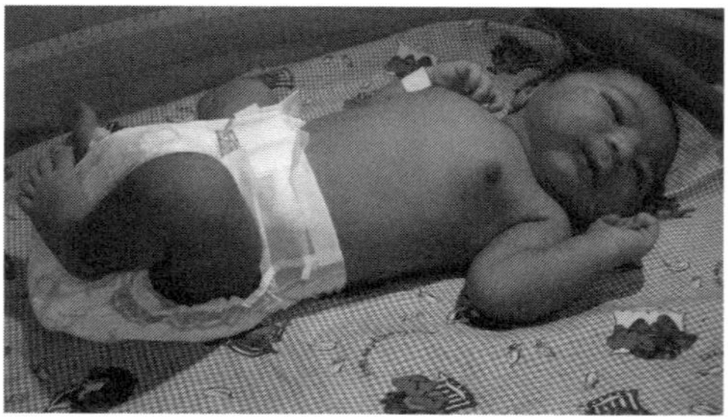

normal birth passage (see **Chapter 34**, *Foetal growth problems: too small or too big*).

- **Polyhydramnios:** The water surrounding the baby (amniotic fluid) may also increase significantly due to diabetes and this can lead to preterm labour and birth.
- **Respiratory distress after birth:** There is an increased chance of the baby developing breathing difficulties (respiratory distress) after birth. The lungs do not mature on time in the baby of a diabetic mother and may cause significant difficulty in breathing.
- **Hypoglycaemia:** When your blood sugar levels are high, the baby also gets extra sugar. To deal with this, she produces extra insulin. Immediately after birth, the baby continues to produce extra insulin for a while. This extra circulating insulin can cause low blood sugars or hypoglycaemia. The baby must be monitored, and treated if the blood glucose level drops too low.
- **Newborn jaundice (hyperbilirubinaemia):** For some reason, newborn jaundice occurs more often in babies of women with diabetes. This is not an infection but a build-up of jaundice pigment in the blood. To treat this problem the baby is placed under special lights that help the jaundice pigments get absorbed faster. This is called phototherapy (see **Chapter 49**, *Your new baby*).
- **Stillbirth** (delivery of a baby that has died before birth) is rare in diabetic women receiving good antenatal care, with good control of blood sugar levels. It is more common in women whose diabetes was not well controlled before and during pregnancy.

Will my baby have diabetes at birth?

Having gestational diabetes does not mean that the baby will have diabetes at birth. However, your baby has a 1–3 per cent risk of developing diabetes later in life. The risk increases if your husband is also a diabetic.

How does diabetes affect you?

Gestational diabetes is not an immediate threat to your health. Most women who develop diabetes in pregnancy, after 20 weeks, and whose blood sugar levels are kept within the normal range, deliver their babies without complications.

Women with diabetes in pregnancy have a greater risk of developing high blood pressure in pregnancy (gestational hypertension and preeclampsia: see **Chapter 37**, *High blood pressure in pregnancy*).

If you have gestational diabetes, you are more likely to develop gestational diabetes in future pregnancies. You are also at a higher risk of developing type II diabetes (non-insulin dependent diabetes) later in life.

Managing diabetes in pregnancy

The key to a good pregnancy outcome is strict maintenance of blood sugar levels in the normal range. The aim is to keep

- Fasting blood sugar level at or below 95 mg/dL
- 1 hour postprandial (after a meal) level at or below 140 mg/dL
- 2 hours postprandial (after a meal) level at or below 120 mg/dL

Managing sugar levels uses a two-pronged plan:

1. Diet and exercise are the cornerstone of diabetic therapy
2. Medications: Oral drugs or insulin

Diet

It's good to keep in mind that a diabetic diet is an extremely healthy diet. Combined with exercise, there is a good chance that this alone may keep your blood sugar levels strictly under control.

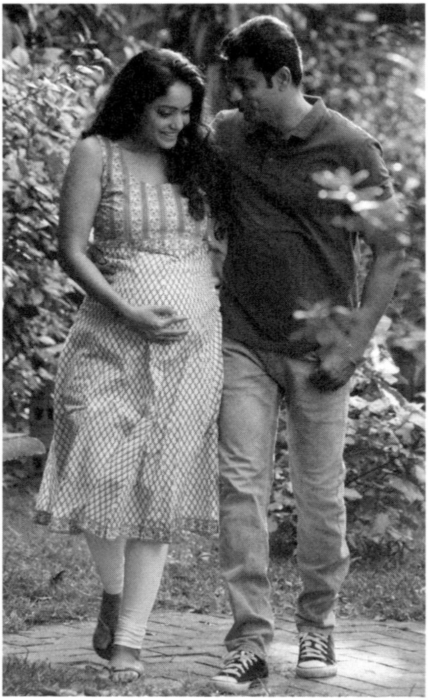

Dietary modification and exercise will help to control blood sugars initially. If this alone is not enough, then medications may be needed.

Exercise

Any activity that keeps you moving, and gets your heart rate up (what is referred to as aerobic activity), is helpful as it makes your body's insulin work better. Walking for a minimum of 30–45 minutes daily is necessary. This can be done at any time, morning or night, or can be

Kirti's mother asked: My 30-year old daughter is pregnant for the first time and is now 7 months. Last week she was told she has developed diabetes. Since she was living alone in Bangalore with her husband, I asked her to move back and stay with me so that I can take care of her. I am very worried. Please tell me what food I can give her. Will this affect her baby?

My answer: I can understand your concern for your daughter and her baby. She has been diagnosed with gestational diabetes, in the second half of pregnancy. With good sugar control, this usually has very little effect on the baby.

A diabetic diet is basically a very healthy one. In pregnancy, it is based on the mother's weight. Usually a diabetic mother is advised to have 30 calories per kg per day, if she has a normal weight to begin with. For women who are overweight, this is reduced. Your daughter's doctor will ask you to see a dietician who will calculate the dietary requirements for her.

Let me break this down for you. If your daughter weighs 60 kilos, and her BMI is normal (23-25 kg/m^2) she should consume 30 x 60 i.e.1800 calories in a day. It is important that the food be divided into 3 meals (breakfast, lunch and dinner) with 2 mid-meal snacks and a glass of milk at bedtime. Of course, the most important thing is calorie restriction. Will your daughter starve and therefore, will the baby starve? Absolutely not! When the correct amount of food is consumed, the normal weight gain in pregnancy will also continue.

Since the body cannot handle sugar in diabetes, it is important to stop all sugars, including honey and jaggery. Vegetables with high sugar content like sweet potatoes, carrots and beetroot should also be avoided. Fruits that are allowed are apple, guava, grapes that are not too sweet, or a small cup of pomegranate. Mangoes, bananas and coconut are loaded with calories and have to be avoided. Fruit juices are not recommended because they are high in fruit sugars. Rice should be included in only one meal. Oats, wheat and millets are good substitutes for rice.

The fact that your daughter is now staying with you worries me for only one reason. You might get a little overprotective and tell her to take it easy. Letting her rest too much, watching TV and reading magazines is the worst thing you can do! One of the most important factors in controlling blood sugars is exercise. The more physical work your daughter does, the better the control of blood sugar levels. She should help with the household chores and also take a brisk walk twice a day, for at least 45 minutes to an hour.

split up. If you are on insulin, have a discussion with your doctor before you start a vigorous exercise programme.

Medications: Oral drugs or insulin

If diet and exercise have not helped, you may be placed on oral medication or insulin shots.

Gestational diabetes: Two oral drugs (metformin and glyburide) have been found to be safe in pregnancy. However, some doctors prefer insulin shots especially if your sugar levels are not coming under control easily.

Pregestational diabetes: Insulin is preferred over oral drugs.

Insulin

If your blood sugar levels remain high in spite of diet and exercise, your doctor may decide on daily insulin injections for you. You might need to be admitted for a few days to the hospital initially to adjust the dose of insulin. Your obstetrician will usually refer you to a physician or endocrinologist who deals with diabetic patients on a regular basis.

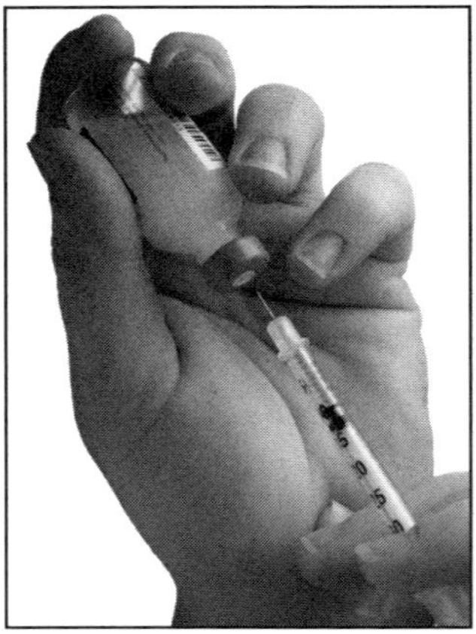

The amount of insulin needed to control glucose levels throughout the day varies from woman to woman and depends on many factors. Your doctor will tell you how to use insulin and how many daily injections you will need. The number of injections and dose of insulin you need may change as the baby grows. When insulin is needed to control diabetes during pregnancy, the diet and the insulin dose must be balanced at all times to prevent harmful levels of glucose. If you need to take insulin, you can easily be taught how to take it yourself.

Low sugar (hypoglycaemia)

Sometimes, on insulin, you can have low blood sugar if you have not eaten enough. Common symptoms of this are weakness, shaking, hunger and sweating. For women taking insulin, it is a good idea to keep a snack handy at all times in case low blood sugar develops.

Will insulin affect the baby? Not at all. The insulin does not cross the placenta and enter the baby's blood stream. On the other hand, good control of your blood sugar levels with insulin will ensure that your baby will be healthy.

Testing your blood sugar levels

It is very important to have the blood sugar levels normal throughout the day. For this, your doctor may order multiple blood tests as soon as the diagnosis is made. Once the sugar levels are under control, you may be asked to check your levels less frequently.

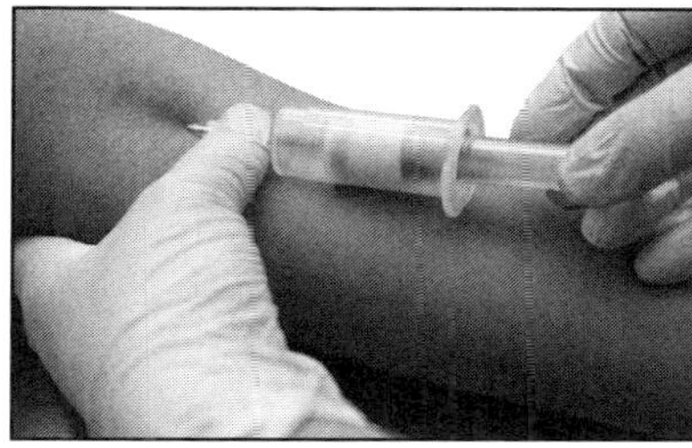

Generally, the sugar levels are tested before and after breakfast, lunch and dinner—that is 6 times a day. This gives the doctor an idea of how your sugar levels fluctuate. This is particularly important when insulin is prescribed. Less frequent testing is required once the dose of insulin is stabilized.

Home glucose testing kits (glucometers) are available that allow you to monitor your glucose levels. These usually involve taking a tiny blood sample with a pinprick device. The blood is put on to a strip and inserted into the glucometer, which gives the blood glucose level.

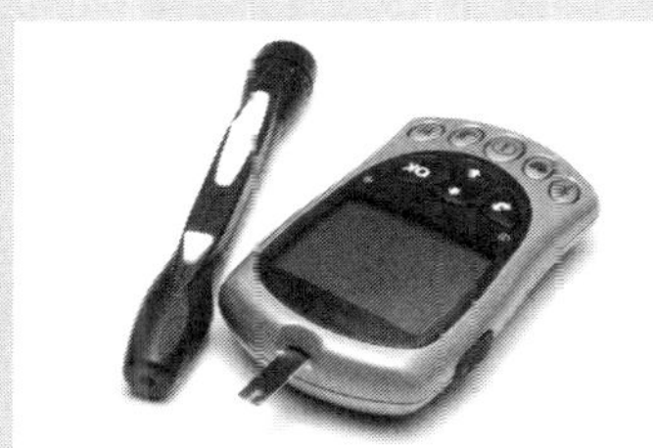

Monitoring the baby's health

Ultrasound examination of the baby is performed at regular intervals to make sure the baby is neither too big (macrosomic) nor too small (growth restricted). The fluid around the baby will also be monitored closely.

Non-stress test and bipophysical profile (see **Chapter 16**, *Tests of foetal well-being: is the baby tolerating pregnancy well?*) may be performed regularly after the 32nd week, particularly if you have pregestational diabetes, or are on insulin.

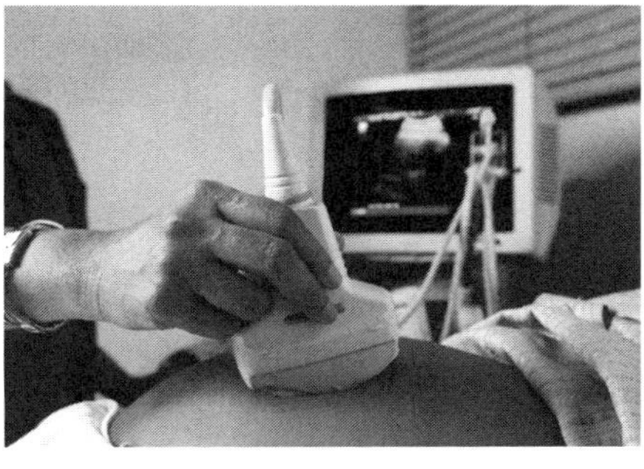

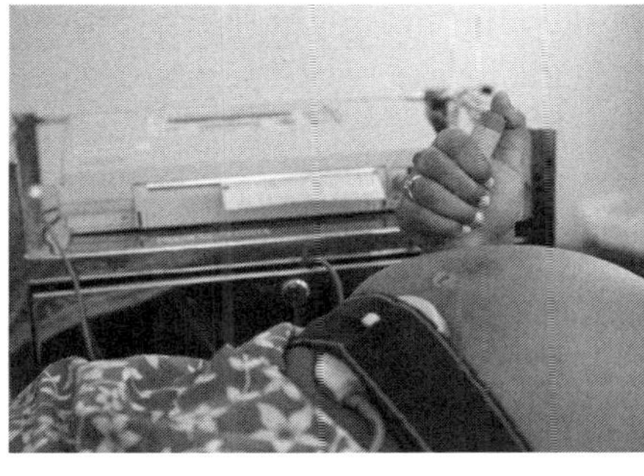

Delivery

The mode of delivery depends on the mildness or severity of the diabetes, how well the sugar levels have been controlled and any accompanying complications in the pregnancy.

- Diabetes well controlled with diet and exercise: Await normal labour
- Diabetes well controlled with diet and exercise but baby has a problem: Caesarean section
- Diabetes well controlled with insulin and baby size is normal: Labour induced at 38 weeks
- Diabetes well controlled with insulin but the baby or you have complications, or the baby is large: Caesarean section

Your blood sugar levels will be monitored and kept under control during labour and delivery.

After delivery

If you are a gestational diabetic, your sugar levels will come back to normal instantly, the minute the baby and placenta are delivered! You will only be asked to check your blood sugars 6–8 weeks after the baby is born.

If you were already a diabetic before you became pregnant (pregestational diabetic), your insulin requirement will come down significantly. You may be able to control your blood sugar levels with diet and exercise alone.

Breastfeeding

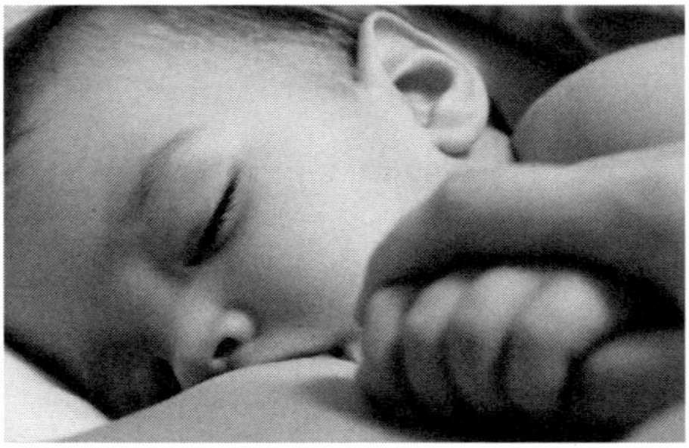

Breastfeeding is not only good for your baby, it is also good for you because breastfeeding uses up more calories. During the first weeks at home with the baby, you are likely to be tired and stressed from lack of sleep. If you are still on insulin, it might be a little difficult to get back on schedule. Low blood glucose is a real danger.

To help prevent low blood glucose levels due to breastfeeding:

- Have a snack before or during nursing
- Drink enough fluids
- Keep a snack next to you to treat low blood glucose when you nurse, so you do not have to stop feeding to treat hypoglycaemia

Birth control

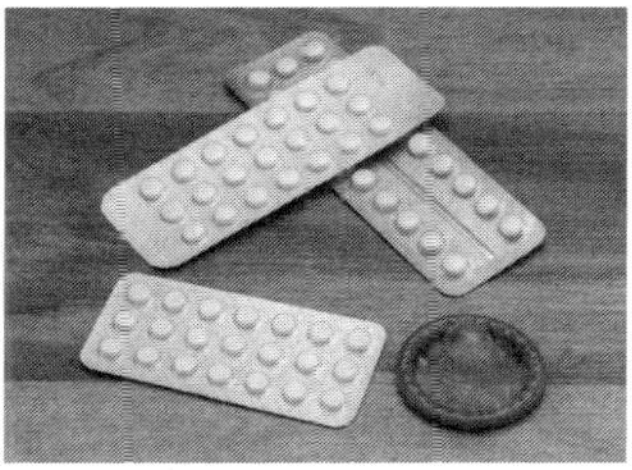

If you are a diabetic or developed gestational diabetes, you should plan future pregnancies with care. It is smart to begin using a form of birth control following delivery. In general, women with diabetes can use most of the available methods (see **Chapter 50**, *Methods of birth control*). At your first postnatal check-up, discuss with your obstetrician which method would be best for you.

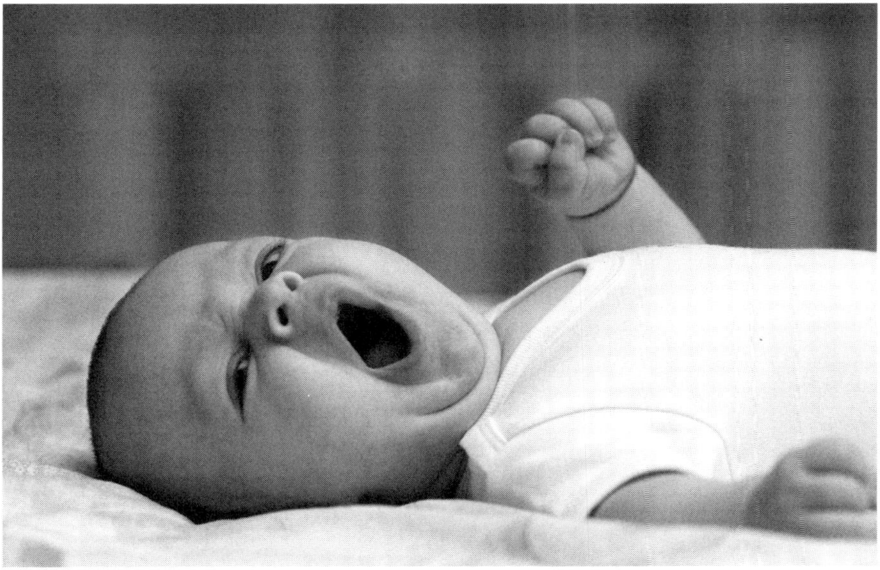

CHAPTER 39

Rh factor and your pregnancy

Srinidhi is pregnant for the first time. She is aware that she is Rh negative. When she went for her first antenatal check-up, her obstetrician tested her husband and found that he was Rh positive. Srinidhi and her husband had many questions. Would this difference in their Rh factor affect the baby? Would she have to take any precautions? Would this affect her next pregnancy? Srinidhi and her husband need not worry.

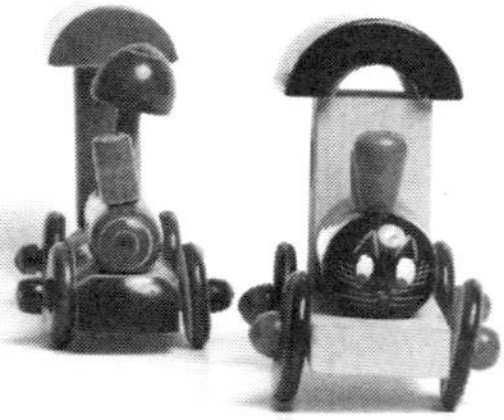

39

Rh factor and your pregnancy

If you have ever had your blood group tested, you will belong to one of four blood groups: **A, B, AB,** and **O**. Each of the four blood groups is additionally classified according to the presence of another protein (antigen) on the surface of red blood cells that indicates the Rh factor. If this antigen is present, you are classified as being **Rh positive**. If this antigen is absent, you are considered **Rh negative**. If you have not been tested earlier, you will have your blood group and Rh factor tested at your first antenatal visit.

> They must have asked for your blood group for your driver's license. If, for example, you filled in B positive, it means you belong to the B blood group and have the Rh antigen.

About 85 per cent of Indians are Rh positive. This percentage varies in some ethnic communities.

What is the Rh factor and why does it matter?

If a woman who is Rh negative and a man who is Rh positive conceive a baby, a problem called **Rh incompatibility** may arise. This can potentially affect the baby while it is still inside the womb. Luckily, in the 21st century, you live in a time when these problems have been almost completely eliminated by available treatments.

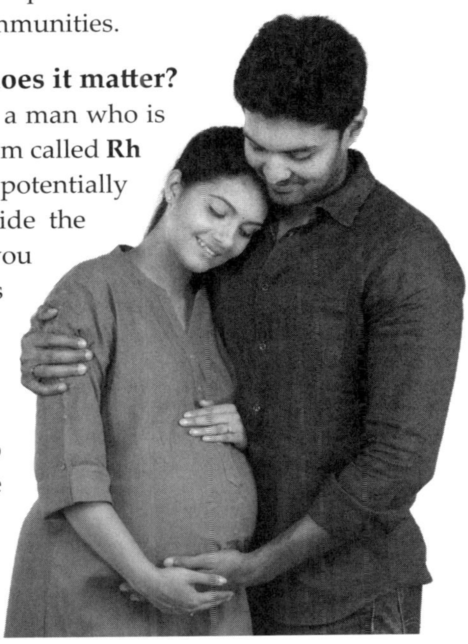

If both the mother and the father are Rh negative, there is no possibility that the baby will be Rh positive. The mother therefore does not run the risk of developing antibodies and there can be no Rh incompatibility.

Rh incompatibility explained

During delivery (or a miscarriage), a tiny bit (5–15 ml) of the baby's blood can enter the mother's blood stream through the blood vessels of the womb. When even a miniscule amount of the baby's Rh positive blood enters the mother's blood stream, her body immediately identifies the Rh antigen as 'foreign tissue'. Her immune system mounts an attack against these 'foreign' cells and produces **an antibody** to destroy the few cells that have entered her blood.

> Since Rh antibodies are produced only after the first pregnancy, Rh incompatibility usually does not lead to a problem in the first pregnancy. Problems however can arise for the second, and subsequent babies.

These antibodies do not affect the mother in any way. They are, however, permanent and stay in the mother's blood stream all her life. When she becomes pregnant for the second time and the baby happens to be Rh positive, these antibodies recognize the 'foreign cell' again. The mother's antibodies mount an attack on the baby's red blood cells and are intent on destroying them.

The amount of harm to the baby depends on the level of antibodies in the mother's blood stream.

- If she has low levels, only a few of the baby's red blood cells will be destroyed and he will have mild anaemia. If the condition is mild, the baby may do well during pregnancy but may develop anaemia and jaundice after birth. This is called Rh disease of the newborn
- If the antibody levels are high, the baby can end up with severe anaemia in the womb and the subsequent complications could be life threatening

Pinky asked: I am Rh negative and went for the first visit with my obstetrician. Why has my doctor asked me to do a test for Rh antibodies?

My answer: All Rh negative women (with Rh positive partners) will be asked to get tested for Rh antibodies. This simple blood test is called an indirect Coomb's test (ICT). If a woman has antibodies in her blood, the test will be reported as positive. If she has no Rh antibodies, then the indirect Coomb's test will be negative.

The level of Rh antibodies predicts if the baby will be affected or not. It will be checked for each of your pregnancies. Even though the chances of having Rh antibodies are very low in a first pregnancy it will be checked anyway so that a complication is not missed.

What if the father is Rh negative and the mother Rh positive?
If the father is Rh negative and the mother is Rh positive, the question of Rh incompatibility does not arise. There is no effect on the baby.

Other situations that can result in Rh antibodies
Rh negative women can be exposed to the Rh antigen in situations other than delivery:

- Blood transfusions with Rh positive blood
- Miscarriage or induced abortion
- Ectopic pregnancy
- Invasive prenatal procedures like chorionic villus sampling (CVS) or amniocentesis (see **Chapter 15**, *Diagnostic tests in pregnancy*)
- Significant bleeding during pregnancy

Preventing the formation of Rh antibodies

One of the great medical advances has been the invention of an injection to prevent problems arising from Rh incompatibility. The complications resulting from Rh incompatibility have come down drastically in the last few decades.

An injection of **Rh immunoglobulin (Anti-D)** prevents the formation of Rh antibodies. Rh immunoglobulin is a blood product that can prevent an Rh negative mother from responding to Rh positive blood cells of the baby, thus stopping Rh antibodies from forming in almost all cases.

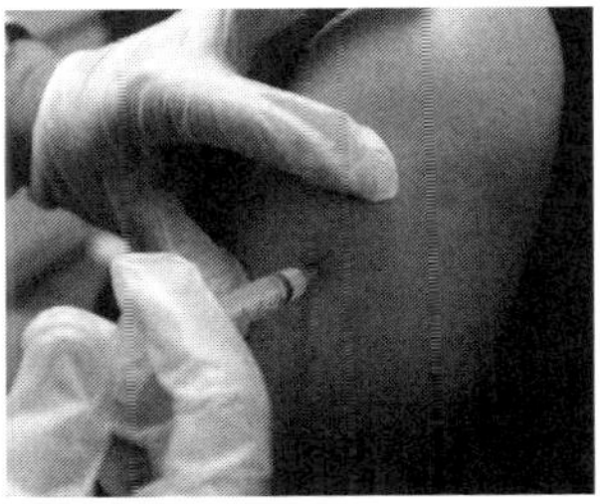

Rh immunoglobulin will not be effective if the mother has antibodies.

Timing of Rh immunoglobulin (Anti-D)

During pregnancy and after delivery
If you are Rh negative and do not have Rh antibodies, the doctor may suggest that:

- You receive an Anti-D injection around the **28th week of pregnancy** to reduce the risk of Rh antibodies forming for the rest of the pregnancy.

Because of the cost of the injection (Rs 3500 or more), and the very minimal advantage to giving it at 28 weeks, it has been suggested that the 28th week dose can be optional in developing countries like India.

This prevents problems in the small number of women who can become sensitized during the last three months of pregnancy. However, this is an unnecessary expense in women whose babies turn out to be Rh negative

- Immediately after birth the blood group and Rh status of your baby are determined. If he is Rh positive, you will be given a dose of Anti-D **within 72 hours of birth.** In almost all cases, this prevents you from making antibodies. *The injection is not needed if the baby is Rh negative*

The Anti-D injection given during a particular pregnancy is only effective for that pregnancy. Any subsequent pregnancies must be treated in the same way.

In other situations

If you are Rh negative, an injection of Rh immunoglobulin must be given if you have had

- A miscarriage
- An induced abortion
- An ectopic pregnancy
- Significant bleeding during pregnancy

Is Rh immunoglobulin required after sterilization?

Your doctor will help you decide if you need Rh immunoglobulin if you are planning to undergo sterilization (a permanent procedure to prevent further pregnancies). After sterilization, you will not get pregnant again so it is possible to avoid the cost of the expensive Anti-D injection.

Some doctors may however advise you to take the injection even after sterilization for the following reasons:

- You may decide later to have the sterilization reversed
- Rarely, the sterilization may fail and you may get pregnant again

Rh disease and its consequences

Rh disease of pregnancy is due to Rh antibodies destroying the red blood cells of the unborn baby. Rh antibodies may form if Anti-D was not given or unusually, even if Anti-D was given. Fortunately, with advances in obstetrics, this complication has become very rare. Even when it does occur, the pregnancy can be managed and a healthy baby delivered.

Rh disease can result in severe anaemia, jaundice, brain damage and heart failure in a newborn. In extreme cases, it used to cause the death of the unborn baby.

Diagnosing and treating Rh disease

If you have been tested with the indirect Coomb's test (ICT) and have been found to have a significant level of antibodies, you will be monitored regularly during the pregnancy. A Doppler ultrasound is used to determine if the baby is developing anaemia. It is done usually after the 18th week of pregnancy. If the Doppler ultrasound shows that the baby may be developing severe anaemia, a foetal blood sampling is done. A fine needle is inserted into the baby's umbilical cord and a blood sample is obtained. When the anaemia is confirmed, blood transfusions are given to the baby. This is successful in 90 per cent of cases. This is a specialized procedure and can only be done in some centres equipped to handle these cases. With the Anti-D injection being available to most mothers, the need for these sort of procedures is coming down.

Newborns with Rh disease

If you are near term and tests show that the baby is developing anaemia, your labour may be induced early, before too many foetal blood cells are destroyed. After delivery, some cases of Rh disease are so mild that the baby does not need any treatment. If the baby has jaundice, he may be placed under special lights (phototherapy). In more severe cases, the baby may need an exchange blood transfusion.

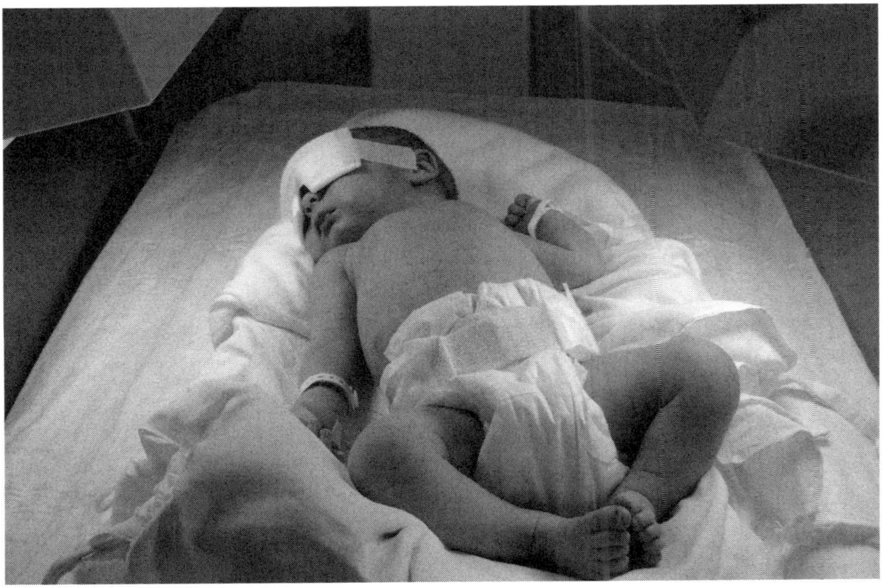

Baby under phototherapy for newborn jaundice due to Rh disease. The baby's eyes are covered to protect them from the light

CHAPTER 40

Pregnancy after 35

Sanjana is 36 years old. She and her husband are now ready to go ahead with a pregnancy.

Smriti and her husband have been married for the past seven years. She has conceived now after treatment for infertility. She is 37 years old.

Shyamala is 35 and pregnant for the second time. Her first child is 13 years old.

Will being 35 or older cause a problem in pregnancy?

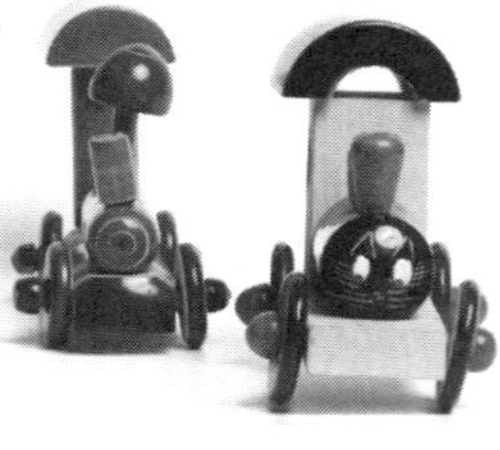

40

Pregnancy after 35

If you are 35 or older and are planning a pregnancy or are already pregnant, you have joined a large number of women who are having babies later in life. It might be a personal choice, it might be a career-driven decision or it may have been that your body did not cooperate with you when you wanted to get pregnant. Whatever the reason, for you this is the right time to be pregnant. You have the advantage of being mature enough to be able to handle the pregnancy.

Most women in their mid-30s and early-40s can look forward to having a healthy pregnancy and a healthy baby. The anxieties and concerns that plague all pregnant women are magnified when a woman has a child later in life. It is, therefore, important for a couple to be aware of the mild risks involved and stay informed about the consequences of a pregnancy at an older age.

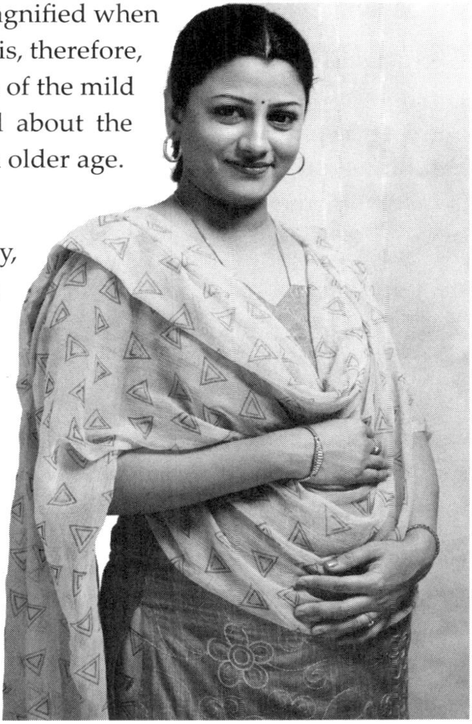

Age and fertility

If you are planning a pregnancy, you should be aware that you might have a little difficulty in getting pregnant. There are no hard and fast rules and there are plenty of women over 35 who conceive immediately when they start trying. However the fact is that there is a gradual decrease of fertility starting in the early 30s. A woman in her mid-30s or older may take longer to conceive than a younger woman.

Though the following problems are more common in women who are 35 or older, it does not mean that you will face every one of these setbacks. You may sail through the pregnancy without any complication. However, it is prudent to be aware of what you may face and be mentally prepared for it.

Given the special concerns about pregnancy past 35, it is especially important for couples to seek preconceptional counselling from their obstetrician before embarking on this very important step in their lives.

Being over 35 makes you less fertile because the eggs you were born with, are now as old as you. You may also produce an egg (ovulate) less frequently, maybe skipping two or three months in a year. As you grow older, you may also develop medical conditions that may interfere with pregnancy. For example, women over 35 are more likely to have endometriosis, which may contribute to decreased fertility.

If you are over 35, it would be a good idea to consult your gynaecologist if you have not conceived after six months of trying. About one-third of women between 35 and 39, and about half of those over 40 have problems conceiving. Many fertility problems can be treated successfully.

Chances of twins

Paradoxically, women over 35 may have difficulty in conceiving but have a greater chance of having twins. The chance of having twins increases naturally with age. The other contributing factor for a multiple pregnancy is that women over 35 are more likely to undergo fertility treatment, and this may increase the chance of twins and triplets.

Risk of miscarriage

At any age, most miscarriages occur in the first three months of pregnancy. The rate of miscarriage in older women is significantly greater than in younger women. This is mainly because of the increasing risk of chromosomal abnormalities due to older eggs. Approximately 10–15 per cent of pregnancies in women in their 20s end in miscarriage The risk rises to about 20 per cent at ages 35–39, 50 per cent by ages 40–44, and about 80 per cent above 45.

Pre-existing health problems and pregnancy

At any age, when planning a pregnancy, a woman should consult her obstetrician before trying to conceive. A preconception visit helps ensure she is in the best possible physical condition before conception. Diabetes and high blood pressure are two conditions that are common in Indians and much more common in women in their late 30s and early 40s. Moreover, women over 35 are twice as likely as women in their 20s to develop high blood pressure and diabetes for the first time during pregnancy.

Careful medical monitoring is required and the appropriate medications must be started before conception and continued throughout pregnancy. This can reduce the risks associated with these conditions and, in most cases, result in a healthy pregnancy.

Risk of birth defects in women over 35

The risk of bearing a child with chromosomal disorders increases as a woman ages. This is again due to the older eggs. The most common disorder is Down syndrome, a combination of intellectual disability and physical abnormalities caused by the presence of an extra chromosome 21 (see **Chapter 12**, *Could my baby have a problem?*).

Age related risk of Down syndrome	
Age 25	1 in 1,250
Age 30	1 in 1,000
Age 35	1 in 400
Age 40	1 in 100
Age 45	1 in 30
Age 49	1 in 10

Prenatal screening for Down syndrome is recommended for all pregnant women. It is particularly important for women who are 35 or older at the time of delivery. Fortunately, prenatal testing to rule out Down syndrome and other chromosomal problems is more commonly available now. A blood test along with an ultrasound will be done to assess the risk of you having a baby with Down syndrome (see **Chapter 14**, *Screening tests in pregnancy*).

If the test comes back positive, prenatal tests like amniocentesis and chorionic villus sampling (CVS) may be offered (see **Chapter 15**, *Prenatal diagnostic tests in pregnancy*). Most women who have these tests will be relieved to find that their baby does not have a chromosomal problem.

Risk of pregnancy complications

While women in their late 30s and early 40s are quite likely to have a healthy baby, they do face more complications along the way. It is important to keep in mind that many of these risks can be managed effectively with good prenatal care and most women will have a happy outcome.

Preterm baby

Women over 35 are 20 per cent more likely to have a preterm delivery (born at less than 37 weeks of pregnancy). Women over 40 are 40 per cent more likely than younger women to deliver prematurely. Preterm babies are at an increased risk for health problems in the newborn period (see **Chapter 32**, *When the baby comes too early: preterm labour and birth*).

Low birth weight baby

Women having their first baby at 35 or later, are 20–40 per cent more likely than younger women to have a baby who has a low birth weight. Women in their 40s may also have a greater chance of having a low-birth weight baby. The placenta may not function well and may result in poor growth of the baby. The baby's growth has to be monitored carefully both with regular check-ups and ultrasound scans (see **Chapter 34**, *Foetal growth problems: too small or too big*).

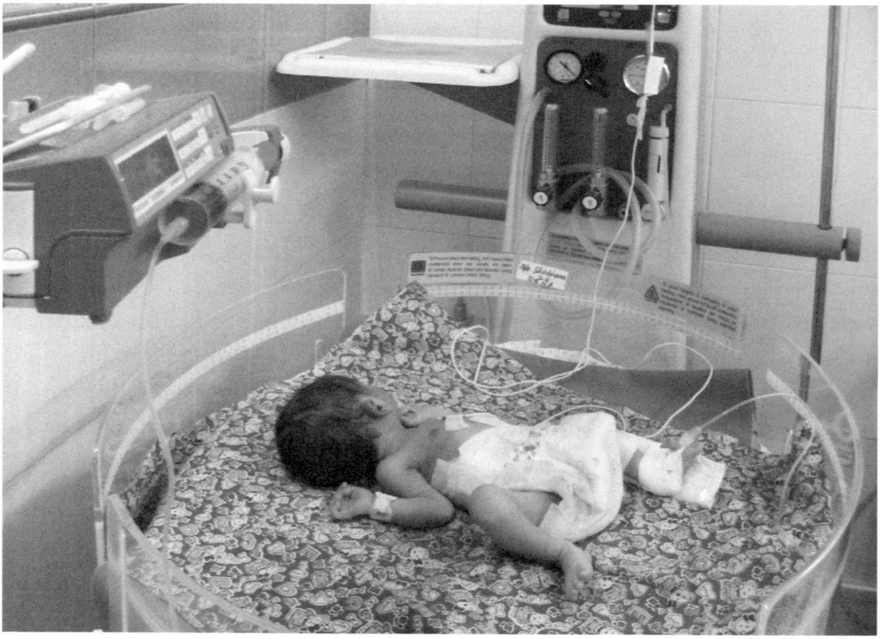

Placenta praevia

If you are over 35, there is an increased risk of having placental problems including placenta praevia. This risk triples in women in the 40s.

High blood pressure in pregnancy

Pregnancy-induced hypertension and preeclampsia are more common in women over 35 (see **Chapter 37**, *High blood pressure in pregnancy*).

Diabetes in pregnancy

Gestational diabetes (diabetes developing for the first time during pregnancy) develops twice as often in women over age 35 as compared to younger women (see **Chapter 38**, *Diabetes in pregnancy*).

Unexplained stillbirth

The rate of stillbirth (delivering a dead baby) doubles in women over 40 but the reasons for this unfortunate event in the over-40 age group are not known.

Problems in labour and delivery

First-time mothers over 35 are more likely than women in their 20s to have difficulties in labour. This may account, in part, for the increased rate of caesarean sections among women over 35. First-time mothers over 40 have the highest chance of having a caesarean section.

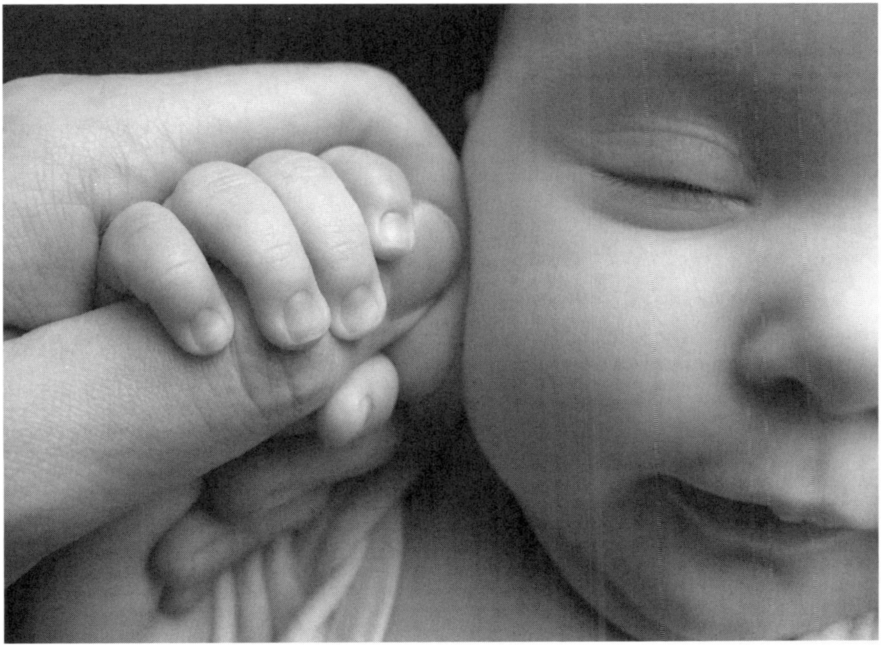

CHAPTER 41

Pregnancy in women with fibroids

Sara just had her first ultrasound in pregnancy. She is 2 months pregnant. She was told that she has a 3 cm fibroid in the wall of the uterus. She and her husband are very concerned. Will the fibroid cause problems for the baby? They need not worry. There is no reason to expect any problems from the small fibroid.

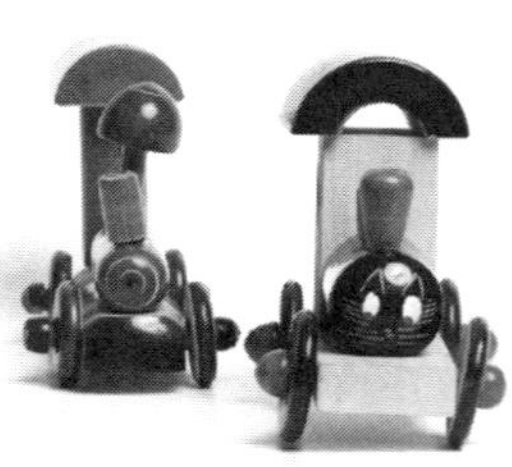

41

Pregnancy in women with fibroids

Fibroids in the uterus are very common. Many women are unaware they have fibroids because they don't have any symptoms. Up to 20–30 per cent of women in the childbearing age group will have fibroids. Do you know that 50 per cent of women will have fibroids by the time they are 50 years old? It is that common! It is as ordinary as having 'beauty marks' or moles on the skin.

Because fibroids are so common, 5–10 per cent of pregnant women will have fibroids. Fibroids during pregnancy are more likely to be encountered in women who are 35 years of age and older, and in women who are having difficulty in conceiving.

> The vast majority of women who are pregnant and have fibroids will have no problems. They will have full-term, healthy babies without encountering any difficulty.

What are fibroids?

Fibroids (also called myomas) are the most common non-cancerous muscle growths found in the uterus. They are round, slightly hard muscle growths that can be found in any part of the uterus. They can be of different sizes, and can be as small as a pea or as large as a coconut. A few women can have even larger fibroids. Depending on where they are located, they are called *submucous* (inside the uterine cavity), *intramural* (in the wall of the uterus), or *subserosal* (on the surface of the uterus).

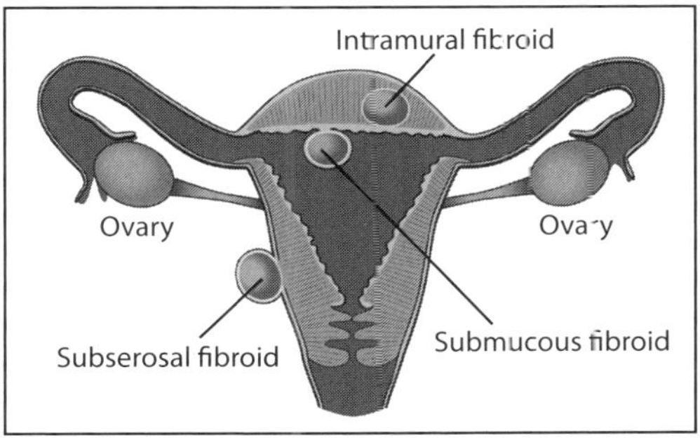

Fibroids have become a major healthcare problem across the world. This is not because they pose a major threat to the health of women but because they have become the cause for thousands of hysterectomies being done, many of them unnecessarily. **Fibroids are non-cancerous** and they do not always require surgery. Yet, absurdly, they are the commonest reason for surgery in women.

Can fibroids prevent you from getting pregnant?

Up to 20–30 per cent of women in the childbearing age group will have fibroids. In spite of this high incidence of fibroids, there is not much scientific evidence that they contribute significantly to infertility. In the majority of cases, women may find out they have fibroids after they get pregnant. This is because fibroids are usually without any symptoms. You might find out you have a fibroid during the routine ultrasound scan done in pregnancy.

What types of fibroids can cause infertility?

Fibroids that are within the wall (intramural) but do not change the shape of the cavity, or those that bulge outside the wall (subserosal) do not decrease fertility, and removal of these types of fibroids does not increase fertility.

However, some fibroids may sometimes interfere with your getting pregnant. The location of the fibroid, rather than the size of the fibroid plays a role in preventing pregnancy.

Submucous fibroid

Submucous fibroids lie very close to the inner lining of the uterus or actually inside the uterine cavity. This kind of fibroid may not allow a pregnancy to get implanted. Even if a pregnancy occurs, there is a slightly greater chance of miscarriage.

The good news is that if you are having trouble getting pregnant, a good quality ultrasound scan will be able to define the position of the fibroid.

Laila asked: I am 26 years old. I was married 8 months ago. I had abdominal pain for which an ultrasound was done. The scan shows that I have a fibroid 4 x 4 cms in size in the wall of the uterus. My doctor wants me to undergo an operation to remove it. Is the operation necessary? Will I not be able to get pregnant because of the fibroid? Will the fibroid affect the baby if I do get pregnant?

My answer: You have a reasonably small fibroid. If the fibroid is in the wall of the uterus or is growing from the outer surface of the uterus, it will have absolutely no effect on your ability to get pregnant. You, therefore, **do not need to undergo surgery for the fibroid.** The fibroid will not interfere with your pregnancy once you get pregnant.

A 3-D ultrasound is particularly useful in this situation. If a submucous fibroid is lying inside the cavity, it can be removed by a minor surgery called **hysteroscopic resection.**

Large fibroid

Even very large fibroids may not have any effect on fertility. Sometimes a large fibroid may grow in the wall of the uterus and press into the uterine cavity. If this distorts or almost obliterates the uterine cavity, it can interfere with the implantation of the embryo and may prevent pregnancy.

What happens to fibroids in pregnancy?

Many women feel concerned that a fibroid will also grow along with the baby. This is one of the common misconceptions about fibroids.

Fibroids respond differently in individual women and it is difficult to predict their growth. Most small fibroids will remain unchanged or may grow slightly. Large fibroids usually remain unchanged or may even become smaller. After the delivery, as the uterus shrinks, most fibroids will shrink along with it. The good news? The majority (90 per cent) of fibroids detected in the first trimester will shrink within 3–6 months after delivery.

Problems caused by fibroids in pregnancy

It is a reassuring fact that most women do not have any problems in pregnancy from the fibroid itself. Of those who do, pain is the most common problem. There may also be a slightly increased risk of obstetrical complications such as miscarriage, preterm labour and delivery, and abnormal position of the baby.

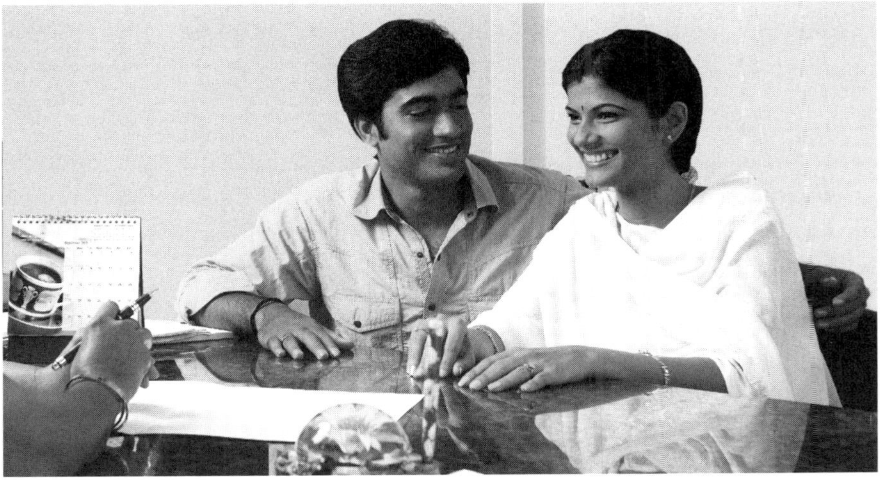

Miscarriage

It is important to remember that the vast majority of women with a fibroid during their pregnancy will not miscarry. The size of a single fibroid does not seem to have an affect on miscarriage risk. A submucous fibroid (that is inside the uterine cavity) may cause a miscarriage if the pregnancy implants on it. If there are multiple fibroids (more than 3) larger than 4 cm each, the risk of miscarriage increases slightly.

Dharma asked: I was married 6 months ago. I missed my period and had a positive home pregnancy test. When I saw my doctor, she found that I have a 6.0 x 5.0 cm fibroid, on the outside wall of the uterus. I have been now advised to abort the pregnancy because she says the fibroid will harm the baby. My husband and I are deeply disturbed because this is our first pregnancy and we don't want to have an abortion. Please advise.

My answer: Having a fibroid is no reason to abort a pregnancy. The chances of your undergoing a miscarriage may be slightly increased, only if the fibroid is pushing into the cavity of the uterus. **Aborting the pregnancy is not recommended just because you have a fibroid.** Countless women have gone through pregnancy with small and large fibroids. If you miscarry or have a complication with the pregnancy *clearly related* to the fibroid, then you may consider having the fibroid removed *before your next pregnancy*.

Pain during pregnancy

Pain is the most commonly reported complaint associated with uterine fibroids during pregnancy. Pain occurs most often in women with large fibroids (> 5 cm) during the second and third trimesters of pregnancy. During pregnancy, an occasional fibroid may grow quickly, causing intense pain.

Why does pain occur?

A condition called **red degeneration** can occur in a fibroid that suddenly grows in pregnancy. The central part of the fibroid does not get enough blood supply and this is the reason for pain. There may be fever along with the pain.

How is the pain managed?

Though you might be anxious because you know you have a fibroid and are worried that the pain may harm the baby, you should know that the pain can be treated with simple medication like paracetamol. If the pain is not responding to paracetamol, you might be given ibuprofen. Rarely, if you are having trouble handling the pain, you might be admitted for bed rest, painkiller injections and hydration with intravenous fluids. The pain usually subsides in a day or two. This will not affect your baby.

Will fibroids affect the way you deliver?

Most women with fibroids in pregnancy will be able to have a vaginal delivery without any problems. Even if you have large fibroids, if your baby is in the head-down position and your labour pains start naturally, your likelihood of having a successful vaginal delivery is high.

Reasons for a caesarean section

Occasionally, a large fibroid may be placed low on the uterus, close to the cervix (mouth of the uterus). In this case, the fibroid may come in the way of a normal vaginal delivery and may require a caesarean section.

Rarely, if the fibroid is very large, it may prevent the baby from getting into the head-down position for delivery. In that situation you will have a caesarean delivery.

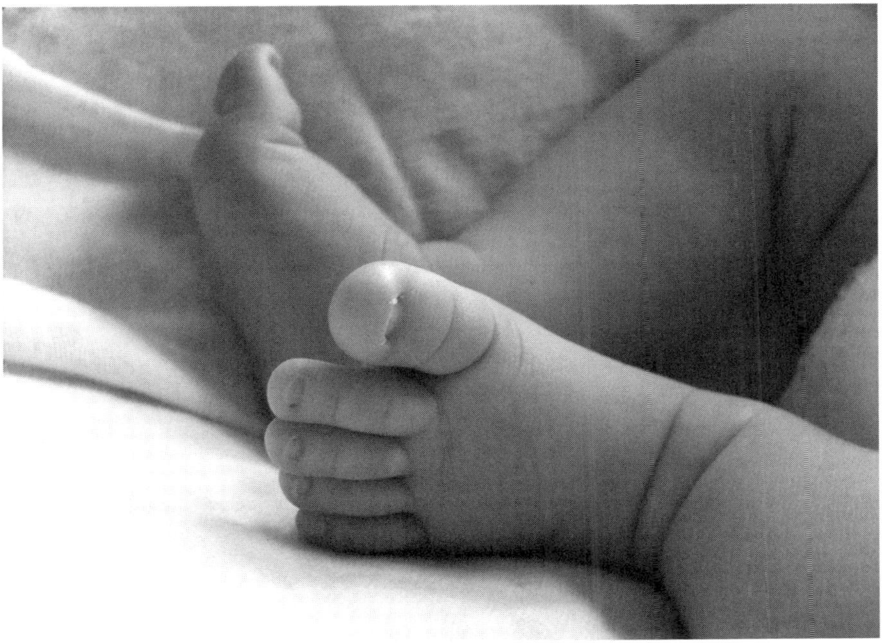

CHAPTER 42

Handling pregnancy loss

Sheela was 11 weeks pregnant when she suffered a miscarriage. Having already shared the news with everybody she knew, Sheela was terribly upset about the miscarriage.

Shravanthi was 32 weeks pregnant when her obstetrician did an ultrasound and told her that the baby's heartbeat had stopped. She and her husband are heartbroken that the baby has died in the womb.

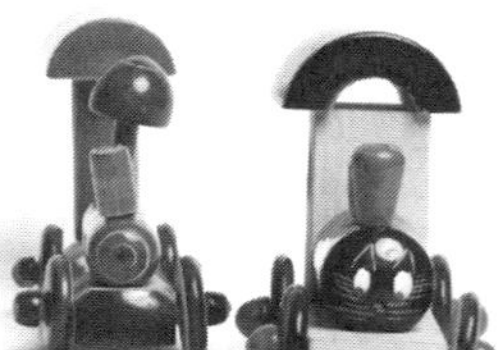

42

Handling pregnancy loss

Sunita is 20 weeks pregnant. An ultrasound has revealed that her baby has a major birth defect because of which the baby may not survive if born. Her obstetrician has suggested termination of the pregnancy.

Sabira had gone to the hospital in labour. Unfortunately, the labour ended with a stillbirth. Her world came crashing down. She and her family are in shock and are struggling to cope with the tragedy.

One of the lessons life teaches us, however reluctant we are to learn the lesson, is the necessity of dealing with loss. A loss of a pregnancy can be devastating. Even though most couples go on to have a successful pregnancy subsequently, the feeling of loss and grief may linger for a long time.

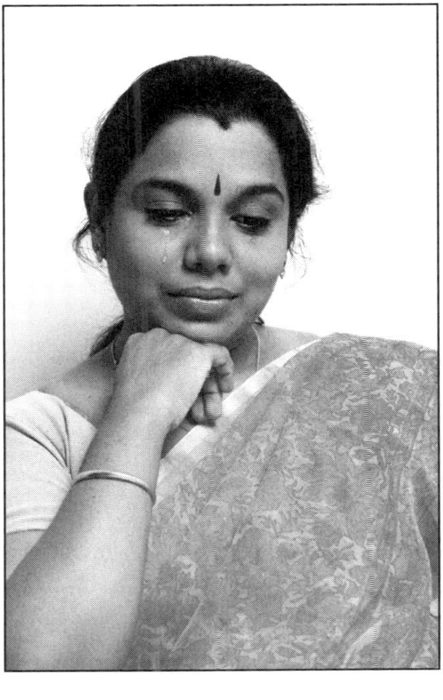

A pregnancy is something that girls and women may dream about for years. Becoming a mother and the thought of motherhood is often a part of a woman's mental makeup. To face an abrupt end to your dreams, even though temporary, may be overwhelming.

Grieving is often complicated by feelings of self-blame and unnecessary guilt, particularly when there is no medical explanation for the loss. Some women internalize the blame and are inconsolable. This is compounded by well meaning relatives, or even strangers, asking the mother if she had done something to cause the pregnancy loss. It is important to remember that there is not much a woman can do to prevent a miscarriage, a birth defect, intrauterine demise or stillbirth. Blaming oneself is a useless exercise and will only prolong the grief.

It is normal to experience grief and go through a grieving process after a pregnancy loss. Emotional healing after a pregnancy loss can take some time. For some, the grieving may only last a few days, while for others, it can take a few weeks or months. Although it can be difficult, it is important to deal with your loss rather than ignore the emotions you may be feeling.

How much grieving is normal?

There are no hard and fast rules and no timelines for grieving. Some couples with an early miscarriage, may take it in their stride. They may understand that it was Nature's way of not allowing an abnormal baby to survive. They are thankful that they did not have to face a problem later in pregnancy. They are sad for the loss but balance it with the optimism that the next pregnancy will be healthy.

You may have your own way of handling grief. You may be surprised at how deeply affected you are. Or you may find yourself able to handle it with optimism. If you find yourself sad and crying a lot, that is fine too. Your dreams for a baby were crushed and it is very normal to grieve.

There are many factors that can influence the amount of grieving you may undergo.

Having previously experienced one or more miscarriages

It is difficult enough dealing with a single miscarriage. When you have repeated miscarriages, you feel the misplaced guilt of being unable to carry a pregnancy. It is hard to understand why these repeated miscarriages happen, even if your doctor is reassuring.

Losing the pregnancy in later months

It is especially tough if you have felt the baby move and formed an emotional attachment to the tiny one inside you. All your energies and thoughts were focussed on the baby. You may have already chosen a name. You may have started dreaming of taking your little one to school.

Losing the baby in labour or immediately after delivery

This is probably the toughest situation to face because of its unexpectedness. Labour may have started normally but then something goes wrong. The loss is so sudden that it takes a long time to process it.

Having conceived the pregnancy at an older age
Losing the pregnancy is all the more difficult because you feel constrained by your biological clock.

Having conceived the pregnancy after undergoing treatment for infertility
Couples who have to undergo expensive and complex treatment for infertility already have been through an emotional roller coaster to conceive. When after all that effort, the pregnancy does not go normally and ends with a loss, the grief can be intense.

The family and social implications of having lost the pregnancy
Cultural and social pressures often equate motherhood with womanhood. The intense social stigma associated with pregnancy losses can be overwhelming. This is where a supportive husband is crucial for deflecting uncalled for blame.

How do grief and healing evolve?

Immediately after the event, your emotions may range from anger to despair. You may actually find yourself being jealous of other women with babies. Remember that grief is not a sign of weakness. It is a natural human emotion experienced by everyone after a significant loss. Do give yourself the time you need to mourn and accept what has happened. Sometimes, it may take weeks or months to recover.

Grief, in all individuals, follows a few well described stages. You may or may not pass through each stage but the last stage is the most important one to reach.

Common stages of grief

Denial
Faced with the news, you may refuse to believe it. You may seek opinions from another obstetrician or ask for another ultrasound scan to confirm the diagnosis. You may bargain with a higher power to make the bad news go away.

Anger
You may be angry at yourself, your husband or a higher power for letting this happen.

Guilt
As a woman, you may wonder if you could have avoided the pregnancy loss by being more careful. Don't blame yourself. There is very little a woman can do to avoid an unexpected pregnancy loss.

Depression

Your pain and sorrow may lead to symptoms of depression. These feelings usually resolve in time with strong support from your husband, family and friends. About 10 per cent of women may end up with clinical depression. If your depression is prolonged, it might be prudent to seek professional support.

Acceptance

Each step in the grieving process brings you closer to acceptance. You will always carry the memory of your baby, but acceptance may ease your pain. Slowly, time and day-to-day living will help you overcome the acute pain.

There will be certain days and occasions when the memories will come flooding back and overwhelm you. You may surprise yourself by the anger and jealousy you might feel towards other women who are happily pregnant. Seeing a newborn baby or another mother with a baby may trigger feelings of sadness. Again, these are not unusual emotions to experience; after all, you are only human. Just don't let these feelings consume you—you will only hurt yourself more. Remember that eventually these feelings will pass. Let your mind heal and learn acceptance even if it is a tough lesson to imbibe.

You do not have to be alone

There is no need for you to keep your feelings bottled up. Your husband and you should be able to talk it over with each other. You have to be the most important support system for each other because no one else can feel the intensity of loss as much as the two of you. Your relationship with your husband might be particularly strained during this time. Remember, he is also grieving. However, he may not be able to express what he is feeling, which can make you feel he is not sharing your grief.

At the same time, do not exclude your parents from the grieving process. They also have lost a grandchild. The older people in the family have experienced life and may be able to provide you with wisdom and support in dealing with this sorrowful life event.

Discuss the loss with your obstetrician. Try to find out what are the causes, if any, for the loss. Find out how soon you can plan the next pregnancy. Taking positive steps like this will help you resolve your feelings of loss.

If you have friends or relatives who keep bringing up stories about other women who have lost a pregnancy or tell you what you should have done

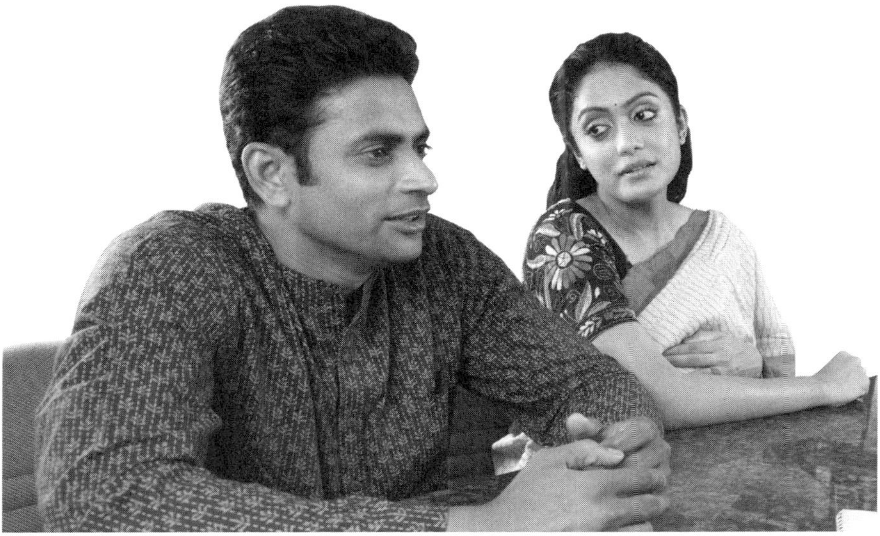

to avoid this loss, stay away from them. You do not need the aggravation of people who are insensitive or thoughtless at this time. Be direct and let them know when you don't want to discuss your pregnancy loss with them.

Sometimes close friends may not know what to say to you at this time of loss. Don't get angry with them and push them away. It may just be enough to have them around you for emotional support.

Planning your next pregnancy

Even though it seems good sense to plan another pregnancy immediately so that you can 'forget' the pregnancy loss, it may not be such a good idea. Give yourself time to recover physically. More important, you need to heal emotionally. This emotional healing may take a few months.

Only when you are fully recovered can you go through the next pregnancy with confidence. If you get pregnant immediately, your pregnancy may be overshadowed with anxiety and fear.

Talk to your obstetrician about the best form of birth control till you decide on your next pregnancy.

The healthy path to healing

Be compassionate to yourself and accept support from family, friends or a spiritual advisor. Loss can also affect you physically. It is not unusual for

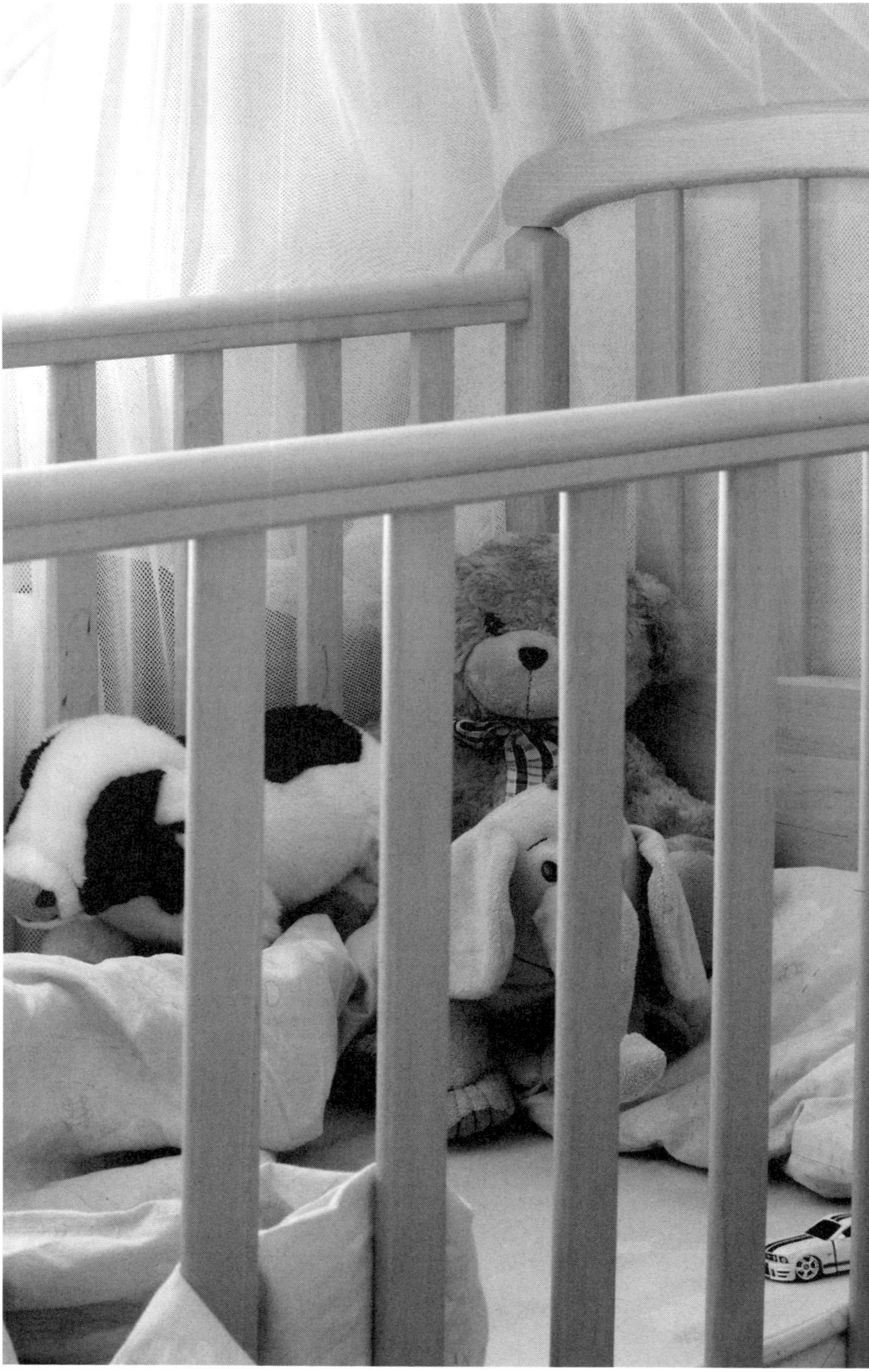

When grief overwhelms us

Be on the lookout for signs that will warn you that you are not moving towards acceptance and healing. Entering the dark tunnel of grief and coming out at the other end unscathed or at least, minimally scarred, requires enormous focus and a lot of support from those closest to you. Warning signs that you are not on the healthy path to dealing with grief include

- Working hard to the point of complete exhaustion to avoid being overwhelmed by your emotions
- Suppressing your emotions and resenting those who try to help you
- Remaining depressed well past the normal healing period and being unable to function normally

One of the commonsense pieces of advice given to those who are grieving is, 'Running away from grief postpones sorrow; clinging to grief prolongs pain; neither leads to healing.'

someone who is grieving to have shortness of breath, palpitations, stomach pain, and sleep irregularities. Sometimes, it may be difficult to see that the physical pain is tied to the emotional, but they often go hand in hand.

Reaching equanimity and acceptance

Although you will not forget your loss, and there will always be a tender spot in your heart, the intensity of the pain will diminish over the years. Time really is a great healer.

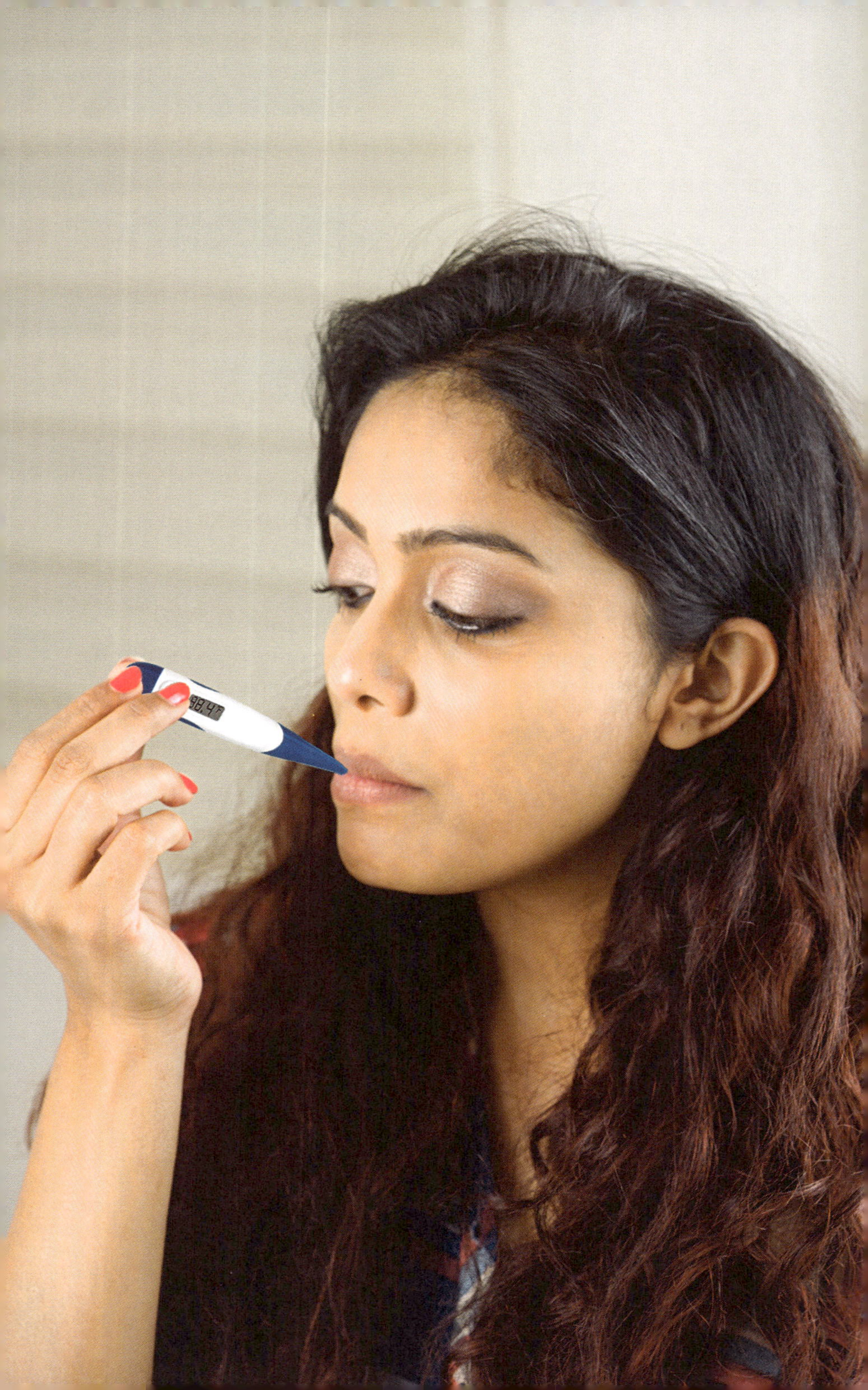

Common illnesses

CHAPTER 43

Fever and infections in pregnancy

Shamini is running a high temperature. She is six months pregnant. Her husband is anxious. Will the fever affect the baby? Will the tablets she is taking for the fever have any harmful effect on their growing baby?

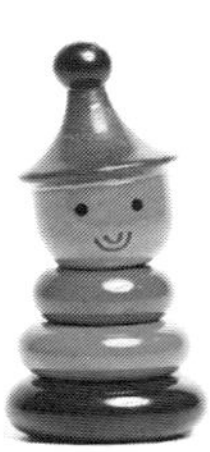

43

Fever and infections in pregnancy

You were quite prepared to put up with the discomforts of pregnancy. But you may not have bargained for a miserable cold, or the flu. If you have a young one going to kindergarten, he seems to be bringing home every variety of viral infection. Or the office canteen seems to be the meeting point for all the bugs floating around among your co-workers. It seems that every illness feels worse in pregnancy! This is quite understandable because your immunity is slightly compromised in pregnancy and your body has to fight that much harder to get rid of the infection.

The common causes of fever that you might encounter in pregnancy are

- Cold and cough
- Influenza ('the flu')
- Typhoid
- Malaria
- Chickenpox
- Measles and Rubella (German measles)
- Urinary tract infection (see **Chapter 44**: *Urinary tract infection in pregnancy*)

Cold and cough in pregnancy

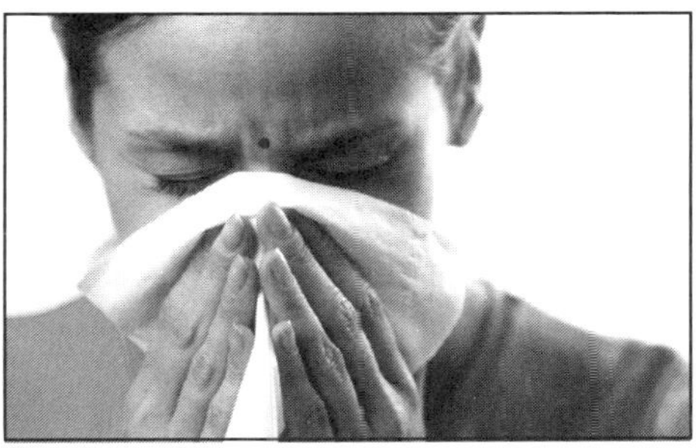

Colds are so common that it would be unusual for you to go through your pregnancy without catching a cold at least once. Colds, coughs, and most fevers lasting less than 5 days, are usually due to a viral infection. In the majority of cases, *there is no need for antibiotics.* They can be treated with medications that are safe in pregnancy and will relieve the symptoms.

Coughs, colds and viral fevers may make you feel tired and miserable but do not have any effect on the baby. Even when you have a severe cough, the coughing will not in any way disturb or harm the baby.

If the cough persists for more than five days or is accompanied by a large amount of yellow or green phlegm, you might want to see your doctor to rule out a lower respiratory infection. Do not take an antibiotic unless a physician prescribes it. Women who have had sinusitis earlier may need to take specific medication to relieve the symptoms.

There is no benefit at all to taking an antibiotic when you actually have a viral infection. More dangerously, you are promoting antibiotic resistance. That means that when you actually need antibiotics, they will have no effect on the infection. Common viral infections that do not benefit from antibiotic treatment include:

- Cold
- Flu
- Bronchitis
- Most coughs
- Most sore throats
- Some sinus infections
- Viral gastroenteritis (diarrhoea and vomiting)

Immediate home remedies

- Drink plenty of fluids, as this will help to thin out the secretions. Water, juices, warm milk and hot tea are good for you
- Steam inhalation will help clear a stuffy nose and also help in relieving coughs
- Sleep in a reclining position with plenty of pillows under your head so that breathing is easier
- Hot water gargles are soothing for a sore throat
- Use mentholated lozenges that help to relieve throat pain and irritation

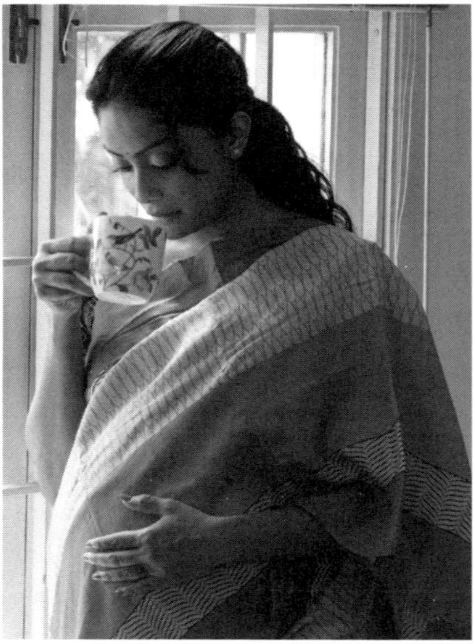

Medications to relieve symptoms

Decongestants: This group of medications is used to treat colds or allergies. They relieve stuffiness of the nose.

Cough suppressants and expectorants: Dextromethorphan, a common ingredient found in cough and cold medications, suppresses cough and is effective for a dry cough. Guaifenesin is an expectorant in many cough and cold medicines and helps bring out phlegm.

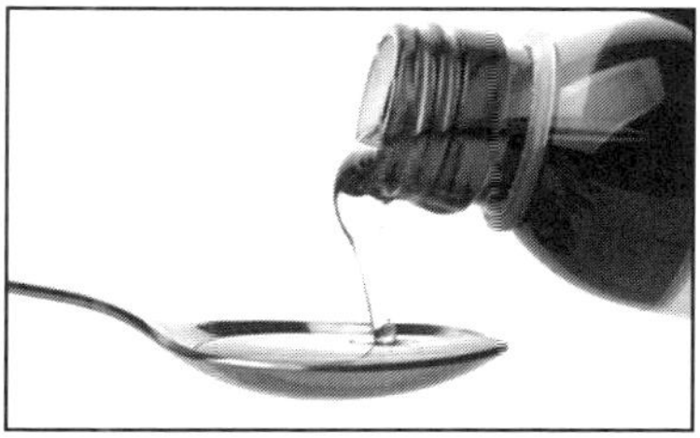

Antihistamines: Cough syrups and cold remedies may also contain an antihistamine. Check with your doctor which antihistamine is safe in pregnancy.

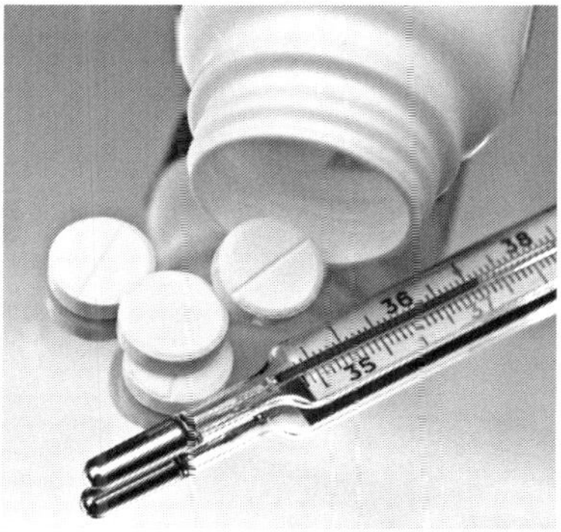

Painkillers and anti-inflammatory agents: It is safe to take paracetamol for headache and also to bring down a fever. Body pain can be treated with ibuprofen (however, ibuprofen should be avoided in the last three months of pregnancy).

Food

Having a cold, cough or fever does not mean that you cannot eat a normal diet. Make sure you drink plenty of fluids and don't get dehydrated. You do not have to avoid cold drinks, juices or curds. They do not aggravate fever or cold. If drinking something cold makes your throat hurt, then you may choose to avoid it.

It is best to avoid high fevers in pregnancy, especially in the first three months. If your temperature is 38°C (100°F) or more, take paracetamol to keep your temperature as near normal as possible. Paracetamol is available in both 500 mg and 650 mg strength. It is safe in pregnancy and can be taken every 4 to 6 hours to keep your temperature below 38°C.

Influenza ('the flu')

Influenza causes more symptoms than a bad cold. It usually comes on suddenly and may present with fever, headache, fatigue, severe body pain, coughing, and sore throat. Having the flu can be very tiring in pregnancy. The best thing to do is to drink plenty of fluids, eat a healthy diet and rest till you feel better. The body pain will respond to paracetamol, which is safe in pregnancy. The fever can also be kept under control with paracetamol. Remember that the flu is caused by a viral infection and does not require antibiotics.

Ibuprofen is a great painkiller for body ache but should be avoided in the last 3 months of pregnancy.

Pregnancy makes you more susceptible to the complications of flu. There is a higher risk of pregnancy complications, such as *preterm labour and preterm birth,* with the flu. Pregnant women are also more likely to be hospitalized as compared to non-pregnant women because of complications.

H1N1 influenza ('Swine flu')

H1N1 influenza epidemics are becoming more common in India. It is now recommended that **all pregnant women should receive the flu vaccine** that provides protection against H1N1 flu.

H1N1 can be particularly hazardous in the second and third trimesters. Due to the susceptibility of pregnant women to complications arising from H1N1 infection, hospitalization is more common in pregnancy. Pregnant women with suspected H1N1 influenza should be started on antiviral therapy at the earliest.

If you have been in contact with someone who has been diagnosed as having H1N1 flu, contact your doctor so that you can be started on anti-viral medication immediately.

Lower respiratory infection

Sometimes, a common cold or cough (which is called an upper respiratory infection) can progress to an infection in the lungs (a lower respiratory infection). You might start bringing up yellow or greenish phlegm that may sometimes have a bad odour.

Drink plenty of fluids to loosen up the phlegm. Steam inhalations will also help. Cough syrups can be used to suppress annoying, incessant coughing.

If the infection does not respond to the usual cold and cough remedies, your doctor might prescribe an antibiotic if she feels it is due to a bacterial infection. The antibiotic prescribed should be carefully chosen to make sure that it does not have any adverse effect on the baby.

Should you be worried about Zika virus?

Zika virus has been making headlines all over the world. In early 2017, the first three cases of infection with Zika virus have been reported in India. Infection with the Zika virus in pregnancy is associated with birth defects, especially a problem called microcephaly. In this condition the baby's head and brain are very small and the baby will have intellectual disability.

Diarrhoea and vomiting

You attended a friend's wedding and now you have developed loose motions. The nausea is bad and you think you may vomit. You have developed gastroenteritis. Sometimes when the vomiting is intractable, you are convinced that you have 'food poisoning'.

The commonest cause of gastroenteritis is a viral infection. If you are having a fever along with it, you might have a bacterial infection. What is the difference? Viral infections don't require antibiotics.

Immediate home remedies

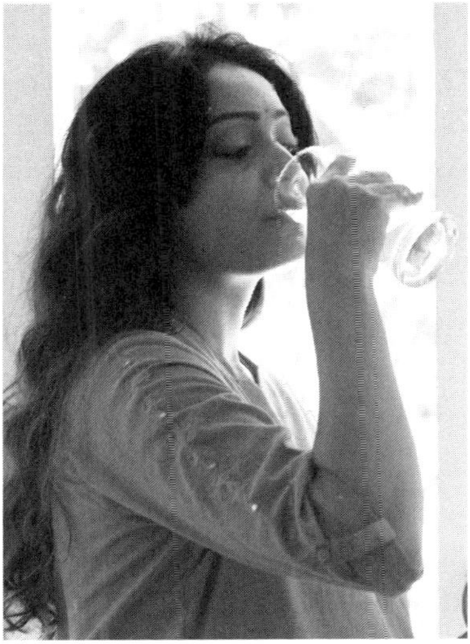

- Drink plenty of fluids, as this will keep you hydrated
- Water, buttermilk, tender coconut water, juices are all good fluids to drink. **Avoid glucose drinks**
- Add a pinch of salt and a pinch of sugar to whatever you are drinking. This is **oral rehydration therapy** and will prevent dehydration. There is no need for electrolyte solutions when you do this

Medications to relieve symptoms

Antacids: An antacid will help soothe the irritation of the stomach lining (gastritis).

Antispasmodics: This group of medications helps relieve the cramping that can accompany diarrhoea. Check with your doctor what you can take.

Antidiarrhoeals: These slow down the movement of the intestines. These should be taken only if your doctor prescribes it. They should not be taken if you have fever along with the diarrhoea.

Antiemetics: These are medications that decrease the nausea and vomiting. Ondansetron is safe in pregnancy and your doctor will prescribe it for you if needed.

Most diarrhoeas do not require antibiotics. If your doctor suspects a bacterial infection, antibiotics may be prescribed. The usual antibiotics prescribed for diarrhoea are not safe in pregnancy so don't take them without checking with your doctor.

Food

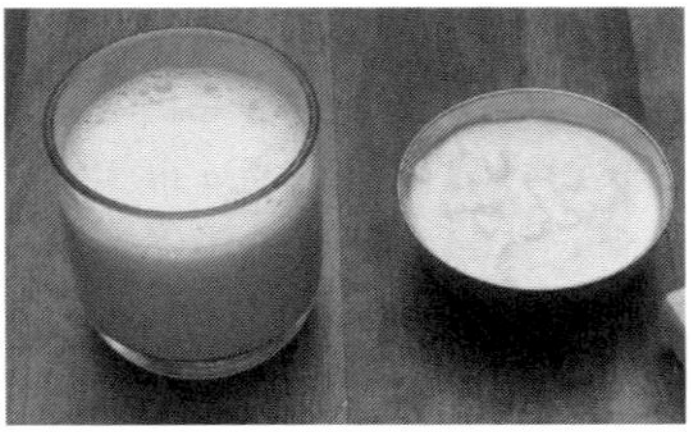

Eat a bland diet till your appetite is back. Idlis and khichdi are easily digested. Curds and buttermilk will soothe your stomach. Once your appetite is back, you can resume a normal diet.

Typhoid fever

Typhoid fever spreads through the consumption of contaminated food and water or through close contact with someone who is infected. Typhoid is suspected when high fever persists beyond 5 days.

Once signs and symptoms do appear, you are likely to experience fever, often as high as 39^0 to 40^0 C (103^0 to 104^0 F), headache, weakness and fatigue, sore throat, abdominal pain, diarrhoea or constipation.

Cause of typhoid fever

Virulent bacteria called Salmonella *typhi* cause typhoid fever. These bacteria spread through contaminated food or water and occasionally through direct contact with someone who is infected. In India, where typhoid is endemic (present all the time), most cases result from contaminated drinking water and poor sanitation. S. *typhi* is passed in the faeces and sometimes in the urine of infected people. You can contract the infection if you eat food handled by someone with typhoid fever who has not washed carefully after using the bathroom. You can also become infected by drinking water contaminated with the bacteria.

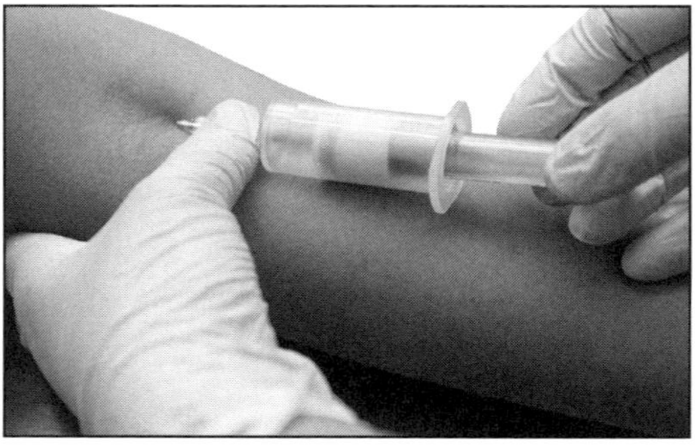

Diagnosis of typhoid fever

Typhoid is diagnosed by a blood test. The blood test will come back as positive only after the 5th day of fever.

Treatment of typhoid fever

Typhoid is treated with antibiotics that should be given for a duration of 10–14 days.

Testing for typhoid before the 5th day of fever is **not** useful. The report will not be positive for typhoid if it is done too early.

Recommended diet during typhoid fever

- *Drinking fluids:* This helps prevent the dehydration that results from prolonged fever and diarrhoea. If you are unable to drink enough fluids, you may be given fluids intravenously
- *Eating a healthy diet:* Low fibre, non-bulky, high-calorie meals can help replace the nutrients you lose when you are ill. You will have a very poor appetite so you have to make sure that you keep up nutrition for you and the baby

To prevent infecting others

These following measures can prevent others in your family from getting infected with typhoid:

- Wash your hands often. This is the single most important thing you can do to keep from spreading the infection to others. Use plenty of hot, soapy water and scrub thoroughly for at least 30 seconds, especially before eating, and after using the toilet
- Avoid handling food. Avoid preparing food for others until your doctor says you are no longer contagious
- Keep personal items separate. Set aside towels, bed linen and utensils for your own use and wash them frequently in hot, soapy water. Heavily soiled items can be soaked first in disinfectant

Malaria

Malaria is an infectious disease caused by a parasite that is transmitted by the bite of the female anopheles mosquito. Pregnancy reduces a woman's immunity to malaria and makes her more susceptible to repeated episodes and more serious forms of malaria.

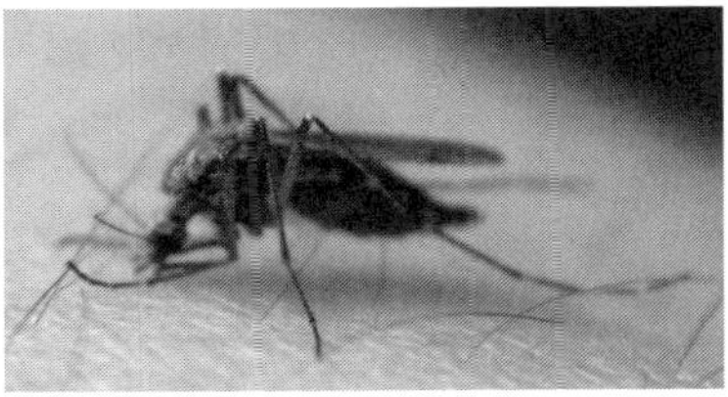

Symptoms

A malarial infection is generally characterized by recurrent attacks of high fever with moderate-to-severe shaking chills and profuse sweating as body temperature drops.

Tests and diagnosis

A blood sample and a blood smear can usually confirm the presence of the malaria parasite and which type it is.

Treatment and drugs

A malarial infection requires prompt evaluation and treatment. In most cases, doctors can treat malaria effectively in pregnancy with tablets of the anti-malarial chloroquine.

Avoiding malaria

- Use mosquito repellent
- Use mosquito netting

Rubella ('German measles')

Rubella is a highly contagious viral infection that has now been mostly eradicated due to vaccination. Rubella may present with very mild symptoms. Almost half of Rubella infections will go unnoticed. There will be fever, redness of the eyes and a rash. The rash can be missed because it lasts less than 3 days and is vey mild. The rash typically starts on the face and spreads down on to the body.

The worry with Rubella infection is that when it occurs in the first three months of pregnancy it can cause major birth defects. The baby can be born with deafness, cataracts and heart defects. Fortunately, Rubella is very rare now.

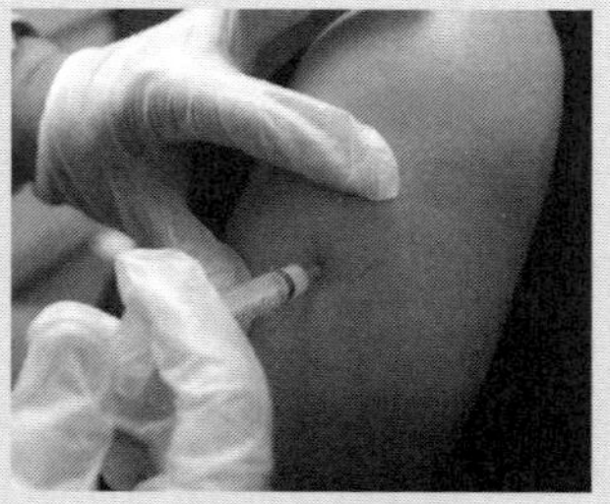

The MMR vaccine protects against Rubella infection. Make sure that you have had this vaccine. If you are not sure that you have had the vaccination in your younger days, it is prudent to take it 3 months before you start planning a pregnancy. You should wait at least 1–3 months after getting the vaccine to become pregnant. **You should not take the vaccine if you're already pregnant because of the real risk of the baby getting infected.**

Chickenpox

There are periodic epidemics of chickenpox. It is much more common in children. However adults who get chickenpox have more complications. If you have come in contact with someone who has had chickenpox, immediately contact your doctor. An injection (Varicella-zoster immune globulin) can be given that can protect you against the infection.

If you get chickenpox in pregnancy, it is recognized by the typical clear fluid-filled blebs that appear first on the abdomen and spread rapidly.

Treatment and drugs

Chickenpox in pregnancy is treated with an antiviral drug for 5–7 days. It is most effective when started within 24 hours of getting the infection. It decreases the severity of the infection.

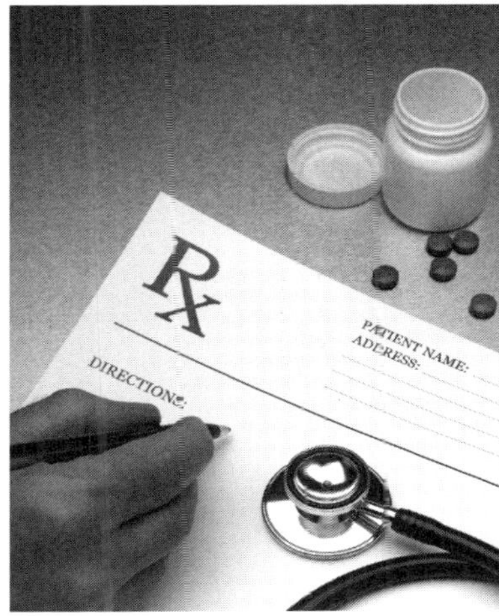

You may be prescribed an antihistamine to control the itching that accompanies chickenpox. Once crusts form, you are no longer infective.

Effect of chickenpox on your baby

Fortunately, it is very rare for chickenpox to affect your baby.

Food

Make sure that you keep yourself well hydrated. There are no food restrictions. Eat a healthy diet and keep up your energy.

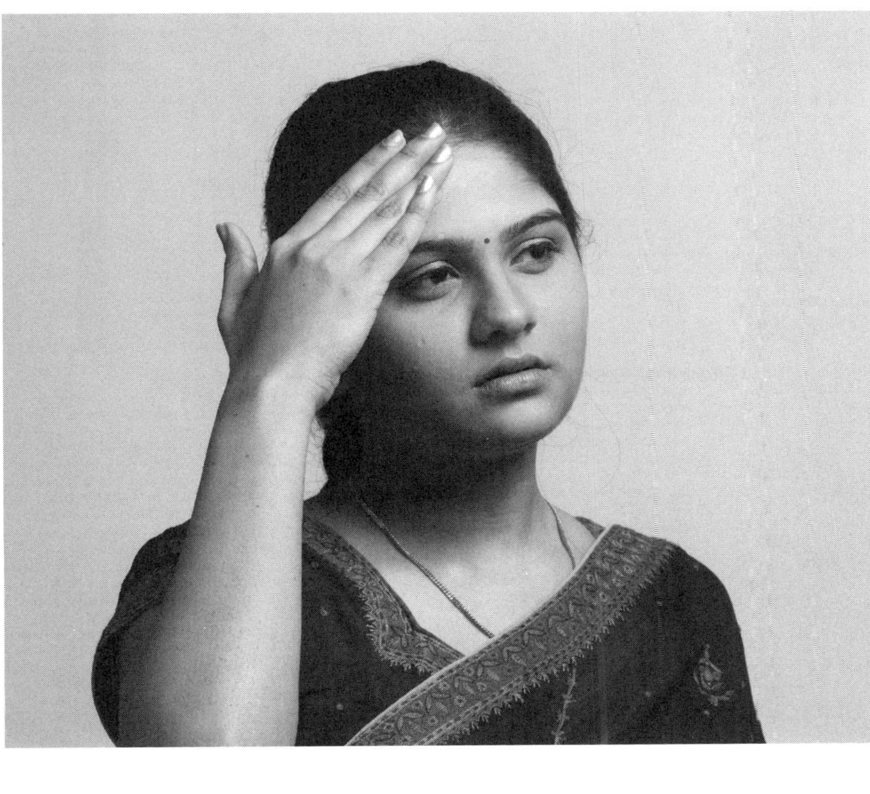

CHAPTER 44

Urinary tract infection in pregnancy

Shabana has been running to the bathroom every five minutes. There is severe burning when she passes urine. She is having pain in the lower part of the abdomen and she is running a mild fever. Does she have a urinary infection?

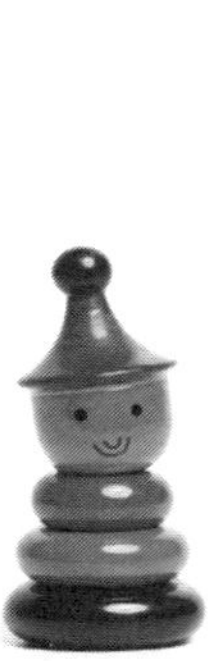

44

Urinary tract infection in pregnancy

A urinary tract infection (UTI) can be very distressing. You may suspect that you have a urinary tract infection when you have an urge to pass urine very frequently but pass only small quantities or just a few drops every time. Burning or pain may accompany this. You may also have pain in the lower part of your abdomen.

Did you know that UTI is one of the most common infections in pregnancy? This is because there are physical and hormonal changes that occur in pregnancy that make you more susceptible to UTI. Bacteria are able to enter your bladder easily and can take up residence there, leading to infection.

What can you do to prevent UTI?

- Drink plenty of water and other fluids to flush out the bacteria from your bladder. This is particularly important in the hot summer months

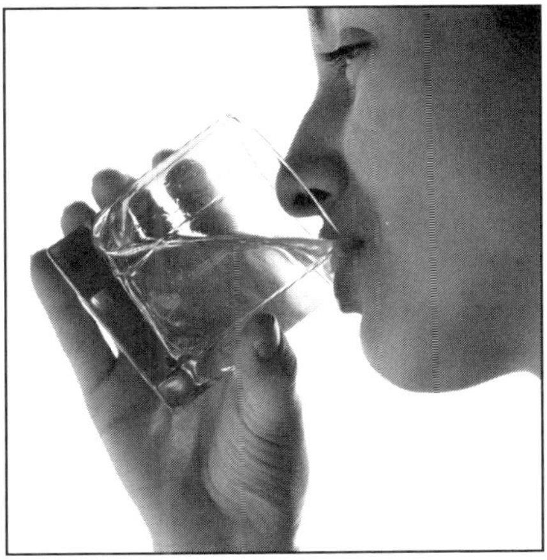

- Don't hold urine in for long periods of time. It is sometimes difficult to find a clean bathroom so women tend to hold it in for a long time. This may lead to an increased risk of infection because bacteria get a chance to stay in the bladder and multiply
- Pass urine before and after having intercourse. This decreases the chance of UTI
- In the later stages of pregnancy, the baby's head may be pressing against your bladder and you may not actually empty your bladder completely. After passing urine, wait for a few minutes and try to pass urine again
- Keep the area clean and wash frequently

Brinda asked: I have some irritation in the area and there is burning when I pass urine. Do I have a UTI?

My answer: It might sometimes be difficult for you to decide whether you have a UTI or a vaginal infection. If you are having burning as you are passing urine or severe pain as soon as you finish urinating, then you probably have a UTI. You will also have the urge to pass urine very frequently.

If the burning happens when the urine splashes down on to your perineum, then you probably have a vaginal infection. Increased discharge and significant itching will also accompany vaginal infection (see **Chapter 45**, *Vaginal discharge and infection*).

When should you suspect a urinary tract infection?

An urge to pass urine frequently, burning or pain at the start or end of urination, a feeling that you need to urinate right after you have just passed urine, are all signs of a UTI. Sometimes you may also pass blood in the urine when the infection is severe.

Types of infection

Cystitis: A urinary tract infection (UTI) confined to the bladder is called cystitis. The bladder will keep contracting and there is a constant urge to pass urine. When you do go to the bathroom, you may pass only a few drops of urine. In severe infection, some women may even pass blood-stained urine. One out of 100 pregnant women have a chance of developing cystitis. Fever commonly accompanies urinary infection.

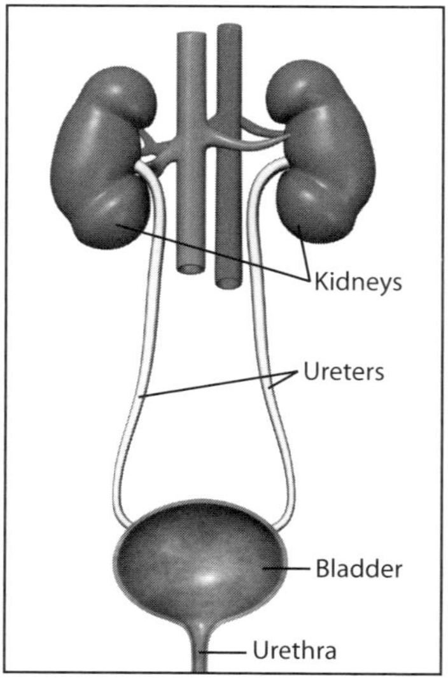

Pyelonephritis: If left untreated, the infection can travel upwards from the bladder and cause infection in the kidneys. This is called *pyelonephritis*. In this case, there will be fever and chills, along with pain in the flanks (over the kidney area).

Pyelonephritis is the most serious medical condition occurring in pregnancy, affecting 2 out of 100 pregnant women. It occurs most commonly in young women pregnant for the first time and tends to present in the 2nd trimester.

Ambika asked: I am 5 months pregnant. For the past two days I have been running to the bathroom every 15 minutes, and having severe burning when I pass urine. I also have a mild fever. My doctor suspects a urine infection and has asked for some tests and given me antibiotics. This is the first time this has happened to me. I used the toilet on the train a few days ago. Is this why I have a urine infection?

My answer: Using the toilet on the train has not caused the infection. There are several bacteria in the vagina and the rectum that can gain entrance into the bladder. Urinary tract infection is more common in women because the urethra is short, making it easy for bacteria to enter the bladder. Normally, the small number of bacteria is not enough to cause an infection. However, since you were on the train, you probably did not drink enough water. Drinking plenty of water and passing enough urine will normally flush out the bacteria before they can multiply and cause a problem.

Does a urinary infection affect the baby?

An infection in the bladder will not affect the baby directly. However, severe bladder and kidney infections are associated with preterm labour and birth (see **Chapter 32**, *When the baby comes too early: preterm labour and birth*).

Diagnosis of urinary infection

When a urinary infection is suspected, it is absolutely essential to get the urine tested before treatment is started.

It is important to confirm the urinary infection with a **culture and sensitivity test** before starting on antibiotics. If the correct antibiotic is not used, the infection will not be eradicated completely and will keep recurring.

When a UTI is suspected, your doctor will ask for two types of tests:

- A microscopic examination of the urine: In women, the presence of more than 10 pus cells is suggestive of a urinary infection. Red blood cells might also be seen
- A culture and sensitivity test will also be performed on the urine. This will tell us the exact type of bacteria responsible for the infection. The test also checks which antibiotic is effective against that particular strain of bacteria

How is a urinary infection treated?

An appropriate antibiotic will be prescribed. Usually the course of antibiotics is for 3–5 days. Your obstetrician will prescribe an antibiotic that

Collecting urine for a culture and sensitivity test

The lab will provide you with a sterile wide-mouth container. Wash your genital area well with water and then pass a little urine into the toilet. Collect the remaining urine in the container. Make sure the container does not touch your skin. This is called a 'mid-stream sample'.

What is a culture and sensitivity report?

For your doctor to confirm that you have a UTI, a colony count should be reported. **An infection is only confirmed if the colony count of the bacteria is more than 100,000 per mL.**

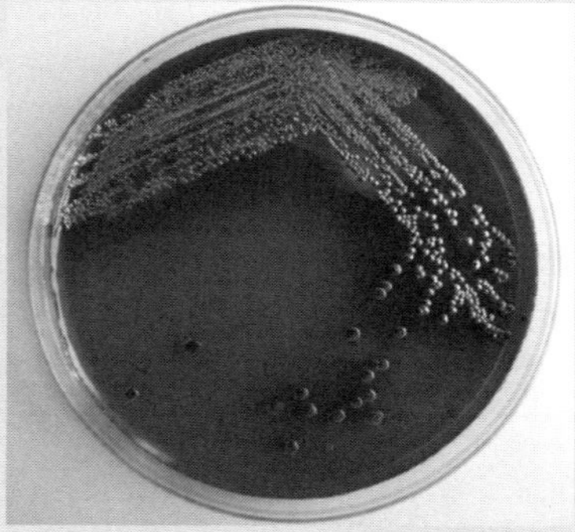

Bacterial colonies growing in the lab

The second part of the report is called the sensitivity report. This matches a number of antibiotics against the bacteria growing in your urine. The doctor will only prescribe an antibiotic that the bacteria are sensitive to. This gives the best chance of eradicating the infection. The doctor will also choose the antibiotic based on its safety in pregnancy.

It usually takes 48 hours to get a culture and sensitivity report back from the lab.

is safe for you and the baby. The choice of antibiotic will depend on the report of the culture and sensitivity test. Sometimes, if the pain and other symptoms are very severe, you might be placed on an antibiotic before the report comes back and this may be continued or changed depending on the report.

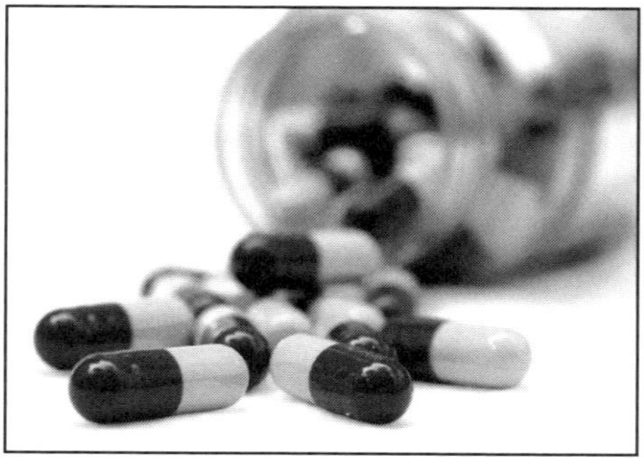

Along with the antibiotic, your doctor may also place you on a tablet that will numb the bladder a bit and decrease the pain of UTI.

You can help by increasing your fluid intake to help flush out the germs from the urinary tract. You can drink plenty of water and also juices, coconut water and buttermilk.

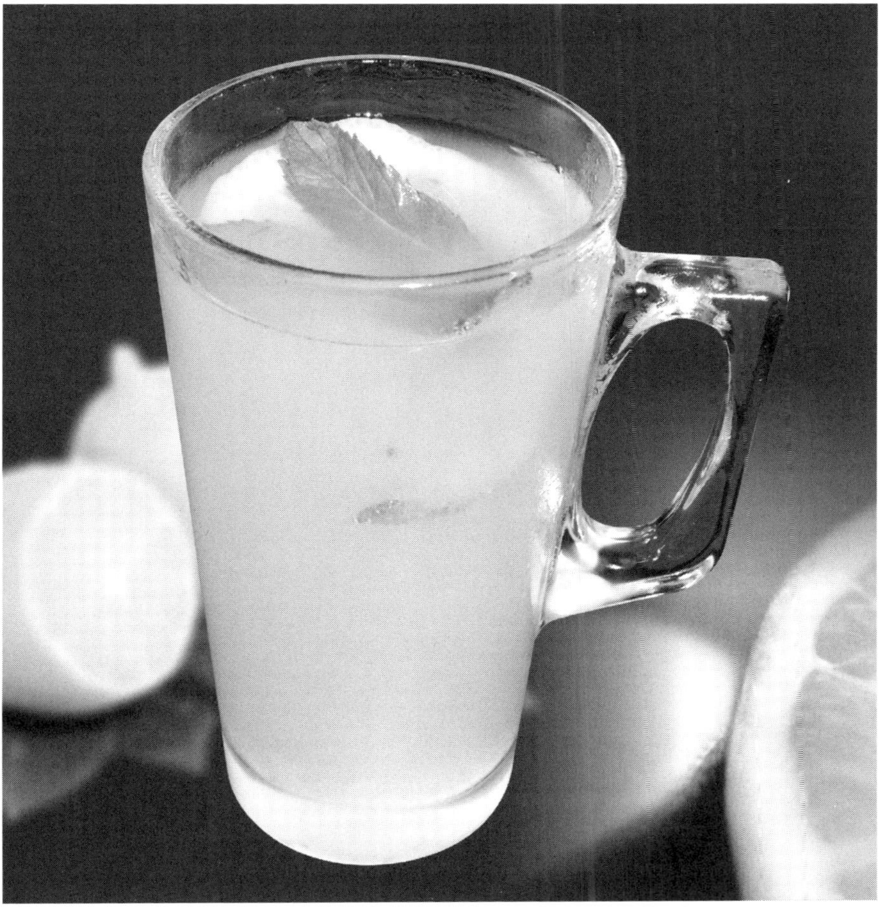

CHAPTER 45

Vaginal discharge and infection in pregnancy

Sona is 5 months pregnant. She has been having a thick discharge for the past two days, accompanied by mild irritation. Since this morning she has been having severe, uncontrollable itching. The inner sides of her thighs are reddened. She has called her doctor for an immediate appointment. Sona has a vaginal infection.

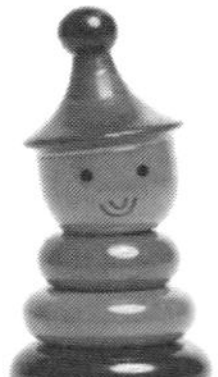

45

Vaginal discharge and infection in pregnancy

Pregnancy brings about many alterations in your body. The surge in estrogen levels makes you susceptible to certain vaginal infections. These infections can be very distressing if the discharge and itching are severe.

Vaginal discharge in pregnancy

Right from the time you became pregnant, you may have noticed an increased amount of mucus discharge from the vagina. As pregnancy progresses, you might find that the amount of discharge may fluctuate from day to day. Sometimes it can be copious enough to require a panty liner. Closer to your due date the discharge may increase because the cervix has softened and has started to open up. Discharge without itching is a normal occurrence in pregnancy.

When the discharge is accompanied by itching, it is an abnormal condition that indicates you have developed an infection.

Vaginal infection or vaginitis

Inflammation or infection in a woman's vagina is called vaginitis. It is quite common for pregnant women to develop vaginitis in pregnancy. Sometimes, the infection may also spread over the skin of the groin area. When there is any abnormal discharge associated with burning or itching, it is best to contact your obstetrician.

The vagina has many organisms, such as bacteria and yeast. These are usually in balance and do not cause any problems. Pregnancy may upset the pH balance in the vagina and one or the other of the organisms may start to increase, resulting in an infection.

To diagnose vaginitis, your doctor will examine you to see what kind of discharge you are having and also the effect it is having on your body. A sample might be taken to check for the kind of organism that is causing the vaginitis.

Treatment will depend on the cause of the vaginitis. Treatment may be either with oral tablets, tablets to be inserted into the vagina or a cream or gel that is applied to the vagina.

Fungal (yeast) infection or candidiasis

Fungal infection or candidiasis is probably the most common types of vaginal infection.

A fungus called Candida causes this infection. Candida is always found in small numbers in the vagina. However, when the pH balance and the balance between the bacteria and yeast in the vagina is altered, the yeast may overgrow and cause symptoms. Do you know that 75 per cent of women will develop a vaginal fungal infection at some time in their life?

Some reasons for a fungal infection

- Fungal infection is more common in pregnancy
- Some types of antibiotics increase the risk of a fungal infection
- Women with diabetes have an increased risk of developing candidiasis

Symptoms

Fungal vaginitis classically presents with a thick, white, and curdy vaginal discharge. The accompanying itching can be intense. The itching and burning can be felt inside the vagina and the area outside the vagina. There may be redness and swelling. You may also find that when you pass urine you may have severe burning on the outside skin when the urine touches it. Having intercourse may be painful.

Treatment

- Your doctor will prescribe vaginal anti-fungal tablets of clotrimazole or micanazole. One tablet should be placed deep inside the vagina every night at bedtime. It is quite easy to push the tablet in with your finger. These tablets must be used for a week to be effective in pregnancy.
- The external itching can be treated with an ointment of clotrimazole or micanazole. Most of the ointments come as a combination with a steroid for quick relief of itching.
- Oral antifungal agents are not safe in pregnancy since they may cause birth defects.

Preventing and avoiding recurrence of fungal infection

Hot and humid weather promotes sweating. This makes you susceptible to fungal infection.

- Keep yourself clean and dry. Dry yourself well after washing the area
- Avoid clothes that hold in heat and moisture. Wear loose cotton clothing. Avoid tight jeans, non-breathable leggings and tights
- Wear cotton panties and avoid synthetics

Trichomoniasis

Trichomoniasis is the second most common vaginal infection in pregnancy. It is caused by the microscopic parasite Trichomonas vaginalis. The diagnosis is confirmed by a simple microscopic examination that will identify the parasite. The only way to get the infection is through intercourse. However, the majority of men with the infection have no symptoms.

Symptoms

Seventy per cent of Trichomonas infections in pregnancy present as a thin discharge associated with itching. The discharge may be yellow-grey or greenish. There may be burning, irritation, redness and swelling of the vulva. Sometimes, there is pain during urination. Intercourse can be uncomfortable.

Treatment

Treatment of Trichomoniasis in pregnancy is with oral metronidazole tablets. It can be taken as a single high dose but that can cause severe vomiting. Doctors usually prescribe it twice daily for 5–7 days. Earlier, metronidazole was not recommended in pregnancy but now there is clear evidence that it does not affect the baby.

Your husband will also be given the same course since the infection may spread back and forth between the two of you (during intercourse) if he is not treated. He most probably will not have symptoms of infection but definitely needs to be treated.

It is important to avoid intercourse during the treatment period and for a week after the course is over.

Bacterial vaginosis

This is another kind of vaginal infection and may present with a thin discharge that has a fishy odour. It is accompanied with itching. It is not a very common infection in Indians though it is the most common vaginal infection in the West. It is treated with 5–7 days of metronidazole.

CHAPTER 46

Medical disorders in pregnancy

Suzanne has had asthma from childhood. Will the asthma affect the baby?

Shabana is on medication for epilepsy for the past two years. She was married eight months ago. She is now pregnant and her doctor has told her to continue her medication. Is this safe?

Sundari's thyroid gland does not produce enough hormone. She takes thyroxine regularly. Her thyroid function tests have been normal. Her doctor has advised her not to reduce the dosage in pregnancy.

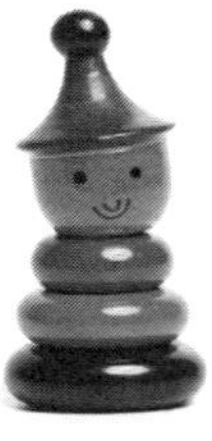

46

Medical disorders in pregnancy

ASTHMA

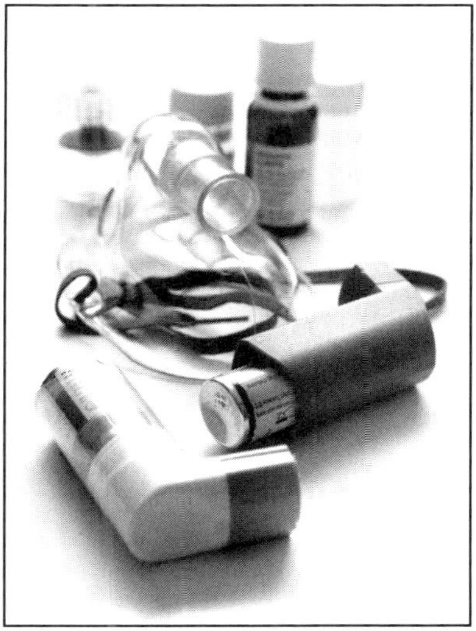

Suzanne has suffered from asthma for many years. From the minute her pregnancy was confirmed, she has been worried. She knows how it feels to be breathless and struggle to get oxygen into her lungs. Will this affect her baby? Will her baby get enough oxygen when she has an episode of breathlessness? Will she be harming the little one with the medications she takes to keep her asthma under control? As long as she continues her medications and carefully avoids the triggers for an asthma attack, she should be able to go through the pregnancy comfortably.

Asthma is the most common lung condition in pregnancy. About eight per cent of pregnant women have asthma. If you have asthma, you should discuss your condition with your physician before becoming pregnant. You should continue your asthma medications. Stopping medications all of a sudden could result in a bad attack of asthma. The risk of poorly controlled asthma is much greater than the risk of taking medications to control the condition.

What causes asthma?

People who have a tendency to have allergies have a greater chance of developing asthma. Substances like dust, mould, pollen and smoke can trigger an episode. The allergic reaction cause the bronchioles (the narrow tubes that carry air into the lungs) to constrict and become very narrow. This results in wheezing, tightness of the chest and a persistent dry cough. You struggle to suck air into your lungs.

Some women develop asthma in the workplace due to exposure to certain chemicals or other substances. Sometimes, asthma is triggered by exercise. **Exercise-induced asthma** is caused by dry air coming into the lungs or a change in the fluid balance of cells. Within 5–10 minutes after beginning exercise, individuals experience asthmatic symptoms such as chest tightness, coughing or wheezing.

Effect of pregnancy on asthma

It is difficult to predict the effect of pregnancy on asthma. The severity of asthma during pregnancy varies from one woman to another. Women who have severe asthma are more likely to face a worsening of the disease in pregnancy. However, it has been clearly shown that well-controlled asthma is the key to a safe pregnancy for both you and your baby.

> During pregnancy as a rule of thumb, asthma worsens in about one-third of women, improves in one-third and remains stable in one-third.

Asthma tends to worsen in the third trimester. This is because the really big uterus is pressing your diaphragm up. Even women without asthma get breathless so it is understandable that this might make an asthmatic uncomfortable. Asthma eases up during the last month of pregnancy.

Effect of asthma on pregnancy

Women who have mild asthma usually go through pregnancy without any major complications. For women with moderate to severe asthma, there is a slight increase in the risk for high blood pressure or preeclampsia. Women with severe asthma that is not well controlled in pregnancy, run the risk of preterm delivery and low birth weight babies.

Medications for asthma during pregnancy

The commonly used drugs that are safe in pregnancy are:

Bronchodilators: These medications rapidly relieve the wheezing by relaxing the airways. Short-acting bronchodilators are safe during pregnancy. They include salbutamol and terbutaline.

Steroids: Most asthmatics will respond well to inhaled steroids. Budesonide and beclomethasone are safe inhaled steroids. Experience shows that the use of steroids by pregnant women is safe for both the mother and the baby. In severe cases, oral prednisone tablets may be given.

Antihistamines: Although antihistamines are not used to directly treat asthma, they may be used to treat the allergies that often accompany asthma.

These drugs include diphenhydramine, chlorpheniramine, cetirizine and fexofenadine. These drugs are safe in pregnancy.

Drugs to be avoided in pregnancy

Taking certain painkillers like aspirin or ibuprofen can aggravate asthma. You should also be aware that certain drugs used in pregnancy can worsen your wheezing. The F-series of prostaglandins, sometimes used in pregnancy to make the uterus contract and control bleeding after delivery, must be avoided in an asthmatic.

Monitoring the baby's growth

Since women with moderate to severe asthma have a greater risk of delivering a low birth weight baby, the baby's growth must be monitored with ultrasound scans.

Labour and delivery

The medications that you are taking will be continued during labour and delivery. Epidural analgesia for pain relief is safe for a woman with asthma. If general anaesthesia has to be given for an emergency caesarean section, the anaesthetist will also give you an injection to prevent wheezing.

Breastfeeding

There is no reason to avoid breastfeeding. On the other hand, there are a number of benefits for both you and your infant.

EPILEPSY

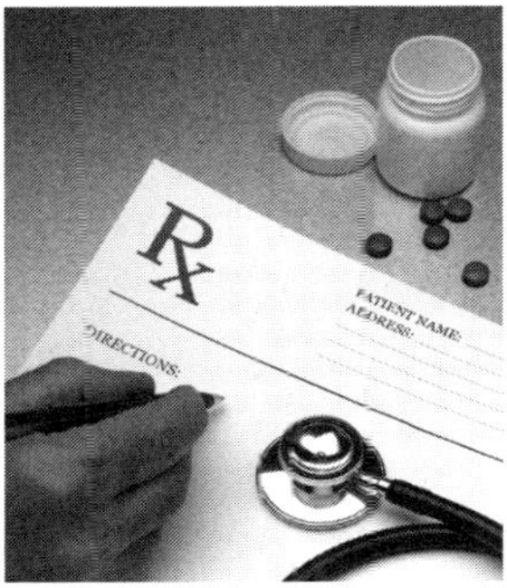

Subbulakshmi was married two years ago. She is an epileptic and has been avoiding a pregnancy because she and her husband are worried the baby might be affected by the medicines she is taking. With good preconceptional counselling and optimal obstetric care, she can have a normal pregnancy and a healthy baby. She can also safely breastfeed her baby.

How common is epilepsy?

There are close to 8 million persons with epilepsy in India. Unfortunately, both in the urban and rural population, people still try to conceal the disease. Girls and women particularly delay seeking professional help. To avoid problems later in the marriage, it is best to have an informal discussion with a doctor by both parties so that all doubts can be laid to rest. There are many cases where a disclosure of epilepsy after the marriage ends up in the woman being sent back to her parents' home, even if she is pregnant.

Epilepsy and pregnancy

The chances of having a normal, healthy child are excellent and are greater than 90 per cent. Both the neurologist and the obstetrician need to be involved in reviewing the anti-epileptic drug that the woman is taking and in deciding whether there is need for a change in medication prior to conception. It is best to be on a single drug rather than a combination of drugs.

Preethi asked: I have been an epileptic since college. I am on an anti-epileptic drug. My husband and I are worried about having a baby with a birth defect.

My answer: Though there is a slightly increased risk of certain abnormalities in the baby due to anti-epileptic drugs, these problems can be prevented by taking folic acid supplementation (5mg/day), particularly prior to conception and in the first three months of pregnancy. A good quality detailed ultrasound at 20–22 weeks can ensure that the baby does not have a birth defect. There may be a need to increase the dose of the antiepileptic drug in pregnancy.

Before conception

If you have epilepsy, it is smart to take certain precautions before you get pregnant, to ensure that you stay healthy and have a healthy baby. See your doctor before getting pregnant to discuss your medication. If there has been no seizure in two or more years, it may be possible to stop the medication gradually. If the medications cannot be stopped, your doctor may suggest that you switch to a medication that is safer for the baby. However, seizures are more harmful to you and your baby than any medication; do not abruptly stop your medication, and make sure your obstetrician and neurologist are in agreement about the medications you are taking.

> Antiepileptic drugs affect the way the body uses folic acid. So make sure you take a folic acid supplement along with your medication.

Risks for the baby

The risk of having a baby with a birth defect is 2–3 per cent in all pregnancies. Having epilepsy increases this risk to 6–8 per cent. This risk may be related to the disorder or to the medication used to treat it. Though rare, the problems that may be seen in babies of epileptic mothers include:

- Cleft lip or palate (the lip or roof of the mouth is not completely closed)
- Heart defects
- Neural tube defects (such as spina bifida)
- Small head
- Low birth weight
- Growth restriction
- Intellectual disability
- Bleeding problems at birth

Children of women with a seizure disorder may also run the risk of developing epilepsy later in life.

Delivery

There is no reason why a woman with epilepsy cannot have a vaginal delivery. Her chance of requiring a caesarean is the same as any other mother.

Postpartum care

After delivery, the medication to control the seizures may need to be adjusted. Just after birth, your baby will be given an injection of vitamin K to prevent any bleeding problems. This is because antiepileptic drugs lower the natural levels of vitamin K (the vitamin that helps with blood clotting) in the body.

Breastfeeding

Women on a single drug can safely breastfeed their babies in consultation with their paediatrician. Antiepileptic drugs are found in small amounts in breast milk, but in most cases this is not enough to affect the baby.

Birth control methods in women with epilepsy

Women with epilepsy can use all available birth control methods. Intrauterine devices provide safe and reliable contraception. It is important to know that some antiepileptic drugs can make birth control pills less effective in preventing pregnancy. It is best to involve both the neurologist and the obstetrician in deciding on the best method of contraception.

THYROID DISEASE IN PREGNANCY

The thyroid gland is butterfly-shaped and located at the base of the neck. The thyroid gland has an enormous impact on your health. Every aspect of your metabolism, from your heart rate to how quickly you burn calories, is regulated by thyroid hormones. You cannot live without your thyroid gland or the thyroid hormones.

Occasionally, the thyroid may not produce enough of the hormone thyroxine. This is called **hypothyroidism**. Sometimes, there is an over production of the hormone. This is called **hyperthyroidism**.

Diagnosis of thyroid disease

Blood tests are done to measure TSH and free T4. If the TSH is raised and the free T4 is low, then you have hypothyroidism. Decreased TSH and raised free T4 are indicative of hyperthyroidism.

Hypothyroidism and pregnancy

Causes of hypothyroidism during pregnancy

The most common cause of hypothyroidism is the autoimmune disorder known as Hashimoto's thyroiditis.

The risks of hypothyroidism to the mother

Most women with mild hypothyroidism may have no symptoms. Untreated, or severe hypothyroidism has been associated with anaemia, muscle pain and weakness, low birth weight infants, and postpartum haemorrhage.

The risks of maternal hypothyroidism to the baby

The thyroid hormone is critical for brain development in the baby. Do not stop your thyroid medication when you find out you are pregnant. It is important that hypothyroidism be adequately treated in pregnancy. TSH and free T4 levels must be checked regularly in pregnancy to monitor if you are getting enough hormone replacement.

> All newborns should be tested for thyroid function on the 3rd or 4th day of life, irrespective of their mother's thyroid status. Children born with *congenital hypothyroidism* (no thyroid function at birth) can have severe intellectual and developmental disability if the condition is not recognized and treated.

Treatment of hypothyroidism during pregnancy

There must be adequate replacement of thyroid hormone in the form of synthetic thyroxine. Thyroxine requirements frequently increase during pregnancy, often by 25–50 per cent. Women with known hypothyroidism should have their thyroid function tested as soon as pregnancy is detected and their dose adjusted by their physician as needed, to maintain the TSH level in the normal range.

> Iron supplements can impair the absorption of thyroid hormone. Consequently, thyroxine and prenatal vitamins should not be taken at the same time and should be separated by at least 2–3 hours.

Hyperthyroidism in pregnancy

Hyperthyroidism is the medical term used to describe the signs and symptoms associated with an *overproduction* of thyroid hormone.

Causes of hyperthyroidism during pregnancy

The most common cause (80–85 per cent) of maternal hyperthyroidism during pregnancy is Graves' disease. This condition occurs in 1 in 1500 pregnant patients.

The risks of hyperthyroidism to the mother

Graves' disease may present initially during the first trimester or may worsen during this time in a woman known to have the disorder. Inadequately treated maternal hyperthyroidism can result in preterm labour and preeclampsia. Very severe hyperthyroidism (known as 'thyroid storm') may also develop.

The risks of hyperthyroidism to the baby

If hyperthyroidism is treated adequately, the risks to the baby are very low. It is important to see your physician before you get pregnant so that the proper medication can be given, in the sufficient dose.

Treatment options for a pregnant woman with hyperthyroidism

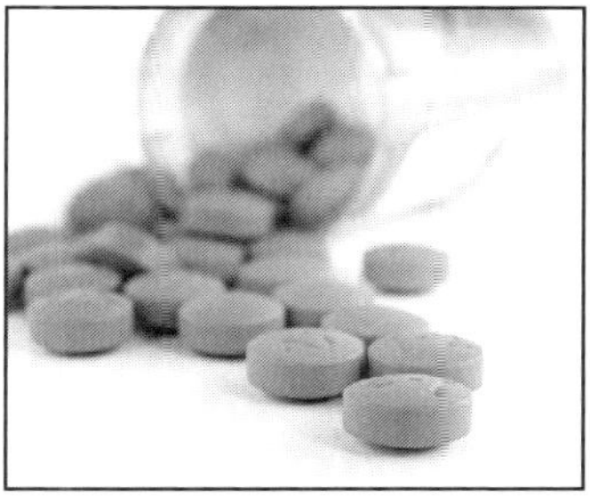

When hyperthyroidism is severe enough to require therapy, anti-thyroid medications are the treatment, with propylthiouracil (PTU) being the drug of choice.

After delivery

Hyperthyroidism typically worsens in the postpartum period, usually in the first three months after delivery. Higher doses of anti-thyroid medications are frequently required during this time. Close monitoring of thyroid function is necessary.

Breastfeeding

It is safe to breastfeed the baby if you are on propylthiouracil (PTU). The baby will require periodic assessment of his thyroid function to ensure maintenance of normal thyroid status.

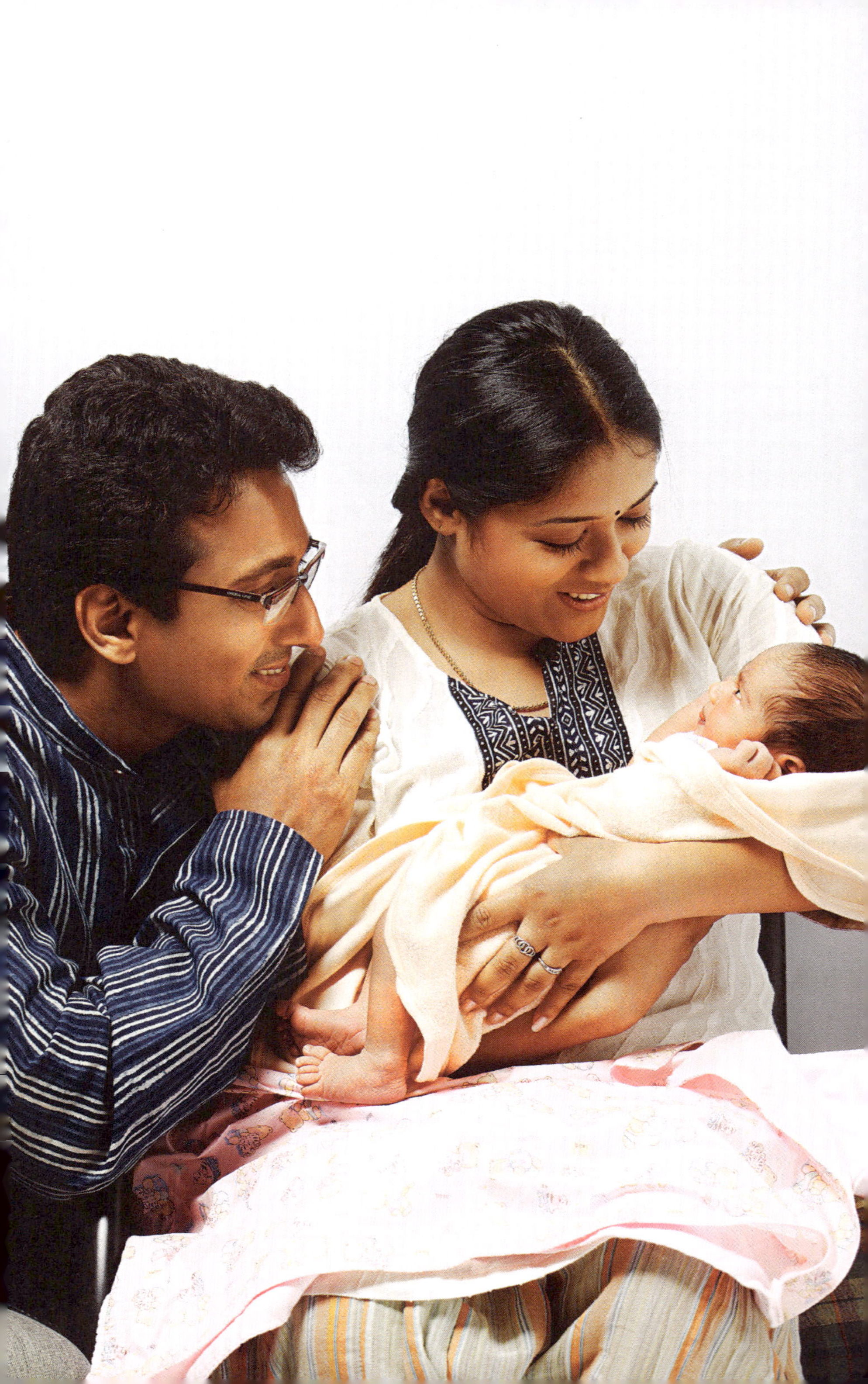

Being a parent

CHAPTER 47

Preparing your child for the arrival of the new baby

Gayatri is the mother of a five-year-old bundle of charm. She has just found out that she is pregnant for the second time. She and her husband, Arjun, want their daughter to be as excited as they are about the new baby. How should they break the news to her?

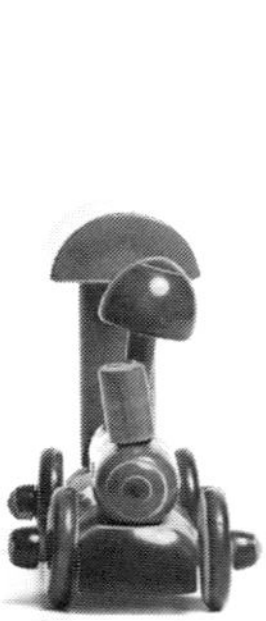

47

Preparing your child for the arrival of the new baby

You and your husband are ecstatic with the positive pregnancy test. You have called your family and shared the great news. Your best friend couldn't stop shrieking with delight on the phone when you told her! You are dying to tell you daughter. Is it too early? Should you wait till you have completed 3 months?

However loved a child is, she will always feel a sense of displacement when she learns that a new baby is on its way. Having been the focus of attention for her parents and grandparents all her life, an older sibling can feel threatened by the new baby and will suffer what is known as 'regression'. She may want to be 'a baby' again, demand to be fed, and may want to be cuddled more often.

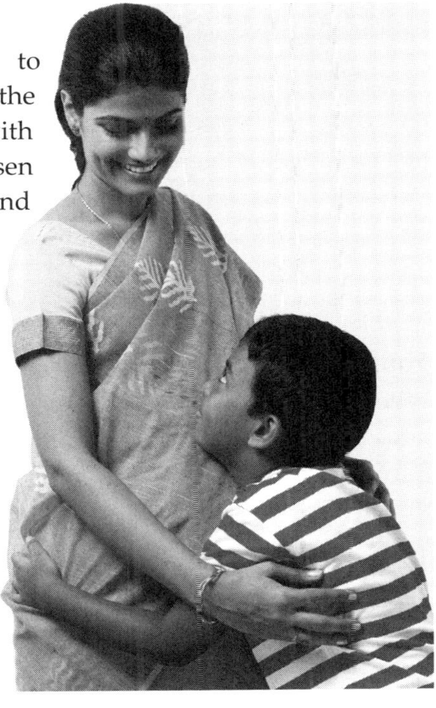

Your child may become difficult to handle and may throw tantrums the way only a child can! Getting angry with her and punishing her will only worsen the problem. Give her all the love and understanding that she deserves. After all, how would you feel if you suddenly had to share your home with a stranger! That is exactly how your child views the new baby–as an usurper of her rightful place in the family.

Remain calm and unflustered. Do not expect your child to behave like an adult and display instant love for the new baby. Ease her into the fact that she is going to be the 'big sister' who will be taking care of the baby.

Make her own arrival special

A good way to make your first child a part of the whole process is to discuss her own birth with her. Explain how excited you were about her coming into the world. Little children are always fascinated by stories of their childhood, especially since they are the main character in the drama that unfolds! Then involve her in the process of the arrival of the new baby. Include her by always saying 'your baby', 'your little one' and 'the baby will expect her big sister to take care of her'. This will give your child a sense of ownership and she will get engrossed in the whole process of your pregnancy.

Telling your child about the new baby

There are no real rules about how you break the news to your child about the new baby. If your first child is still young, he might not quite understand the concept of waiting for a few months till the baby arrives. You might wake up every day to be bombarded by the same question, 'Has the baby come yet?'

If your child is going to school, you can relate the date of delivery with the school calendar or a special holiday. For example, you might say, "The baby will arrive just around the Christmas holidays."

How your child handles the news also depends on the age of the child and the size of the extended family. If your child is used to being in the middle of a large family, he will handle the newcomer better. If the child has been the centre of attention in a small nuclear family, he may find it hard to give up his place. If there has been the birth of another child in the close family and your child has been aware of it and has participated in the fun of a new arrival, he may handle it better.

Your child is not asking for details!

When your 5-year-old daughter asks, "Where do babies come from?" she is not asking for a lesson in reproduction. She will be quite satisfied with the information that the baby is going to come from her mother's tummy and that the doctor will take it out.

As your child gets more involved and is really interested in what is happening, help her understand by showing her what she looked like when she was a baby. Her own baby pictures will help her realize how small the new arrival is going to be.

If your child is old enough, you can share the pictures in this book about how the baby is developing (**Chapters 6 to 8**). You can also take her to see a friend who has had a baby.

Involve your child during pregnancy

If your child is old enough to understand the concept of another baby, tell her around the third month of your pregnancy. Of course, if your child is older and understands your conversations well, tell her when you think she is ready so that she does not feel left out.

Take your child with you to the antenatal check-ups so that she can be involved in the process right from the beginning. Ask your doctor if she can be allowed to hear the baby's heartbeat (which is possible when using a hand-held Doppler). One of the truly delightful moments is when the older sibling's eyes light up when she hears the baby's heartbeat.

Let your child help in picking stuff for the new arrival. Let him give you suggestions about baby names. Don't be surprised when he wants to name the baby after his best friend in school or his favourite teacher!

The age of the child

If your child is **2–3 years** old, she might tend to be more possessive of your affections and might find it hard to 'share' you.

A **4–5 year** old might find it easier to share because he has learnt to deal with other children in school.

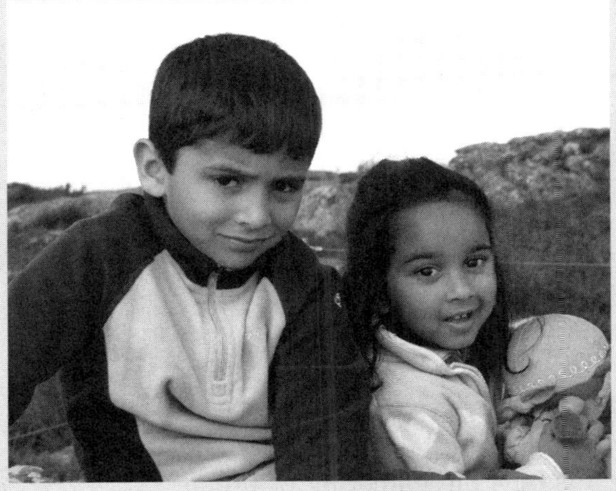

If the child is **six or older**, he might want to be informed about all that is happening and might be interested in helping out with the new arrival.

Pre-adolescents or **adolescents** could swing either way. They might resent this 'usurper' of their place in the family or they might be completely overjoyed with the new one.

Take the focus away from the baby's gender

Either directly or by suggestion, do not influence the child to say that she specifically wants a sister (or a brother). Encourage her to say that she wants a baby and it does not matter whether it is a boy or a girl. When you keep stressing that you want the baby to be of the opposite sex of your child, she might feel that you don't appreciate her or that she was a disappointment. She will then resent the new baby.

You might also want to talk to your parents or other relatives about what to say to your child. Very often, the elders in the family may keep trying to tutor the child into saying that the baby must be a boy (or a girl). This only confuses the child into believing that you can actually choose the sex of the baby. Let everybody encourage the child to wish for a healthy, normal baby.

> Regardless of the child's age, parents have to be realistic and need to know that each child will react differently to the arrival of a new baby. Be patient and most importantly, don't feel guilty about having another child!

Involve your child in the hospital

As you get closer to the due date, and if your first child is old enough, involve him in the preparations you will be making for going to the hospital. He can help you pack the baby's things in the hospital bag.

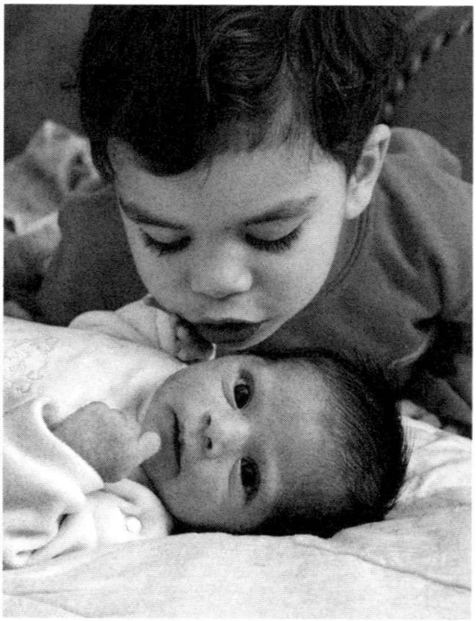

Make arrangements for your child to be taken care of when you are in the hospital. You must also prepare the child for the separation and let him know that he is being very helpful to you by being mature and staying at home.

Let your first child come and visit you as soon as possible. Let this be an intimate time for you, your husband, your child and the newborn. Do not let this be a big gathering of friends and relatives where your first child will feel that all the attention has been taken away from him.

Your child will want to touch and feel the baby. Do not get agitated and angry. Let him gently touch the baby while you are holding her. Calmly explain that the new baby is fragile and needs gentle handling.

Do not be surprised if your first child regresses and wants to be held and cuddled by you. Give him all the hugs and reassurances he needs.

After bringing the baby home

When you come home, reserve some special time for your firstborn. Have someone handle the baby for a while and focus all your attention on the older one.

Visitors will have a tendency to make a big fuss over the newborn. Make sure your first child is involved in introducing 'our baby' to others. Gently remind visitors that your older child may not really be interested in conversations that revolve only round the new baby.

Include your first one in pictures of the baby. Have her help you with the little chores involved in baby care.

If your child sulks and throws a tantrum, be patient and calm. Do not lose your temper or tell her that she is a bad sister. Be firm and allow the child to calm down. Be lavish with your hugs and cuddle her as much as she wants.

If the child continues to be aggressive, make sure that you do not leave him alone with the baby. The aggression will become less eventually—you have to be calm and firm at all times.

> Don't forget that a new baby is as great a transition for your child as it is for you. This may bring on a feeling of insecurity as well as anticipation. Try to make this a positive experience for the entire family.

CHAPTER 48

Your new baby

Deena and Jeffrey can't take their eyes off their new baby. How tiny and perfect he is! They feel a bit anxious and a bit excited. Will they be able to do everything that this little human demands? Will they be able to fulfill his every need? Will they ever feel confident enough? They shouldn't worry. Every parent is filled with doubts but they will do well.

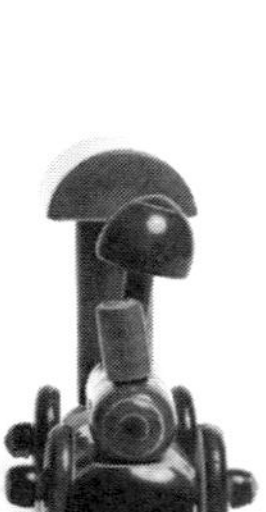

48

Your new baby

As a new parent, you might be filled with trepidation. Newborns do not come with instructions, but like all responsible parents, you will pick up the skills as you go along. Remember, parenting is an instinctive and intuitive process.

You may spend hours looking at every tiny part of your baby—his little fingers and little toes. You will wonder if the shape of the ear is normal or the way that his legs curve indicates any problem. There will be panic when even a tiny spot appears on his body. You will try to interpret every grunt or cry that he makes. In a few days and weeks the initial panic will subside and you will have more faith in your ability to take care of your little one.

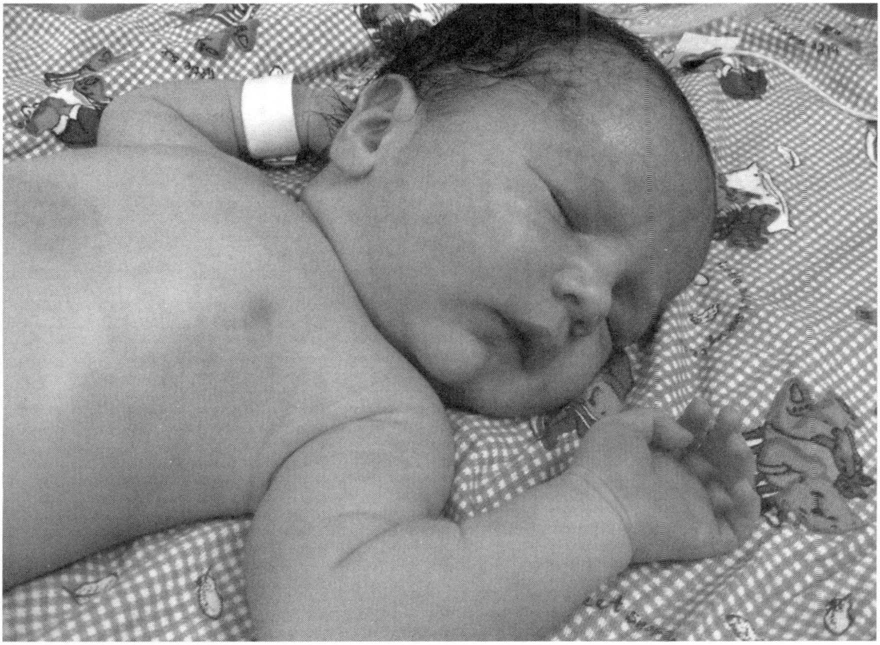

Holding your baby

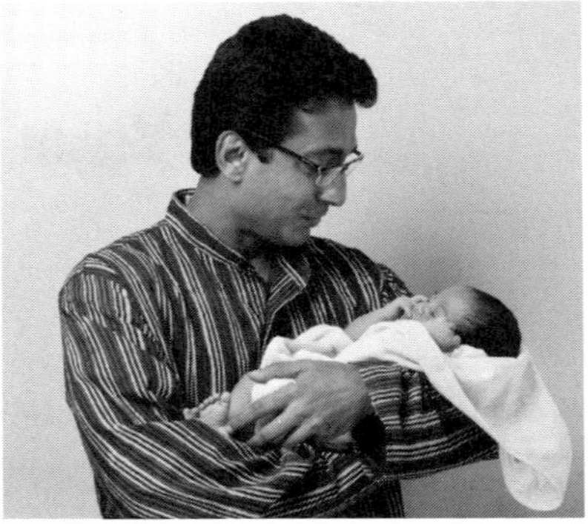

Always make sure you support the newborn baby's neck when holding her. She will feel safe and secure if you support her head and neck with one arm and her bottom and thighs with the other hand. Hold her close to your body for added security.

The baby's skin

When your little one was floating and swimming around in the amniotic fluid in your womb, her skin needed to be protected from getting wrinkled. At birth, your newborn may be covered with a white greasy substance called **vernix caseosa** that protected her skin. The vernix also contributes to her soft skin after birth. This is usually wiped off when she has her first bath. You might still find traces of it in the folds of her body for a few days.

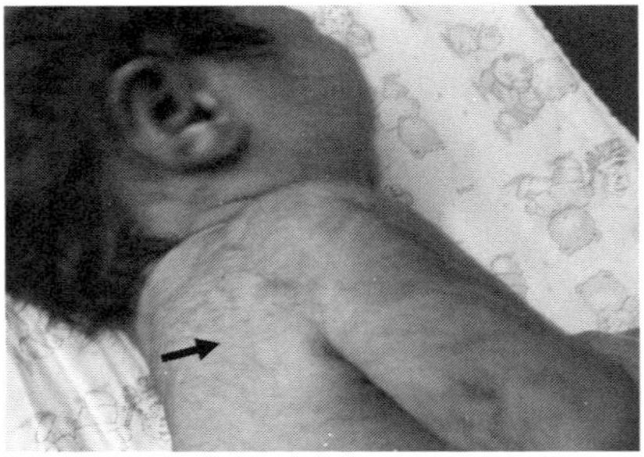

Lanugo hair

The baby's skin may be red and slightly wrinkled at birth. After a few hours, you may notice that the skin colour is patchy—areas of pale skin alternating with pink. This is due to the blood vessels under the thin skin and will disappear as the baby matures.

The skin will also be covered with fine **lanugo hair** which may be found on the shoulders, forehead and sometimes over the legs and arms. This soft hair will soon disappear.

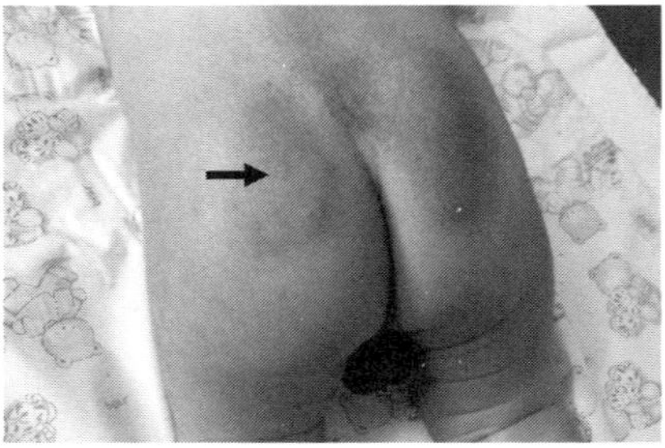

Mongolian patches

The baby may have greenish-black patches over the buttocks or the lower back. These are called **Mongolian patches** and disappear in a few weeks.

In the first few weeks, most babies will develop a pinkish rash over their cheeks, almost like pimples. This is in response to your hormones that the baby is getting through breast milk. This does not require any treatment and may last for two to three months.

The baby may have little white bumps on the nose and face called **milia**. These are caused by blocked oil glands. When the baby's oil glands enlarge and open up in a few days or weeks, the white bumps will disappear.

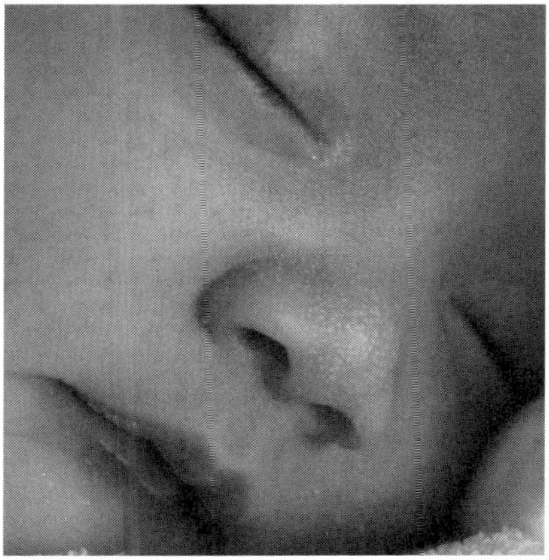
Milia on the baby's nose

Another common newborn rash looks like mosquito bites and can occur anywhere over the body, most commonly over the back. This is called **erythema toxicum.** The cause is unknown, and it resolves without treatment after a few days or weeks.

Dry, peeling skin is often due to a baby being born a few days after the due date. The underlying skin is perfectly normal and soft.

In hot weather, your baby may develop prickly heat or heat rash. They look like tiny raised red bumps on a red patch and are most often found around the neck, on the chest, back and the scalp. This rash is more common if the baby is overdressed. A cool bath and light clothing may help the baby be comfortable.

During a baby's first few months of life, she may develop a **cradle cap**, a condition that looks like dirty, rough skin on the scalp. Washing the scalp daily with soap and water will clear it up in most cases. You can also gently brush the scalp with a soft baby brush or toothbrush. Sometimes, rubbing a little oil into the scalp before washing the head will help. If the condition persists or spreads, see your paediatrician.

A **diaper rash** is very common and usually clears up in three or four days. Diaper rashes can be prevented by frequent diaper changes, increasing air exposure by keeping the diaper off as much as possible, and using a mild soap after bowel movements. A cream containing zinc oxide can be used to protect the delicate skin and this can be applied after every diaper change or if it is not severe, after every two or three diaper changes.

The baby's eyes

The eyes may be puffy at birth. The baby will try to open her eyes but will scrunch her eyes up if the light in the room is bright. Remember that the baby will not be able to focus for several weeks. The eyes may also keep watering because the tear ducts may not have opened up. In a few weeks, this problem will resolve by itself. If there is a sticky discharge in the eyes, wipe the eyes gently with a cotton ball soaked with warm water. If the discharge persists, it is best to consult the paediatrician.

Do not be alarmed if the baby seems to have a squint and appears cross-eyed. This is a temporary condition and once the baby matures enough to focus his eyes, this condition will correct itself.

The umbilical cord

When the baby is born, the umbilical cord is clamped and cut close to the baby's body. About 2–3 cm of the cord will still be attached to the baby's body. Within a day or two, the umbilical cord that was shiny and moist at birth, will shrivel up and darken in colour. This umbilical stump will dry and drop off in 10–15 days. The stump must be kept clean and dry. Fold the baby's diaper below the stump so it is exposed to the air. This will prevent it from being constantly soaked by urine. A wet cord may smell and appear infected. Do not worry; this is normal. When the stump falls off, you may detect a little blood on the diaper, which is normal. Do not apply any ointment, creams or home remedies to the cord or stump.

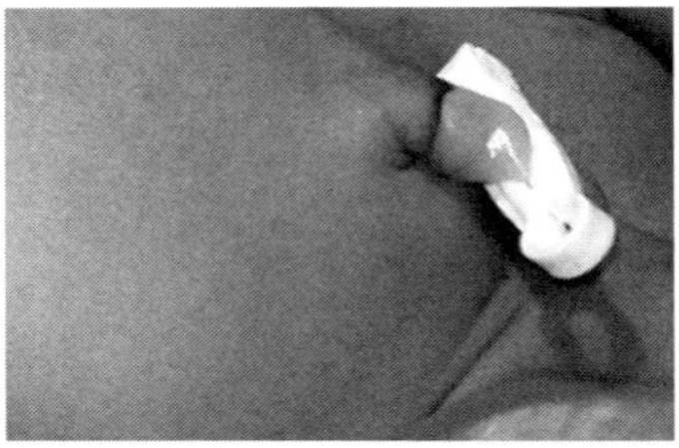

Clamped umbilical cord

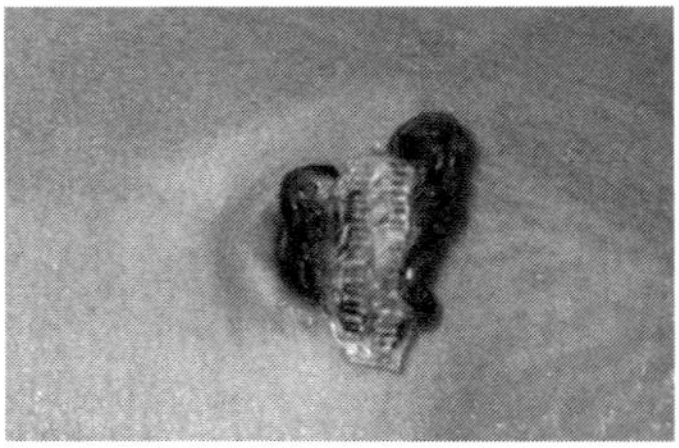

Umbilical cord drying up

Sometimes, the cord will dry but continue to hang from the umbilicus by just a small thread like attachment. Do not pull it off. It will fall off by itself.

Umbilical hernia

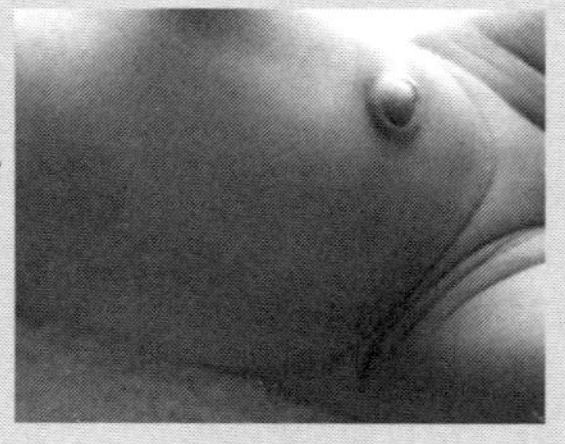

Some babies may have a very prominent umbilicus. Every time the baby cries, the umbilicus and the area around it will bulge out, sometimes alarmingly. The swelling will become less prominent when the baby stops crying or straining. You don't have to worry! This is an umbilical hernia and many babies are born with it. Usually this will become smaller and may even disappear completely within a year. You need to see your doctor immediately if the swelling is hard, appears red and does not go down on gently pressing down with a finger.

Sometimes, after the stump falls off, a pink or yellowish piece of flesh may remain, which will disappear by itself. This is called an **umbilical granuloma**. At times, there is a yellowish discharge or even a small amount of bleeding from this. The paediatrician may apply medication to this to help it dry up.

Regurgitation of milk or spitting up

Is the baby spitting up? As soon as you feed the baby and put him on your shoulders, does he bring up some or all of the milk? Some babies just spit up more than usual. This worries you, doesn't it? You may think that the baby won't put on weight because he's bringing up his food. Calm down!

Most newborn babies will bring up a small amount of milk soon after feeding. This happens because the baby swallows air while feeding. The swallowed air comes up as a burp and part of the milk also comes out along with the air. Burping the baby by holding him upright on the shoulder for 5–10 minutes after the feed relieves the gas and regurgitation (see **Chapter 27**, *Breastfeeding*). The problem will usually settle down in a few weeks.

Stools

During the first two or three days, the baby passes black, tarry stools which are followed by greenish stools for the next few days. With the establishment of regular breastfeeds, the baby will pass regular, semisolid, yellowish stools. Most babies pass 4–8 stools in a day. Remember that some babies pass stools after each feed. This does not mean that the baby is having diarrhoea (see **Chapter 27**, *Breastfeeding*). Some babies pass stools once in 2–3 days. If the stools are hard and the baby cries excessively while passing stools, consult your doctor to rule out constipation.

Straining and grunting

Most babies will strain and grunt almost like they were severely constipated. Your little fellow may go red in the face and grimace alarmingly. This is just a way of passing gas or even passing urine. This straining will usually decrease in a few weeks.

Diarrhoea is diagnosed when the baby is passing large quantities of watery, loose stools at a greater frequency. When the baby is being exclusively breastfed and is not receiving any other top feeds, she is unlikely to develop diarrhoea caused by infection.

Constipation may be suspected if the baby is passing hard, pellet-like stools that cause pain or bleeding. The first thing to do is to make sure the baby is getting enough milk. Your paediatrician may prescribe a medicine to ease the passage of stools.

Urine

Most newborns pass urine within 48 hours of birth. If the baby has not passed urine within 48 hours, the paediatrician will make sure the baby is not dehydrated. If the baby does not pass urine in spite of adequate feeds, tests will be done to make sure that the baby has no kidney problem. A normal baby passes urine about 5–10 times per day. Babies usually cry on passing urine. This does not mean that the baby is having pain. This just helps them push the urine out.

Diya asked: How often should my baby be passing urine and stools?

My answer: If your baby is getting adequate breast milk, he will pass urine 4–6 times during the 3rd and 4th days. This will increase to 6–8 times from day 5 onwards.

Meconium (black-green stools) will change to transitional stools (yellow-brown) within approximately 3 days of birth and the baby will have 4–8 stools per day after day 4.

Sleep

During the first few days of life, most babies keep their eyes closed with occasional attempts to open their eyes. Of course, there are some babies who open their eyes immediately and seem to be quite alert and awake!

Your newborn may sleep during the day and be awake and playful during the night. You might have noticed during your pregnancy that the baby was usually less active during the daytime and up and kicking when you want to rest at night! This sleep rhythm continues even after the baby

Laying your baby down to sleep

When you put your little one down to sleep, move slowly and gently to prevent him from getting startled or waking up. Put his head down first. Always make sure to support his neck. Then gradually lay the rest of his body down. Gently slide out your hand from under his head. Then remove the other hand. Stay by his side, stroking him and speaking or singing to him softly. He will hopefully settle down to sleep.

is born. For new parents it may seem that the baby never sleeps. The good news is that most babies tend to fall into a set sleep pattern in 4–6 weeks.

The best position for sleeping

The best and safest position for the baby to sleep is on his back. Make sure you leave him on a firm mattress or bedding. The sheet or blanket should be tucked in well around him and there should be no loose bedding item. Don't leave stuffed animals in the bed with him.

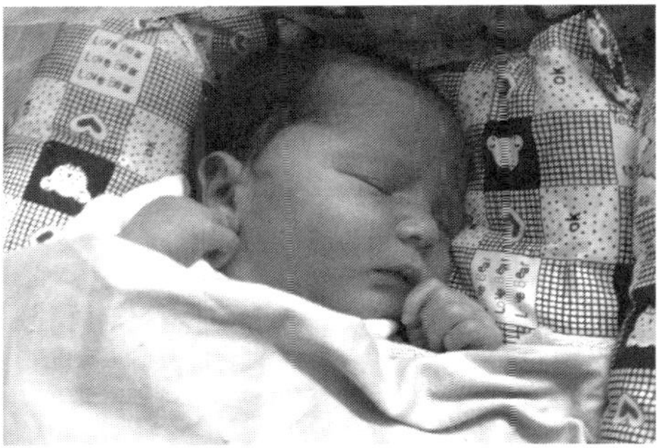

Startle reflex and other reflexes

When a newborn baby is startled by a sudden noise, he responds by arching his back, kicking his legs and jerking his arms. This is known as the **Moro reflex.**

When you place a finger or any object in the baby's palm, the baby will grab on tightly.

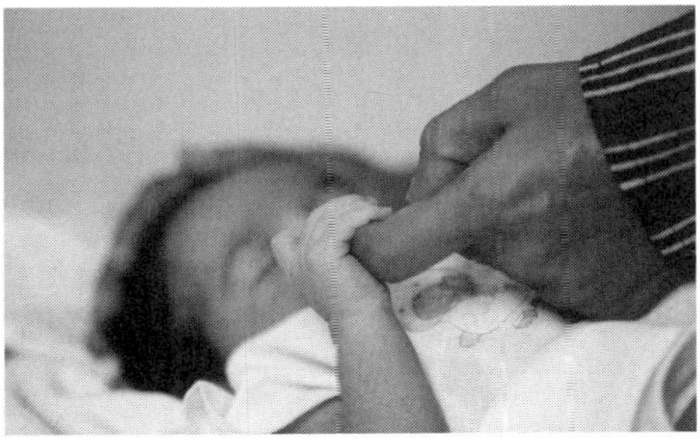

Rooting reflex is when your baby is searching for food. She will open her mouth and turn her head toward your hand if you stroke her cheek.

When your baby is drowsy or sleeping, you may notice her smiling. She is in a dreamy state and this is termed **reflexive smiling**. It will be a few weeks before she will actually be smiling back in response to your smile.

Sneezing

This is very common and usually is a way for the baby to clear her nose. It does not mean that she is getting a cold.

Hiccups

Remember that your baby was hiccupping even inside your womb! When the baby hiccups, it does not mean anything is wrong. It will subside by itself and the baby is really not feeling any discomfort.

Excessive crying in newborns

Most babies cry when they are either hungry or having discomfort such as a wet or soiled nappy.

Presence of continuous crying or a high-pitched cry may suggest infection, and the baby should be taken to the doctor immediately.

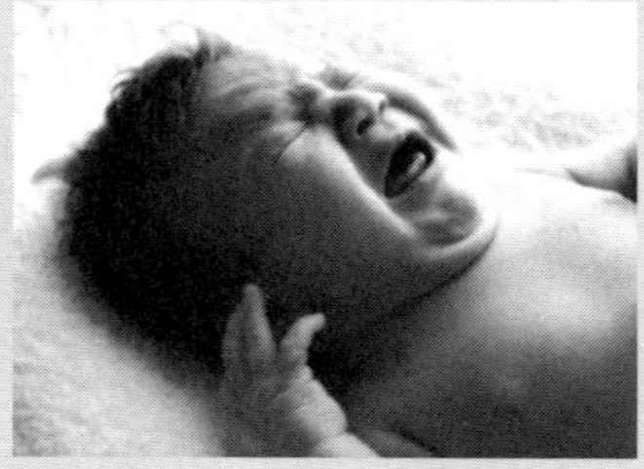

Some babies suffer from colic. Most babies will have a particular time of the day when they will cry inconsolably for 3–4 hours. If you have fed the baby, the diaper is clean and there is no fever, you just have to walk around with the baby or rock her and hope she calms down. An infant with colic may have gaseous distension of the abdomen and usually feels comfortable when placed on her tummy for a few minutes. This helps the baby pass gas. Of course you should be right next to her when you leave her on her stomach. Colic will usually subside in a few weeks and commonly does not persist after the third month.

Bleeding in baby girls

When you feed your baby, hormones that are circulating in your blood stream get passed along to her. Due to the hormones passing from the mother to the baby, little girls may have mucus like discharge or even bleeding from the vagina. This is nothing to be concerned about and will subside on its own.

Fever

It is unusual for a newborn to develop fever. The paediatrician will make sure that the fever is not due to dehydration before checking for an infection. During the summer months, some babies may develop a mild fever during the second or third day of life. If the child is active and feeds well, usually there is no cause for worry. Ensuring proper feeds and hydration, easily treats a rise in temperature due to dehydration.

Giving the baby a bath

Babies have sensitive skin that dries out easily. Till the umbilical cord falls off, it is all right to wipe the baby off with a wet cloth dipped in warm water. Once you are comfortable with giving a bath, you can use a basin to bathe the baby.

Ideally, a bath should be given in the morning or at the end of the day before a breastfeed so that the baby can feed and fall asleep. If the baby is very hungry, feed her but wait for at least 15 minutes before you bathe her so that she does not spit up the milk.

Your newborn does not need to have a bath every day. It does not matter if you skip a day as long as wipe her face, neck and diaper area with a wet towel whenever she is dirty.

Tips for a happy bath time

NEVER leave an infant alone near a tub or bucket of water—not even for a minute!

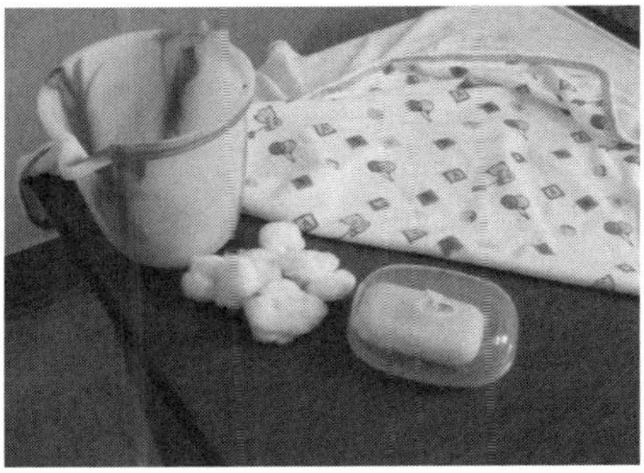

Make sure you have all supplies ready before you begin the bath:

- Towel
- A mild shampoo or soap
- Cotton
- A small, soft hand towel to clean the face

Make sure the room is warm enough and the water is not too hot or cold before putting your baby in the tub. Use only a mild baby soap and shampoo.

Use a small wet towel or your hand to gently wipe the baby's face and ears. No soap is necessary near the eyes.

Using baby powder

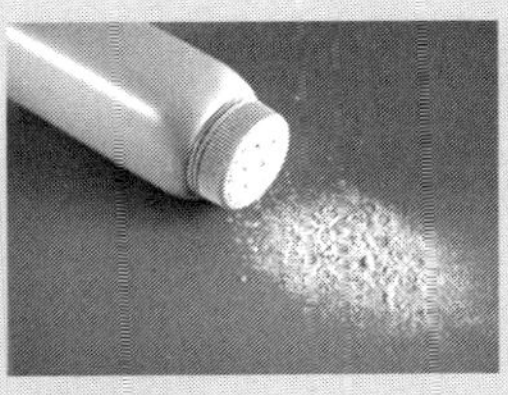

We always associate babies with sweet smelling baby powder. Though our grandmothers and mothers all used powder lavishly on babies, now the recommendation is to avoid powder near the baby's face. The baby may inhale it and this may harm the baby's lungs. If you really want to use powder, use it below the level of the baby's umbilicus. Take the powder on your palm and with the other hand pat it onto the baby.

Baby oil and lotion

It is not essential to apply oil to the baby's body or head. However, in our culture, giving a baby an oil bath is quite a ritual. Lotions are usually not necessary unless the skin is very dry. It may be useful in cold, dry places.

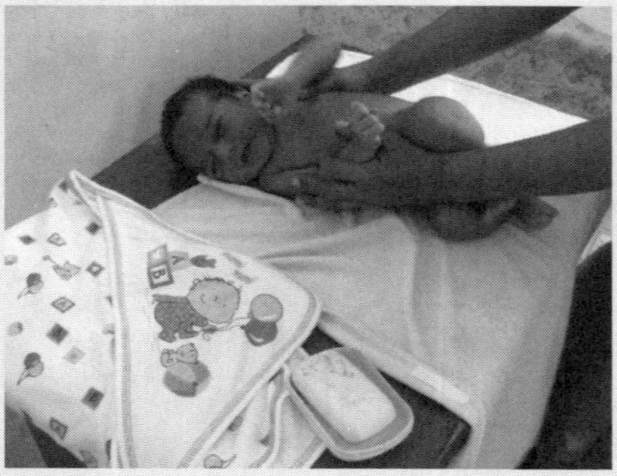

1 *Take your baby's clothes off. Make sure that it is not drafty so that the baby does not feel cold. Keep two towels ready. One is for wrapping the baby and one is to dry him off.*

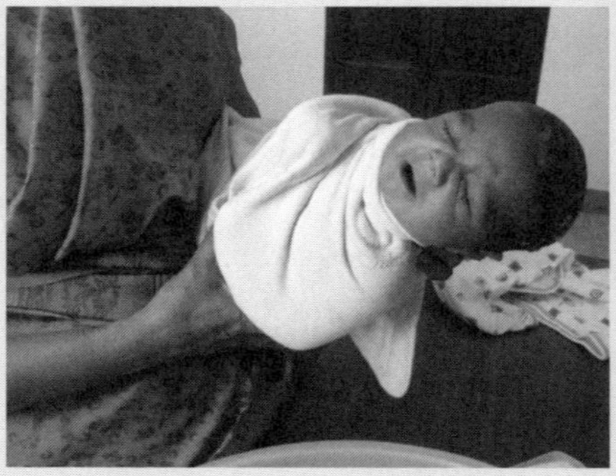

2 *Once you have undressed the baby, wrap the baby in a towel. This helps you hold your slippery baby while you wash his face and hair. Wrap the baby snugly in the towel so that his arms and legs will not dangle while you wash his hair.*

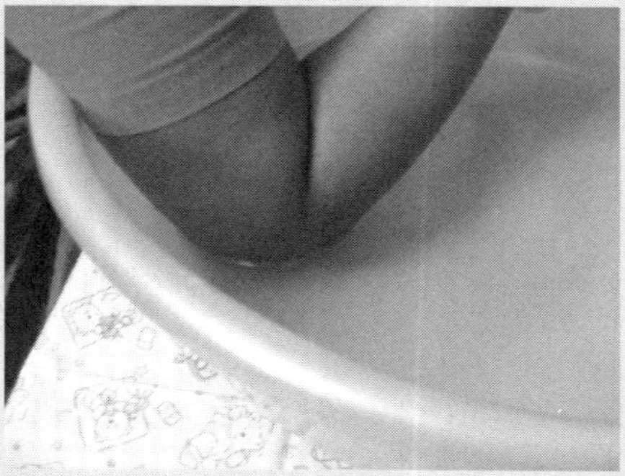

3 *Fill a bowl or basin with warm water: Use your wrist or elbow to check the water to make sure it is just the right temperature. Be sure the water is not too cold or too hot. Very hot water can be dangerous.*

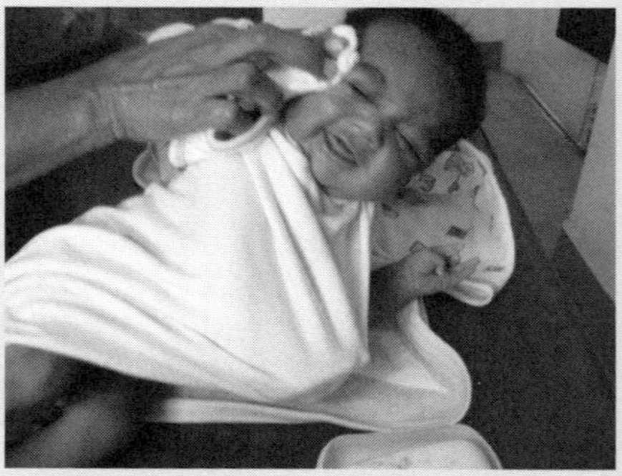

4 *Use damp cotton balls to wipe your baby's eyes. Gently wipe the face with your wet hand and then dry his face with a towel.*

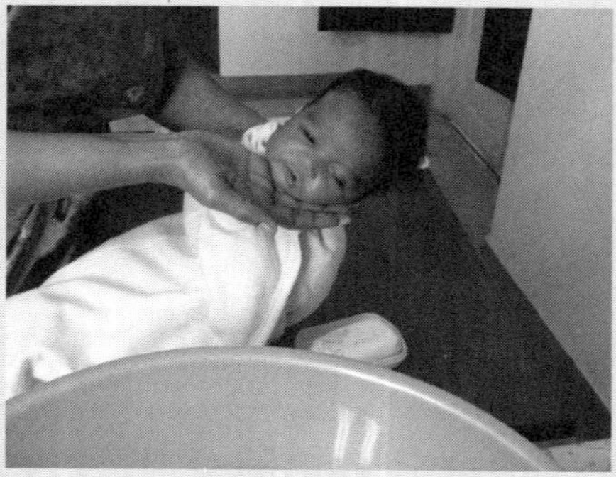

5 *Wash and dry under his neck.*

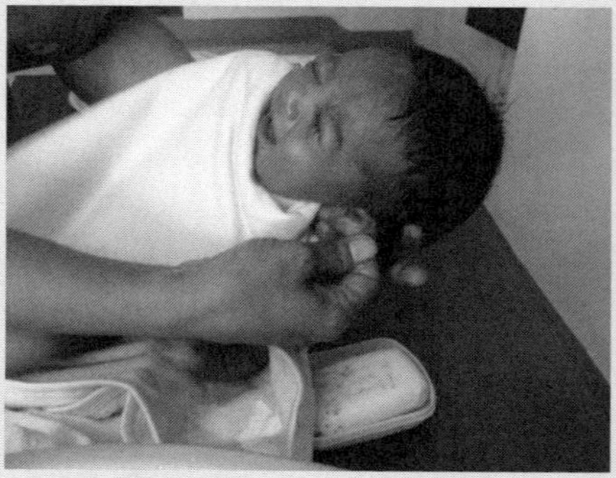

6 *Gently wash the outside and back of each ear and behind his ears.*

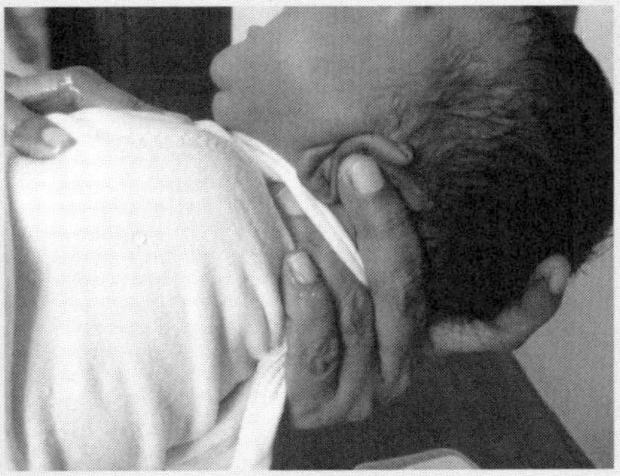

7 Wash your baby's hair and scalp very gently, using soap or a baby shampoo. You need to do this only once or twice a week. To prevent water from entering the baby's ears, gently fold the ears and hold them in place with your thumb on one side and the middle finger on the other.

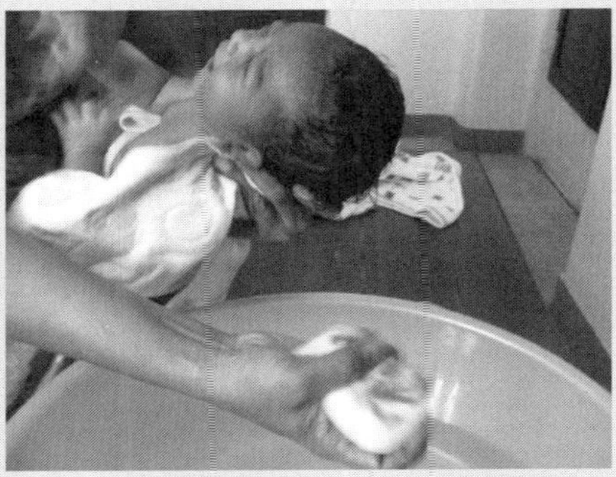

8 Hold his head over the basin and gently pour some water on his head. Hold him firmly like a bundle. Let his bottom rest on your waist, under your left elbow. Cradle his head in your left palm, with your fingers gently gripping his neck.

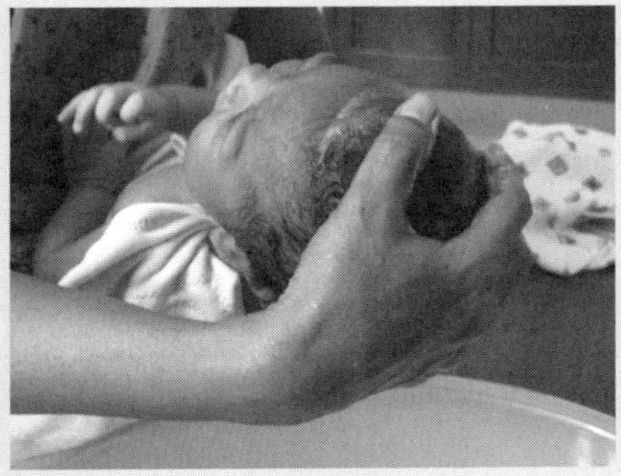

9 Take some baby soap or shampoo in your hand and apply it to his scalp. Rub the soap softly into the scalp till there is a lather. Remember that the baby's scalp will not be that dirty so you do not have to wash his hair every time you give him a bath.

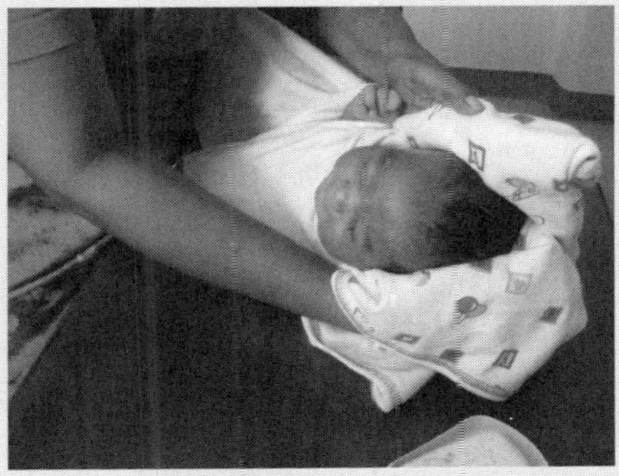

10 Wash off the soap from the hair using your cupped palm or a mug to pour water. Dry the head with a small towel.

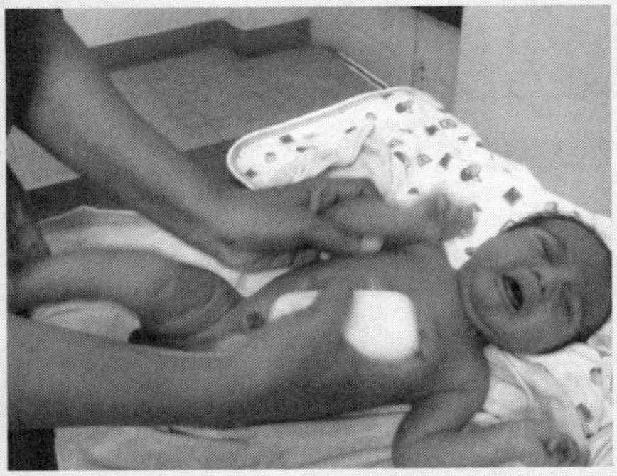

11 Now lay your baby on the table and unfold the towel that was wrapped around him. Rub soap on his body.

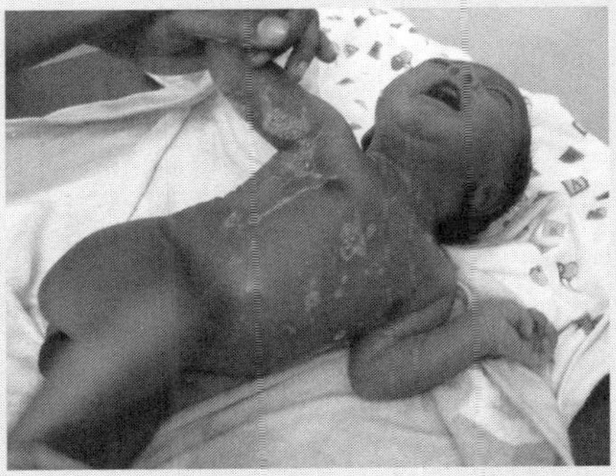

12 Make sure that you don't forget to soap all the folds.

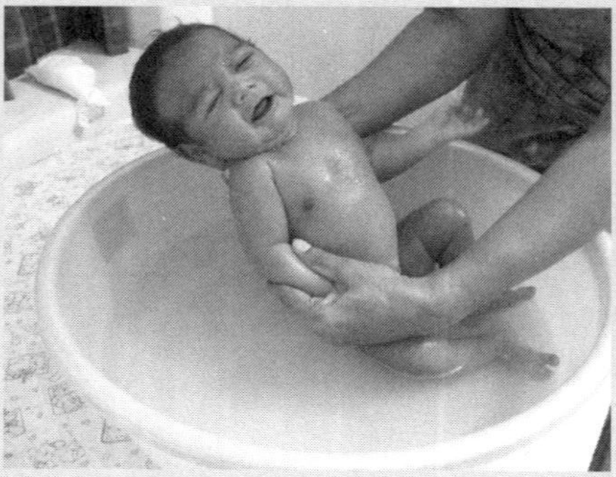

13 *Place him back in the basin, making sure to hold him firmly. A folded towel at the bottom of the basin can provide traction.*

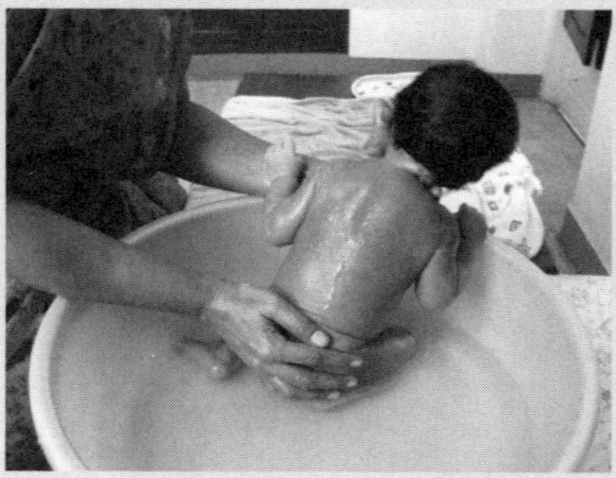

14 *Supporting his chest with your palm, soap his back too. Then rinse him off, pouring water with a cupped pal or with a mug.*

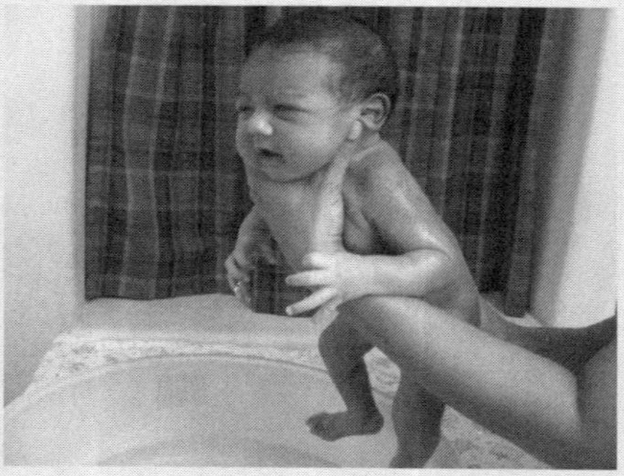

15 *Remember, babies can be slippery so always keep a good grip on him. Don't worry; you will master the art of giving a baby bath very soon!*

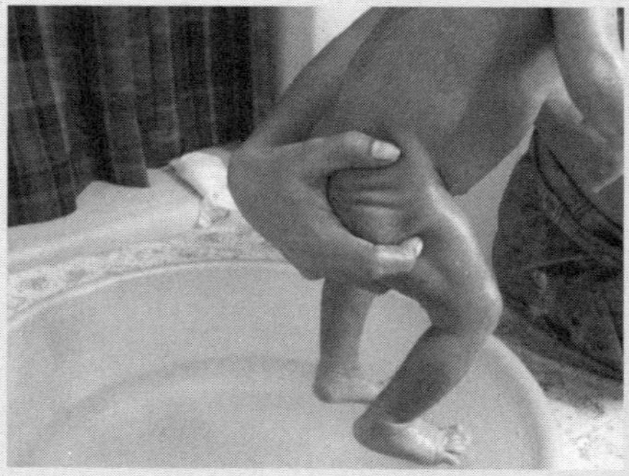

16 *Lift him gently out of the basin, holding him firmly.*

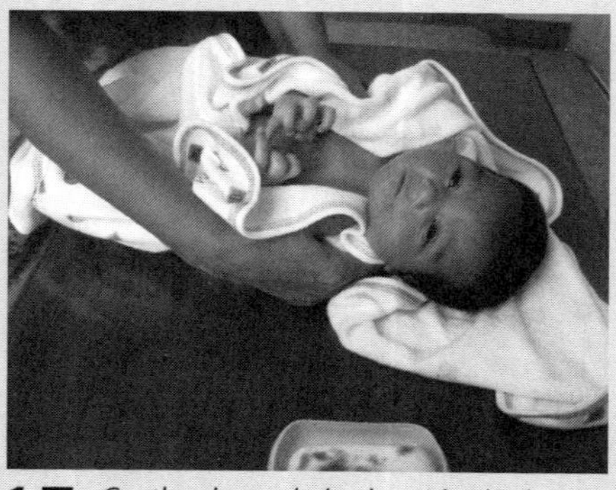

17 *Gently rub your baby dry with a bath towel. Always keep him covered and warm when he is wet.*

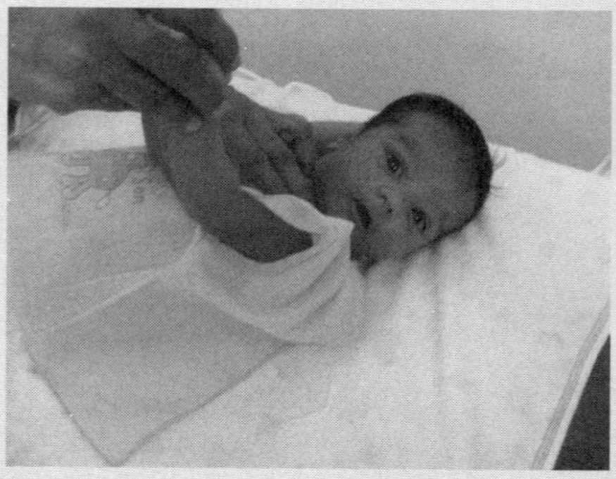

18 *A fresh, clean and sweet-smelling baby!*

The art of changing a diaper

New parents are usually apprehensive about changing diapers. Once you have done it a few times, you will become confident enough to do it fast and with the least amount of trouble!

When you are going to change the baby's diaper, make sure all the things that you need are right next to you.

- A fresh diaper: If using a cloth diaper, you will need diaper pins and waterproof panties. You can also use a cloth diaper which comes with ties
- Cotton and warm water in a mug for cleaning and a small towel for drying the baby
- Zinc oxide ointment if needed (for diaper rash)
- A plastic bag or small plastic disposal basket to throw the used diaper in

Which diaper is best?

Most new parents dread changing diapers and worry that they may not be able to handle this chore! Diapering has become much more easier now with the availability of readymade cloth diapers and also disposable diapers. It does not matter which diapers you use. Just keep in mind that disposable diapers can be much more expensive. You can use cloth diapers for daily use and reserve disposable diapers for going out. Soiled cloth diapers are difficult to handle when you are out.

Disposable diapers

Disposable diapers may be easier to use but they do have a major environmental impact. They are made of plastic that takes hundreds of years to disintegrate. They are one of the major causes of blocked sewage systems. Use washable cloth diapers as much as possible. This is not only very good for your baby but also for the environment.

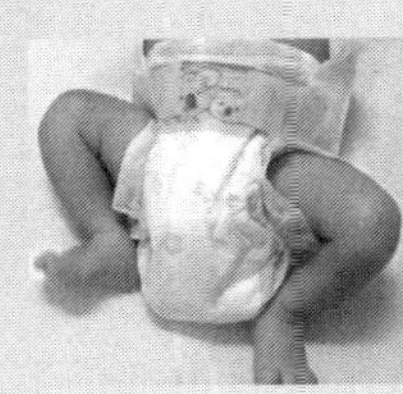

Tips for proper diapering

- Until the umbilical cord falls off, fold the diaper down to expose the cord to air and to keep it from getting wet
- Make sure you soak the cloth diaper in water soon after it gets soiled otherwise it will be difficult to get rid of the stain
- There is no need to add an antiseptic solution to the water which is used to wash the diaper
- Wash your hands with soap and water after changing your baby

Diapering made easy

After unfastening the diaper, use it to wipe away most of a bowel movement, **from front to back**. Then clean away any urine and remaining stools with wet cotton. Pat your baby dry with a towel. While changing a baby boy, hold a fresh diaper over his penis, otherwise he will spray you and himself too!

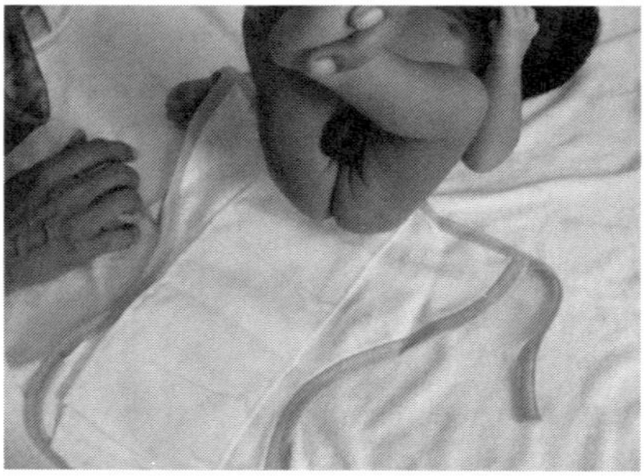

Put on the clean diaper. If you are using a cloth diaper, you may need to fold it to fit snugly around the baby. As your baby grows, the diaper will fit even without folding. Slide the diaper under your baby till the top edge is at the baby's waistline. Bring the front up between his legs, and hold it in place while you fold the sides in toward the centre and fasten with a diaper pin. If the diaper comes with ties, you can knot them in front. Washable cloth diapers are now available with a plastic lining that makes them leak proof (or almost!).

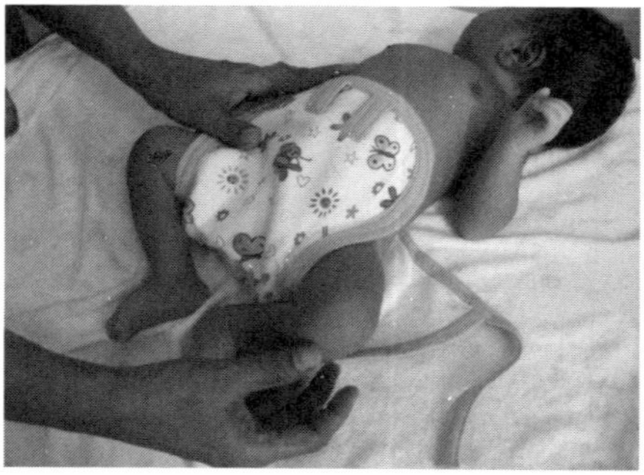

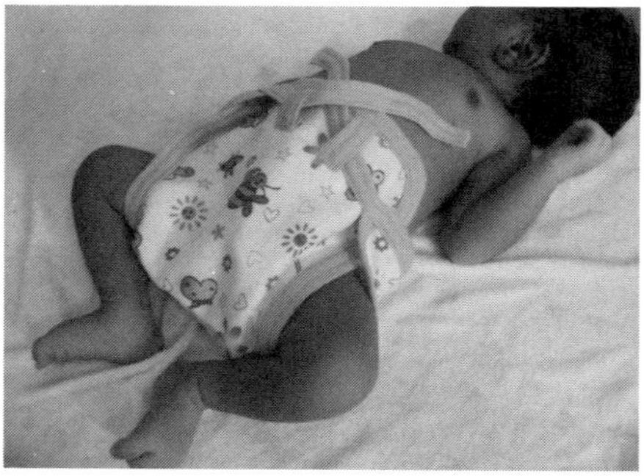

If you are using disposable diapers, lay the diaper flat, with the tabs at the back. Slide the diaper under your baby till the top edge is at the baby's waistline. Bring the front up between his legs and tuck it around his stomach. Unpeel the tabs, pull them firmly over the front flap and fasten the diaper (be sure not to fasten the tape to your baby's skin). The diaper should fit snugly, but it shouldn't be tight.

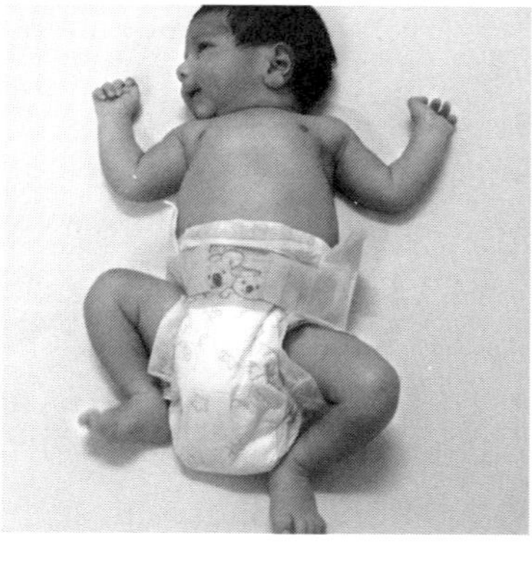

Heena asked: How do I avoid diaper rash?

My answer: The key to avoiding diaper rash is changing the diaper frequently, and meticulously keeping the area dry.

When you clean the baby, **wipe from front to back so that stools do not get near the urethra, especially for baby girls.** This can avoid urinary tract infection. Wait for a few minutes and let the baby's bottom air out before you put on the next diaper. Zinc oxide-based creams are available and they should be applied after every diaper change or at least after 2–3 changes. The cream will protect the baby's soft and sensitive skin from the acidity of urine and stools.

What baby clothes do you need?

Newborn baby clothes, first and foremost, need to be soft and comfortable. They do not have to be elaborate or expensive.

Before you decide to buy baby clothes for your newborn, keep the following factors in mind:

- What climate do you live in and what season of the year is it?
- Do you have help for washing the clothes or do you have a washing machine?
- Do you already have old clothes that you used for your first baby?
- Will your friends or relatives give or loan you clothes for the baby?

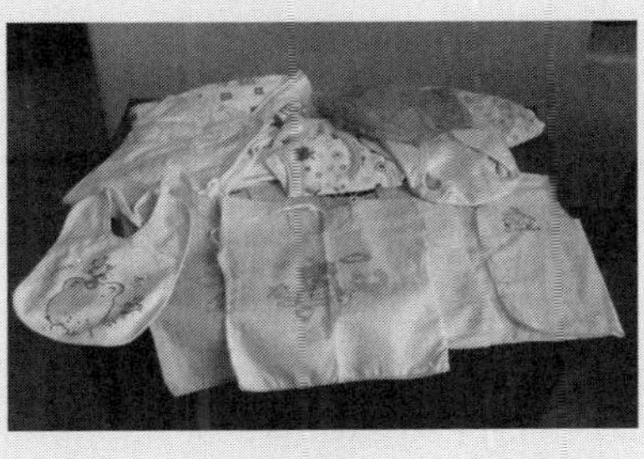

Do not go by the size given on baby clothes. The sizes given are often misleading. For example, a dress marked '2–6 months' may be too small for your newborn. You should buy clothes that are larger than needed because your baby will grow in leaps and bounds and will quickly stopping fitting into them!

You will not go wrong if you buy or stitch cotton clothes, especially in the summer months. If you live in a colder area, you will need warmer clothes for the baby. Try to avoid synthetics that do not let the pores of the child breath.

When selecting newborn baby clothes, you must consider ease of wear and comfort of dressing. The clothing should be roomy and should not be restrictive. Most importantly, the clothes should be easy to put on and remove. To begin with, soft jablas are uncomplicated to use and make it easy for you, as a new parent, to dress your baby.

Baby bibs

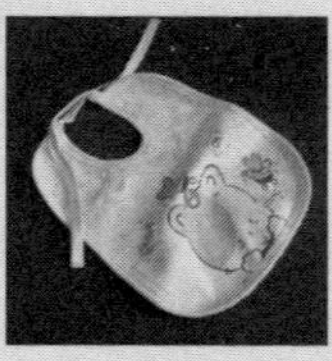

A bib is an essential baby requirement. Bibs soak up the baby's regurgitated milk. They can also be used to quickly clean up the area around the mouth. They help keep the area around the neck dry and this prevents rashes under the chin and in the neck folds. When the baby starts teething in a few months, she will drool a lot of saliva. A bib will soak up the saliva and prevent rashes around the neck.

Newborn jaundice

Most babies will have mild newborn (or neonatal) jaundice. Treatment is required when the jaundice is pronounced.

Jaundice is a yellow discolouration of the skin and the white part of the eyes. It results from having too much of a substance called bilirubin in the blood. Most babies are born with a high amount of red blood cells. Bilirubin is formed when the body breaks down these red blood cells. The liver usually processes and removes the bilirubin from the blood. Jaundice in babies occurs because their immature livers are not efficient at removing bilirubin from the blood stream.

Newborn babies will begin to appear jaundiced when they have more than 5 mg/dl of bilirubin in their blood. It is important to recognize and treat neonatal jaundice. The level of the bilirubin may be treated according to the baby's age. For example, a bilirubin level of 12 mg/dl needs to be treated if the baby is less than 48 hours old but is considered normal when the baby is more than 5 days old.

High levels of bilirubin can cause permanent damage to a baby's brain. This brain damage is called **kernicterus**. Today, because of increased awareness and effective treatment of neonatal jaundice, kernicterus is extremely rare. Kernicterus will usually happen when the bilirubin level crosses 25mg/dl in a baby born at full term. A premature baby may have damage with a lower bilirubin level.

The risk for newborn jaundice increases if:

- The mother's blood group is O and the baby's blood group is A, AB or B. This is called ABO incompatibility
- The mother is Rh negative and the baby is Rh positive. This is called Rh incompatibility (see **Chapter 39**, *The Rh factor: how it can affect pregnancy*).

- The baby is premature
- The mother had diabetes during pregnancy

Treatment of newborn jaundice

Jaundice is most often treated with phototherapy. This involves placing the baby beneath special lights. Two factors help decide whether or not to start phototherapy: the age of the newborn and the level of bilirubin. If the baby develops jaundice within the first few days, phototherapy is definitely started. The level of bilirubin in the blood is assessed to decide when the phototherapy should be started and how long it should be continued. A premature baby will be started on phototherapy earlier than a full-term baby.

The light used for phototherapy is able to penetrate a baby's skin. The light changes bilirubin into a soluble form that is easily handled by the baby's body. The baby's eyes are covered, to shield them from the lights.

When all other treatment has failed to reduce the bilirubin level enough, the last resort is an exchange transfusion. In this treatment, the baby's blood is exchanged with donated blood. This is a specialized procedure and is done only in centres where there are neonatologists who care for critically ill newborns.

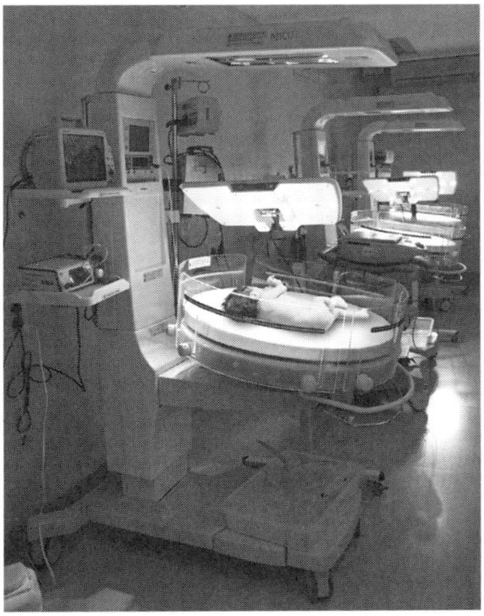

Phototherapy unit

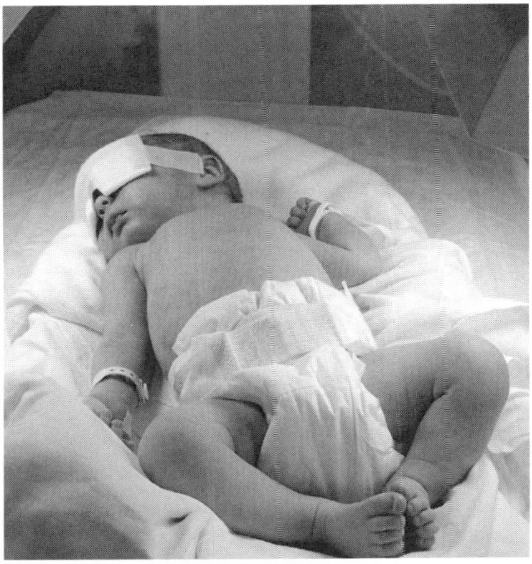

Baby under phototherapy for newborn jaundice. The baby's eyes are covered to shield them from the light

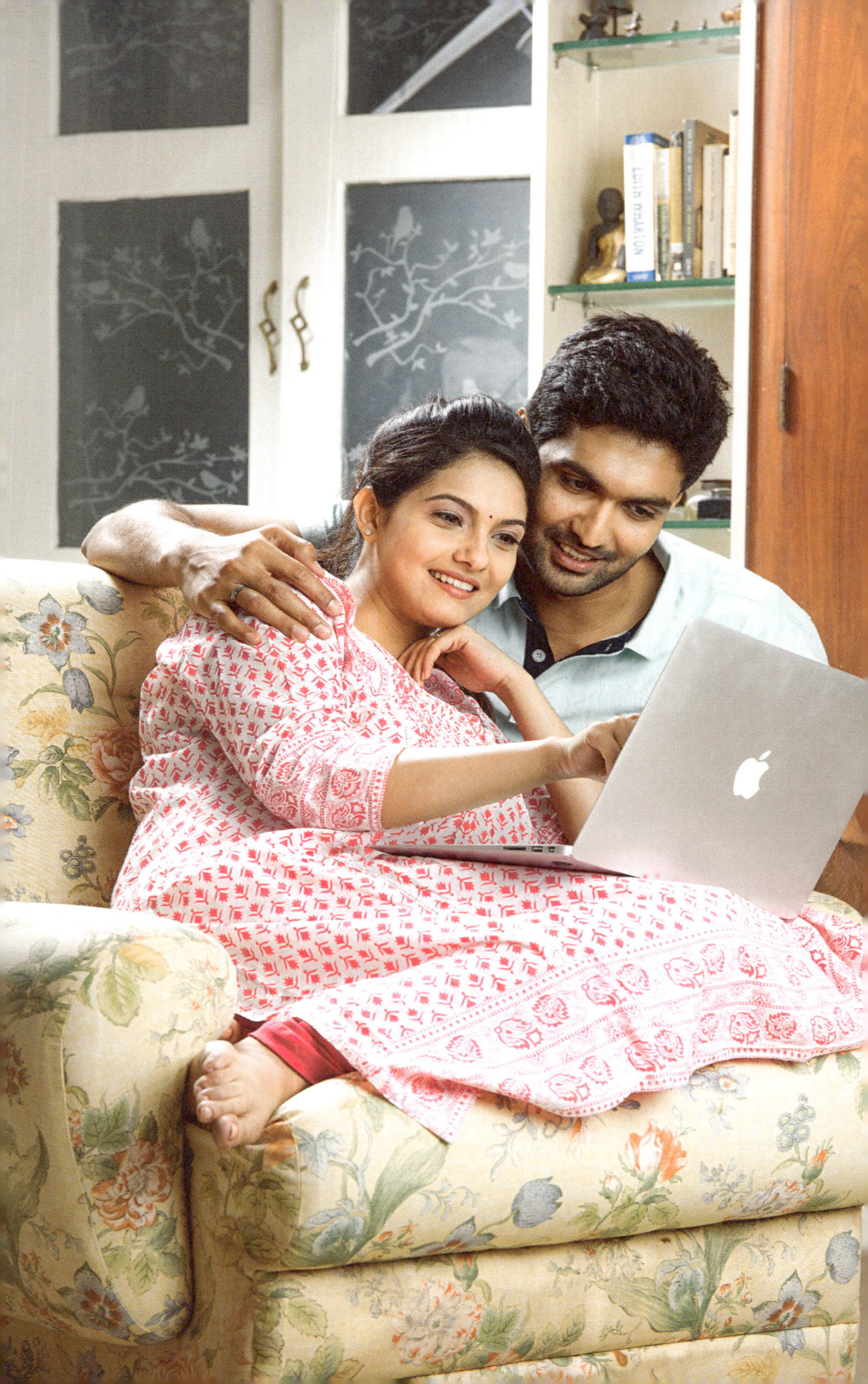
EDITH WHARTON

Birth control

CHAPTER 49

Methods of birth control

Sadhana is looking forward to her wedding with excitement. In the midst of the frenetic preparations, Sadhana has an appointment with her gynaecologist. She and her fiancé have decided to wait for a year before planning a family.

Sumangali has just had a baby. At her postnatal check-up, her obstetrician has discussed birth control with her. Sumangali wants to avoid a pregnancy for a few more years.

Sandra has two children and wants a permanent method to avoid further pregnancies.

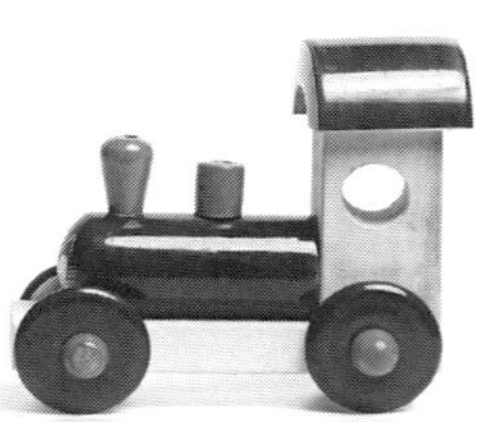

49

Methods of birth control

Your freedom to plan when you actually want to have a baby, the number of children you want, and the gap you want to maintain between pregnancies is a fundamental human right. Did you know that India was the first country in the world to initiate a nationwide family planning programme in 1952? Unfortunately, the number of unintended pregnancies continues to be unacceptably high.

The need for contraception varies with each individual. It is important to choose the right method of avoiding a pregnancy. Today's woman has a variety of birth control options. Each method has its advantages and disadvantages. All of the available methods are safe when used appropriately. Be sure to discuss the pros and cons of each method with your doctor so that you can choose the method best suited for you.

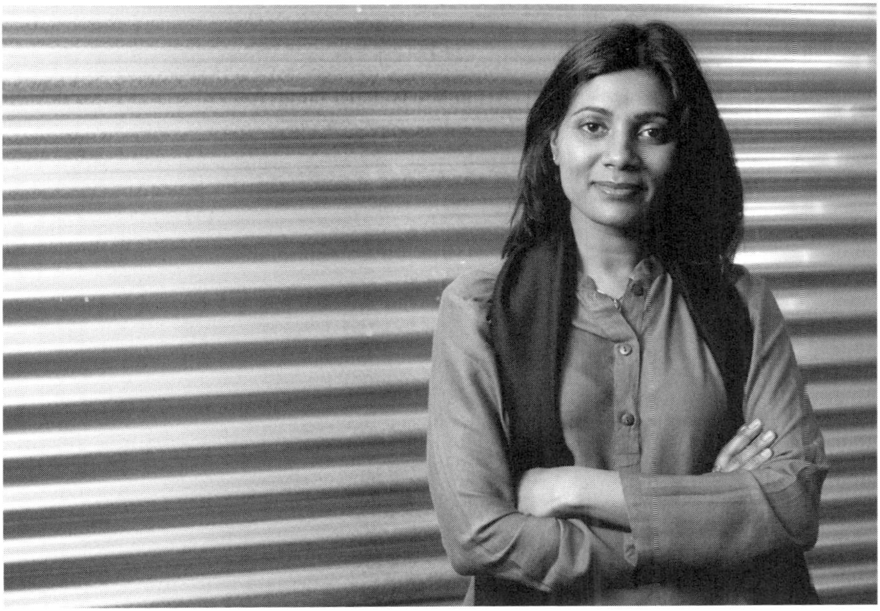

What is birth control or contraception?

Birth control or contraception is the term used for the prevention of pregnancy. There are many ways to prevent pregnancy. Some are much more effective than others. The revolution in contraceptive techniques has empowered women and given them several safe options. Knowing what methods are available will help you decide which option is right for you and your lifestyle.

How does birth control work?

To understand how birth control works, you must understand how a pregnancy occurs. A woman has two ovaries, one on each side of the uterus. Each month, one of the ovaries releases an egg. This process is called ovulation. On an average, ovulation occurs about 12–14 days before the start of the next period.

If a woman has intercourse at the time of ovulation, fertilization can occur. The sperm deposited into the vagina travels up through the cervix, through the uterus and into the Fallopian tubes.

If a sperm encounters an egg in the Fallopian tube, fertilization (union of egg and sperm) can occur. The fertilized egg then moves down the Fallopian tube to the uterus where it attaches itself (implantation).

Temporary methods of birth control

- Natural methods
- Mechanical barriers
- Hormonal contraception
- Intrauterine devices (IUDs)

Permanent methods of birth control

- Female sterilization
- Male sterilization

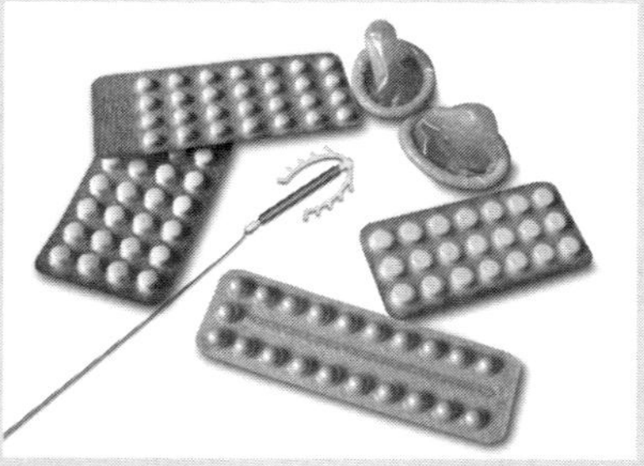

Birth control methods work by interfering with the process of reproduction at different steps of the process. They may:

- Block the sperm from reaching the egg (male or female condoms, female diaphragm, sterilization)
- Kill the sperm (spermicidals)
- Keep the eggs from being released each month (birth control pills, injections, implants)

- Change the lining of the uterus so that the fertilized egg cannot start growing (birth control pills, intrauterine contraceptive devices)
- Thicken the mucus in the cervix so the sperm cannot easily pass through it (birth control pills)

Best choices at different stages of your life

Never had a child, want to avoid or postpone a pregnancy	
Birth control pills	Most effective, 5% chance of pregnancy
Condoms	Less effective, 20% chance of pregnancy
Natural methods	Least effective, 25% chance of pregnancy
Have a child, want to avoid or postpone a pregnancy	
IUDs	Most effective, less that 1% chance of pregnancy
Birth control pills	Very effective, 5% chance of pregnancy
Have completed family, want no more children	
Male sterilization	Failure rate 0.2% or 2 per 1000 procedures
Female sterilization	Failure rate 0.2%–0.5% or 2–5 per 1000 procedures

TEMPORARY METHODS OF BIRTH CONTROL

'Natural' family planning

The 'natural' family planning methods of birth control do not depend on any devices or drugs.

Lactational amenorrhoea method

If you exclusively breastfeed your baby for six months, your hormones will prevent the ovaries from releasing an egg (that is, there will be no ovulation) for the first six months after the baby is born. Many women use this method before switching to a more long-term form of birth control. This method may fail if:

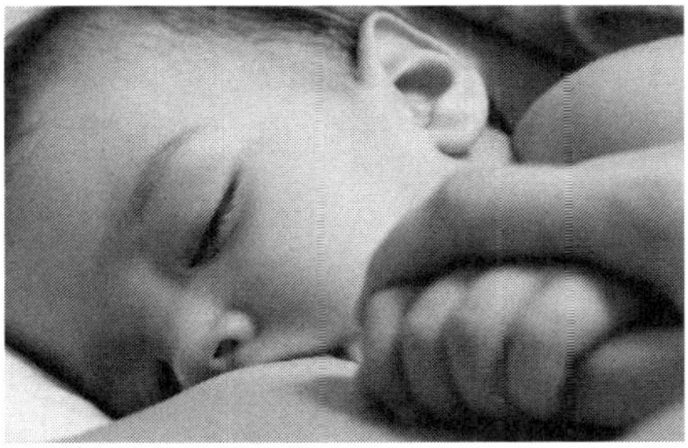

- Your periods resume
- You are not breastfeeding exclusively
- You continue to use this method after the baby is six months old

Failure rate: This method has a failure rate of 2 per cent.

The 'safe' period

This method depends entirely on how regular your periods are. The method involves avoiding sex at the time of the cycle when you are ovulating. To prevent pregnancy with this method, you must have very regular periods (28–30 day cycles) and you must be meticulous about noting the day the period starts.

The 'safe' period includes the first 7 days from the day the period starts (including the days of bleeding) and the last 7 days before the onset of the next period. The rigid adherence to specific days when you can have sex, can take the spontaneity out of a normal marital relationship. It is also not a reliable form of contraception because mistakes can be made in calculating the dates.

Failure rate: The 'safe period' has a high failure rate of 25 per cent.

Using technology to track periods and fertility

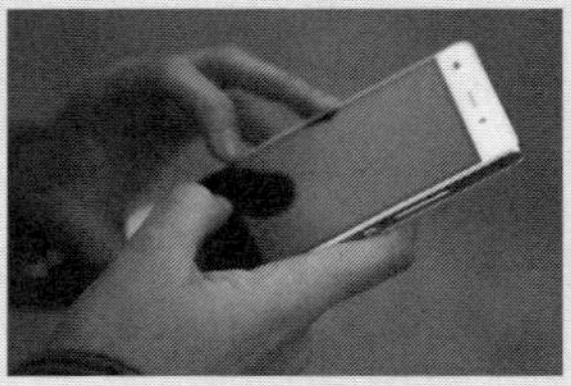

Many apps are available now that track your periods. These apps may be useful to mark the start of your period. They also denote the most fertile time of your cycle. Avoiding the fertile period may help avoid a pregnancy.

A word of caution: 1 out of 4 couples using the so-called 'safe period' method will face an unplanned pregnancy.

The withdrawal method (coitus interruptus)

The withdrawal method involves removing the penis from the vagina just before semen is released (ejaculation). Often the sperms are deposited in the vagina before or during withdrawal, making this method unreliable.

Failure rate: The withdrawal method has a high failure rate of 20 per cent.

Barrier methods

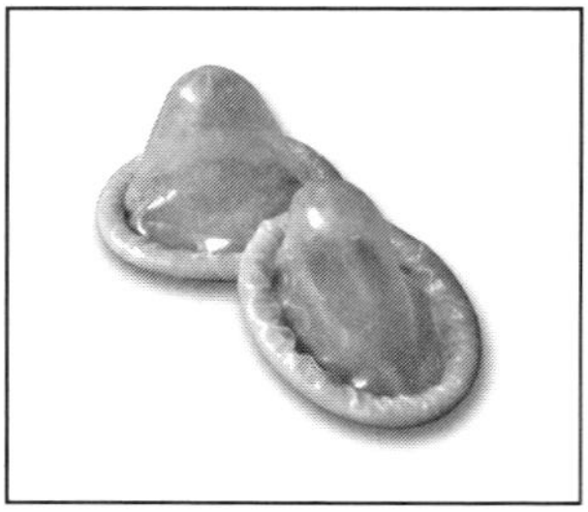

Barrier methods prevent the sperm from coming in contact with the egg by providing a chemical or physical barrier.

Barrier methods include spermicides, condoms, the diaphragm and the cervical cap. The diaphragm and cervical cap are not available at present in India.

Male condoms

The male condom is one of the most popular mechanical barriers used around the world. It is still the only reversible form of male contraception currently available. It is a thin sheath made of latex (rubber). Latex condoms are less likely to slip or break than those made of polyurethane, and they are contoured for a better fit that can provide fairly effective protection. More expensive polyurethane (plastic) condoms are available for men with latex allergies.

Do not use oil-based lubricants e.g., white petroleum jelly (Vaseline) or coconut oil with a condom because these can cause the condom to tear and can cause failure of birth control.

The man rolls the condom over the erect penis just before any contact with a woman's genitals. The condom should be put on before intercourse, well before ejaculation, since the man can discharge sufficient semen to cause pregnancy before ejaculation occurs.

If the woman has some discomfort because the vagina is dry, a pre-lubricated condom can be used. Water-based lubricants like K-Y jelly or Lubic gel can be used for extra lubrication.

Failure rate: Condoms have a relatively high failure rate (20 per cent) and should be used only if an unintended pregnancy will not pose a problem. If preventing a pregnancy is a high priority, some other form of contraception should be used.

Prevention of sexually transmitted diseases

Condoms are not just useful in preventing pregnancy but are very important in the prevention of sexually transmitted disease in both male and female partners. They are protective against gonorrhea, Chlamydia, trichomoniasis, herpes and HIV.

Birth control pills

Birth control pills (oral contraceptives or 'the pill') are a safe and reliable method of avoiding a pregnancy in the majority of women. At least 100 million women worldwide use combination oral contraceptives.

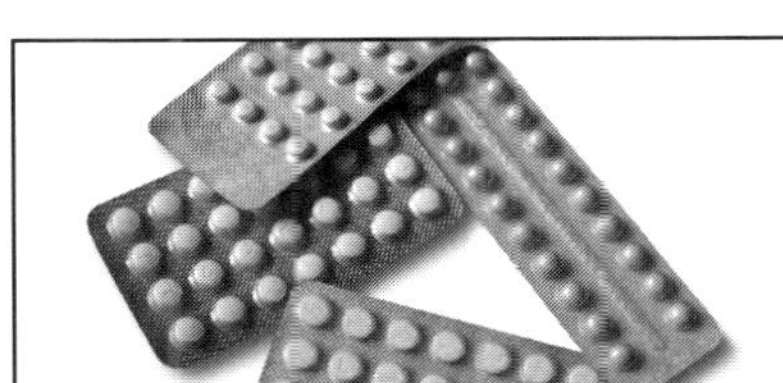

Birth control pills contain synthetic forms of the hormones estrogen and progesterone (progestin). They are called *combination birth control pills* and are the more common type of oral contraceptive. There are progestin-only pills too.

How do birth control pills work?

The hormones in birth control pills work by

- Stopping your ovaries from releasing an egg each month
- Causing the mucus in the cervix (mouth of the uterus) to thicken, which then acts as a barrier to sperm
- Making the lining of the uterus unsuitable so that the embryo finds it difficult to get implanted

Combination birth control pills

Combination pills are sold in 21-day or 28-day packs. Each pill in a 21-day pack contains estrogen and progestin. You take a pill a day for 21 days, and then wait for seven days before starting a new 21-day pack. The period starts in the period-free interval.

> Birth control pills might cause nausea when first started. This subsides in a few weeks. You can ask your doctor for a tablet to decrease the nausea.

28-day packs typically contain 21 hormone pills and 7 inactive pills that do not contain hormones. The period will occur during the days that you take the inactive pills.

Failure rate: Combination birth control pills are 97 per cent effective with a low failure rate of only 3 per cent. Low failure rates and the safety of birth control pills make them an ideal contraceptive method for couples looking for reversible contraception.

Progestin-only birth control pills or 'mini-pill'

Progestin-only pills, which only contain progestins, are always sold in 28-day packs and all the pills are active. Progestin-only pill users will experience very scanty periods or may not have periods at all.

> The progestin-pill is preferred for breastfeeding mothers because they don't reduce breast milk in contrast to combination birth control pills that can reduce the quantity of breast milk produced.

Progestin-only pills must be taken at the same time each day to maintain top effectiveness. If there is a deviation of even three hours, back-up contraception (e.g. condoms) must be used for the next two days. These hormones should not be used by women in their 40s, since they pose a higher risk for adverse effects in this group.

Failure rate: Progestin-only pills have a failure rate of 3–6 per cent.

Kanchan asked: I have a prescription for birth control pills. I am a little confused on how to take them. What if I miss a pill?

My answer: There are 3 methods of starting birth control pills.

- On the first Sunday after your period started (even if it is the next day). Start each subsequent pack on the first Sunday after your period
- On the very day the prescription is given, irrespective of the day of your cycle
- On the first day of your period: this is the best method if they are low-dose pills (20 mcg of estrogen). Start each subsequent pack on the first day of your period

You must use a condom as back-up contraception for the first 7 days when you start on the first packet of the pills. The pills are taken once a day, ideally at the same time of the day, until the pack is used up. If you are on a 21-day pack, you then wait for 7 days before starting a new pack. The period starts in the period-free interval. The contraceptive effect continues even on the days that you are not taking the pill. If you are on the 28-day pack, the period will occur during the days that you take the inactive pills.

If you miss a pill:

- If you have missed 1 pill, take the missed pill when noticed and take the next pill at the usual time (2 pills can be taken on the same day)
- If you have missed 2 or more consecutive pills, take 1 of the missed pills immediately and then 1 every day till the pack is over You will need to use condoms for the rest of the cycle

Advantages of birth control pills

- Worldwide, birth control pills continue to be a popular reversible contraceptive choice. They are among the most effective contraceptives
- Failure rates are very low and are usually caused by not taking the pills regularly
- In women with heavy periods, they reduce the bleeding and so lessen the chances for anaemia
- They greatly reducing the pain associated with periods

Getting married and want to be on the pill?

Try to see your doctor two-three months before the wedding. There will be less of a chance of an unintended pregnancy if you get on the pill at least 2 cycles before the wedding. Whenever you decide to go ahead with a pregnancy, you can stop taking the pills. Your periods and fertility will usually return to normal within 3 months of stopping the pills.

Alpana asked: I want to start on birth control pills but my best friend says I will put on weight. She also told me that her cousin had a baby with a birth defect after taking the pill. I have heard from others that the pill might cause cancer. Is any of this true?

My answer: Over the years, the dose of estrogen in birth control pills has been become very low, making them extremely safe to use. The side effects are also very few. As far as weight gain is concerned, a minimal gain of one or two kilos may occur because of water retention.

The hormones in birth control pills are in no way responsible for birth defects. Genes and heredity cause birth defects. It is not true that you have to wait a few months after stopping the pill to try for a pregnancy.

The risk of uterine and ovarian cancer actually decreases with birth control pills. Only women who have been on birth control pills *continuously for more than 5 years* have a slight increase in the risk of breast cancer.

The intrauterine device (IUD):

The intrauterine device is a small plastic device containing copper or hormones, that is placed inside the uterus and left there for 5 to 10 years. The copper from the copper-containing IUD inactivates the sperm rendering it incapable of fertilizing the egg. The IUD also changes the physical environment of the reproductive tract. This prevents:

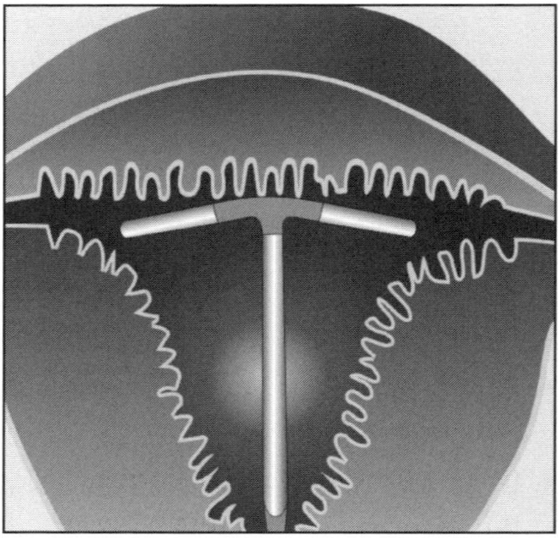

An IUD in position inside the uterus

- The egg from being fertilized
- The embryo from implanting and growing in the uterus

Over the years, several types of IUDs have been available. The ones most commonly available in India are the copper IUD and the hormonal IUD (LNG-IUS).

Failure rate: IUDs have a very low failure rate of 0.6 per cent for the copper-containing IUD and 0.1 per cent for the hormonal IUD.

The copper-containing IUD

The copper IUD is one of the safest, least expensive and most effective contraceptives available. The copper IUD constantly releases a small amount of copper into the uterus. It also inactivates the sperm and reduces its ability to fertilize an egg. The copper IUD can be left in the uterus from 5 upto 10 years, depending on the amount of copper it carries.

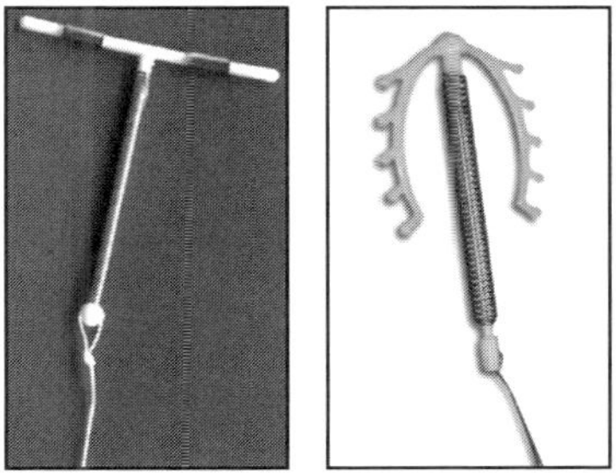

Copper-containing IUDs

The hormonal IUD (LNG-IUS)

The hormonal IUD releases a small amount of the hormone progestin into the uterus. This thickens the cervical mucus, which blocks the sperm from entering the cervix. It also thins the the lining of the uterus, preventing a fertilized egg from attaching on to it. The hormonal IUD can be left in the uterus for 5 years. It has the added advantage of making the periods very scanty. Though the LNG-IUS is very effective, it is more expensive than the Copper-T.

Inserting an IUD

An intrauterine device (IUD) can be inserted at any time, but is best inserted immediately after a period. This ensures that you are not pregnant at the time of insertion. It also makes it easier to insert the IUD. If you have just delivered a baby, the doctor will wait for your uterus to shrink back to its normal size before inserting the IUD. This usually happens about 6–8 weeks after the delivery.

You do not require any anaesthesia for the insertion. It is a simple procedure and is done on an outpatient basis.

After the IUD insertion

There might be some spotting or bleeding for a few days following insertion. You might have some cramping too while the uterus learns to get used to the IUD. A simple painkiller like paracetamol or ibuprofen will help.

Every month, immediately after the period, check whether the IUD is in place. Attached to the IUD are two thin but strong nylon strings. These strings lie in the vagina and can be felt by inserting a finger into the vagina. If you feel the threads, the IUD is in position. The IUD does not interfere with intercourse. You will be advised an annual check-up with your doctor to check on the IUD.

Some women never get used to the IUD and may have to have it removed to relieve the irregular bleeding and/or cramps. This happens in about 10 per cent of women.

Very rarely does infection set in after the insertion of an IUD. If there is severe lower abdominal pain along with fever and a foul smelling discharge from the vagina, an infection might be suspected. Removing the IUD immediately and treatment with antibiotics will usually alleviate the symptoms.

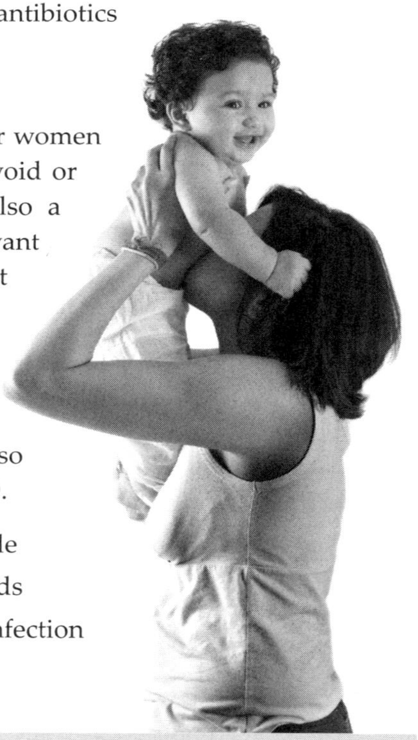

Is the IUD for you?

An IUD is often an excellent choice for women who have had a child and want to avoid or postpone another pregnancy. It is also a good choice for women who do not want any more pregnancies but who do not want permanent sterilization. Women who are unable to use birth control pills (for example, those with heart disease, epilepsy, migraines, severe hypertension or liver disease) may also be good candidates for the copper IUD.

Women who should avoid IUDs include

- Women with heavy or painful periods
- Current or recent history of pelvic infection
- A large uterus distorted by fibroids

If you have never been pregnant, an IUD may not be the best choice for you. Your uterus has not been stretched by a baby and may try to expel the IUD. The very small risk of infection that may block your tubes permanently, is also a good reason to avoid an IUD if you have never been pregnant.

Advantages of an intrauterine device

- The IUD is more effective than oral contraceptives in preventing pregnancy and it is reversible. Fertility returns immediately as soon as the IUD is removed from the uterus
- Unlike the birth control pill, there is no daily routine to follow
- Unlike the barrier methods there is no insertion procedure to cope with before or during sex
- Intercourse can resume at any time, and as long as the IUD is properly positioned, neither you nor your partner typically feel the IUD or its strings during sexual activity
- It is the least expensive form of contraception over the long term

Problems with an IUD

Expulsion: Sometimes the uterus just does not allow the IUD to stay in place and expels it. An estimated 2–8 per cent of IUDs are expelled from the uterus within the first year. Expulsion is most likely to occur during the first three months after insertion. The risk for expulsion is highest during menstruation, so you should check the strings after the period to make sure the IUD is in place.

Perforation is an extremely rare complication where the IUD punctures the uterus while being inserted or later on if the IUD shifts position.

What happens if you get pregnant with an IUD?

Though the failure rate of the IUD is extremely low (1–6 women per 1000 users), a pregnancy may occur. If you want to continue with the pregnancy, there are two options:

- If the strings attached to the IUD are still felt outside the cervix (mouth of the uterus), the doctor will gently remove the IUD as an outpatient procedure, with no harm to the pregnancy
- If the strings are not seen, the pregnancy can be allowed to continue with the IUD in place. The IUD does not come into contact with the baby because it lies behind the placenta and so will not harm the baby

If you do not plan to go ahead with the pregnancy, a medical termination of the pregnancy can be done.

Injectable contraception

Injectable contraceptives are given once every three months. The commonly used injection is depo-medroxyprogesterone acetate (DMPA). Like other

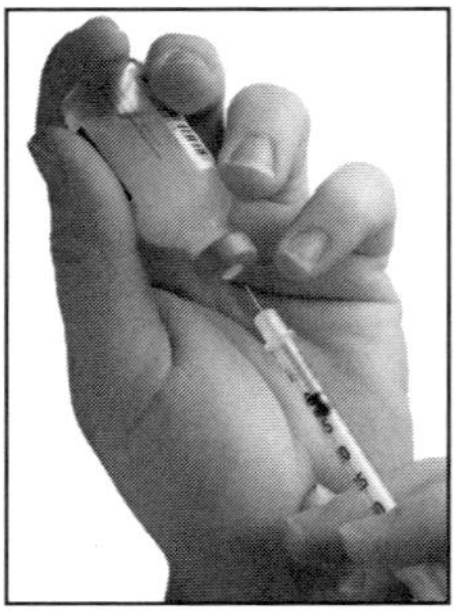

progestin contraceptives, DMPA prevents pregnancy by halting ovulation, thickening the cervical mucus and stopping the implantation of fertilized eggs into the uterine lining.

DMPA is effective in preventing pregnancies. However, it should not be used for more than two years because it can cause thinning of bone (osteoporosis).

How is the injection taken?

The injection is given intramuscularly and repeated every three months. While taking these injections, the periods can become scanty, irregular and may sometimes cease completely. Some women have very heavy bleeding after stopping the injection and that is why this method is not very popular.

Once the injections are stopped, it may take 6 to 10 months for your periods to resume and fertility to be restored. This is one of the disadvantages of this method.

Failure rate: Injectable DMPA has a low failure rate of 0.3 per cent.

PERMANENT METHODS OF BIRTH CONTROL

Sterilization

Sterilization is the surgical closing of the tubes that normally carry the sperm or eggs. **A woman or man who undergoes sterilization will no longer be able to conceive children.**

When a woman is sterilized, the Fallopian tubes that carry the eggs from the ovaries to the uterus, are sealed.

In a vasectomy, which is the sterilization procedure for a man, a surgeon cuts and seals the tubes that carry the sperm. A vasectomy is an easier surgical procedure than female sterilization.

Failure rate: The failure rate with a sterilization procedure is less than 1 per cent in both males and females.

Female sterilization

Female surgical sterilization (also called tubal sterilization or tubal ligation) is a low-risk, highly effective one-time procedure that offers life-long protection against pregnancy. Tubal sterilization is performed in a hospital.

How does female sterilization work?

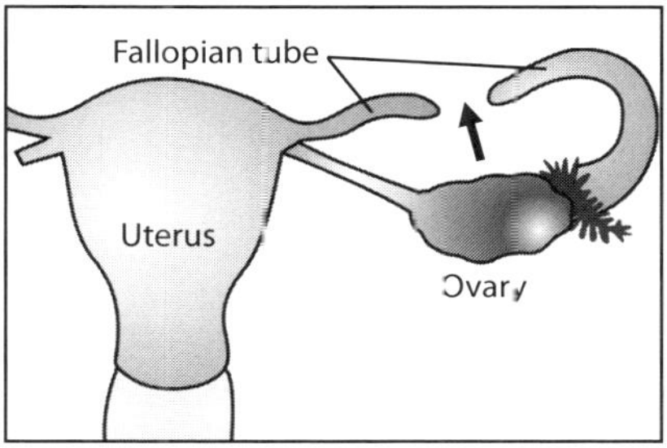

Female sterilization: The Fallopian tube is cut and separated (arrow)

Every month, the ovary will produce an egg. The egg enters the Fallopian tube and when the sperm encounters the egg in the Fallopian tube, fertilization can occur. Female surgical sterilization procedures block the Fallopian tubes and thereby, prevent the sperm from reaching and fertilizing the eggs. The ovaries continue to function normally, but the eggs they release break up and are harmlessly absorbed by the body.

Periods are not affected by the sterilization procedure. You will continue to have normal periods since the hormones in your body are not affected by the procedure. Similarly, libido (sexual desire) is not affected by the procedure. In fact, many women feel so comfortable knowing they cannot get pregnant that they are able to enjoy their sex life better.

Old wives' tales

- Women are concerned that they will put on weight or lose weight after sterilization. **Not true!** Getting sterilized does not have any effect on your weight.
- The eggs that are released every month accumulate inside the body and therefore will cause weight gain. **Not true!** Human eggs are microscopic and disintegrate within a few days of being produced.
- Sterilization leads to 'weakness' and back ache. **Not true!**
- Sterilization causes problems with digestion. **Not true!**

Is female sterilization reversible?

If a woman changes her mind and wants to become pregnant after undergoing a sterilization procedure, a reversal procedure is available, but it is difficult to perform and requires an experienced surgeon. Subsequent pregnancy rates after reversal are between 20–30 per cent. A better option available now is undergoing an IVF pregnancy ('test-tube' baby) rather than reversal surgery.

One-child sterilization

If you want to undergo sterilization after having only one baby, it is probably prudent to wait till the child is 5 years old before you go ahead with permanent sterilization. This will ensure that the baby is healthy and has safely gone through most childhood illnesses.

When can female sterilization be done?

Female sterilization can be done immediately after a delivery (puerperal sterilization) or a few months or years after childbirth, when the woman desires it (interval sterilization).

Once you and your husband have made a decision to proceed with a permanent method of family planning, it is best to discuss this with your obstetrician. Your obstetrician will guide you in this regard and will discuss the options with you.

Are you making the right decision?

Before undergoing sterilization, you must be absolutely sure that you do not ever want to be pregnant again and bear children, even if the circumstances of your life change radically.

Sterilization is an important step in life and it should be done after discussion with your partner. You should also discuss vasectomy for your husband because vasectomy is a simpler procedure that has a lower failure rate than female surgical sterilization and carries fewer risks.

Indian law allows a woman to make the sole decision about being sterilized. You do not require the written permission of anybody else, including your husband, to undergo sterilization.

Puerperal sterilization (done immediately after delivery)

When a woman chooses to undergo sterilization immediately after childbirth, it is done on the second or third day following delivery. Because the uterus has still not contracted down completely after the delivery, the incision is made just below the umbilicus. Both tubes are tied and cut. Either spinal or general anaesthesia is used. This minor surgery only adds another two or three days to the hospital stay.

If possible, it is better to have a paediatrician (child specialist) examine your baby before you go ahead with the sterilization. This will ensure that sterilization is not done if the baby has any major problem.

If you are undergoing a caesarean section, and you and your husband have decided to proceed with sterilization, then the procedure will be carried out at the same time. The procedure adds another few minutes to the operation and does not in any way cause complications. If a paediatrician is available at the time of the caesarean section (most of the times there will be one in the operation theatre during the caesarean), she will examine the baby to make sure that he has no problems. Sterilization is done after the paediatrician gives the go-ahead.

Interval sterilization

Some women choose to wait for a while before they proceed with sterilization. Other women find themselves unexpectedly pregnant and may want to undergo a sterilization immediately following termination of pregnancy. The two methods for interval sterilization are by laparoscopy or by a minilaparotomy.

Laparoscopy

Laparoscopy is the most common surgical approach for tubal sterilization. The procedure begins with a small incision in the abdomen in or just below the umbilicus. The gynaecologist inserts a narrow viewing scope called a laparoscope through the incision. A second small incision is made just above the pubic hairline, and a probe is inserted. After identifying the tubes, the gynaecologist blocks them using different methods. Tubal rings or electrocoagulation (using an electric current to block a portion of the tube) are the commonest methods used.

Laparoscopic sterilization is considered a day surgery and you can be discharged on the same day of the surgery. You can resume normal work in a day or two after the procedure. It is recommended that you avoid intercourse for two weeks after the procedure.

Myth: Laparoscopic sterilization is a reversible and temporary form of contraception. It is not! It is as permanent a method of sterilization as the other surgical procedures.

Minilaparotomy

Though this method is used less often now after the advent of the laparoscopic method, it may be performed for interval sterilization. Minilaparotomy requires a small abdominal incision, usually just above the pubic hairline. The tubes are identified, tied and cut. Women who undergo minilaparotomy typically need a few days to recover.

Male sterilization or vasectomy

A vasectomy is a permanent sterilization technique for men. It requires minor surgery to cut the vas (the tubes that carry sperm). This operation keeps the sperm from being present in the semen when a man ejaculates. Without sperm, fertilization of an egg cannot occur and pregnancy is prevented. Vasectomy is a much simpler procedure than female sterilization.

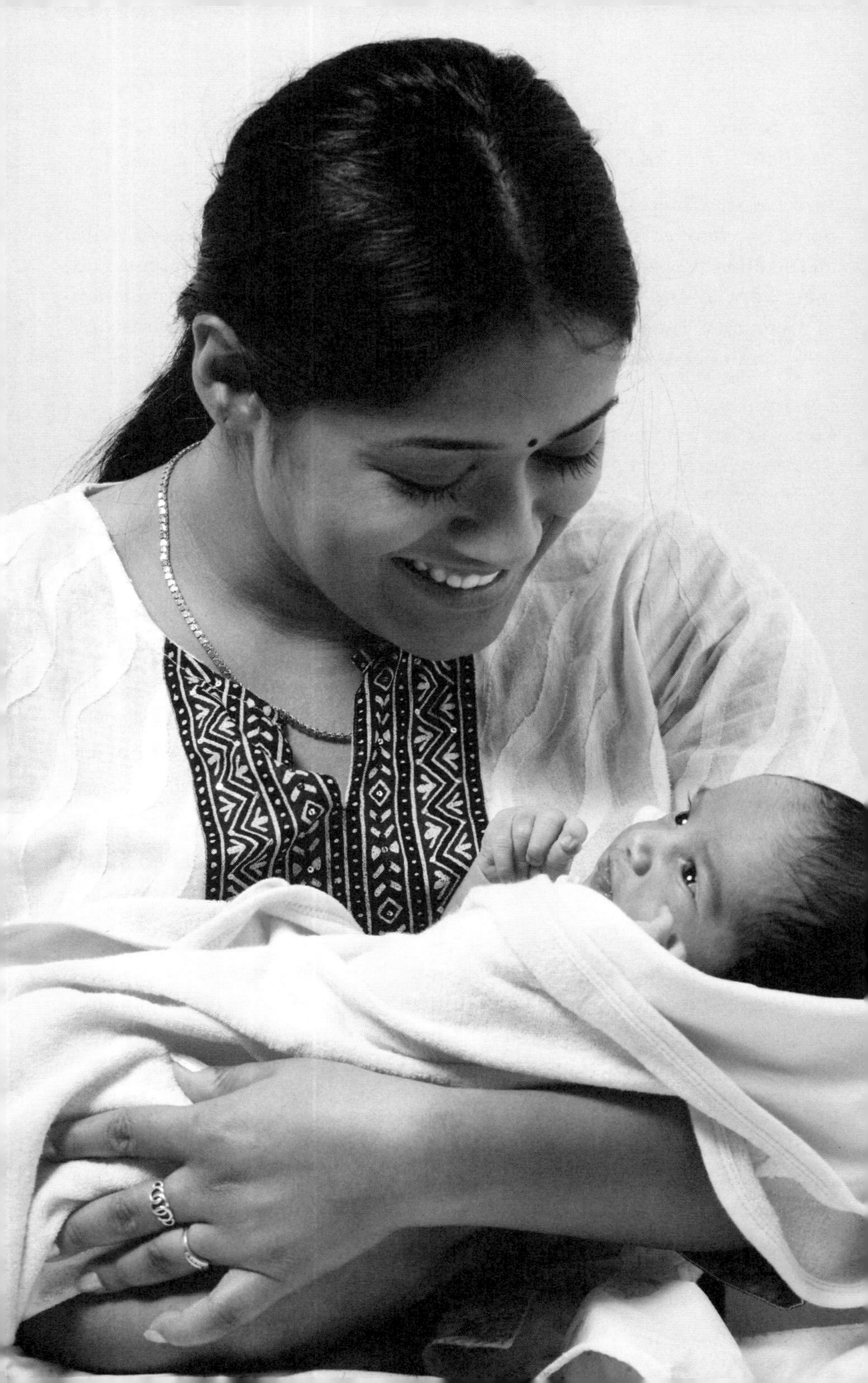

A vasectomy only requires local anaesthesia. The procedure itself takes about 15 minutes.

After the procedure, men are advised to take two days off and perform only light activities for a week. It may take a week for men to feel comfortable enough to resume sexual activity.

Vasectomies are not effective right away. The sperms that were already in the tubes before the operation need to be ejaculated. This may take about a month or 10–30 ejaculations. Using other forms of birth control is important until follow-up sperm counts show complete absence of sperms in the semen.

Myths: It is falsely believed that a man will become 'weak' after having a vasectomy. This is not true at all. Some men are reluctant to undergo a vasectomy because they worry that their sexual desire and performance will be affected. Again, this is a myth and not true.

How well do the various methods prevent pregnancy?

When a couple uses no contraception, the rate of pregnancy is 80 per cent in a year. Apart from permanent sterilization, the the Pill and the IUD are the most effective methods of birth control. The least reliable methods are the 'safe period' and the withdrawal method.

Birth control method	Percentage of women who will get pregnant in the first year of typical use
Natural family planning ('safe period')	25%
Withdrawal	20%
Male condom	20%
Combination birth control pills	3%
Progestin only pill ('mini pill')	3–6%
IUD-Copper T	0.8%
Injection (DMPA)	Less than1%
Female sterilization	0.2–0.5 %
Male sterilization	0.2 %

CHAPTER 50

Emergency contraception

Sahana is extremely worried. She has miscalculated her dates and may have had intercourse during the fertile part of her cycle. She has not been using any contraceptive method to avoid a pregnancy. Her child is only six months old and she definitely does not want to be pregnant again.

Sucharita is anxious. During intercourse, the condom slipped, and she and her partner are anxious because they are not ready for a pregnancy.

Both Sahana and Sucharita need emergency contraception.

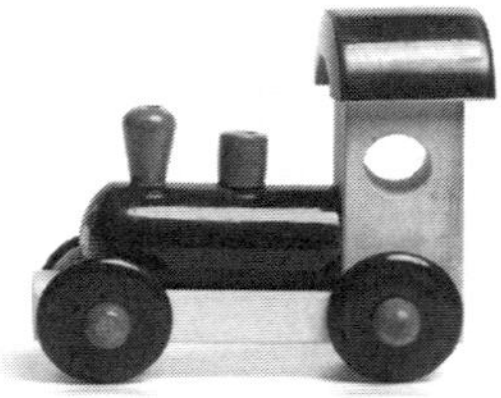

50

Emergency contraception

Emergency contraception (EC) is used to prevent pregnancy after a woman has had unprotected or inadequately protected intercourse. In other words, she has not used any birth control method to avoid a pregnancy. It is also useful for couples that have had a failure of a contraceptive method they have been using. Drugs or an intra-uterine device (IUD) are used as an emergency approach to preventing a potential pregnancy.

Emergency contraception can prevent most pregnancies if taken at the right time after intercourse. This means that only 2 out of 100 women will get pregnant, if emergency contraception is taken correctly within 72 hours after having unprotected intercourse or contraceptive failure.

Emergency contraception (also called the 'morning-after pill') should be not taken regularly or used as a standard form of birth control. If the necessity arises for emergency contraception, it is a good time to revaluate your options and check with your doctor for a reliable form of birth control. This would be the appropriate time to decide whether you need birth control pills or an intrauterine device (see **Chapter 49**, *Methods of birth control*).

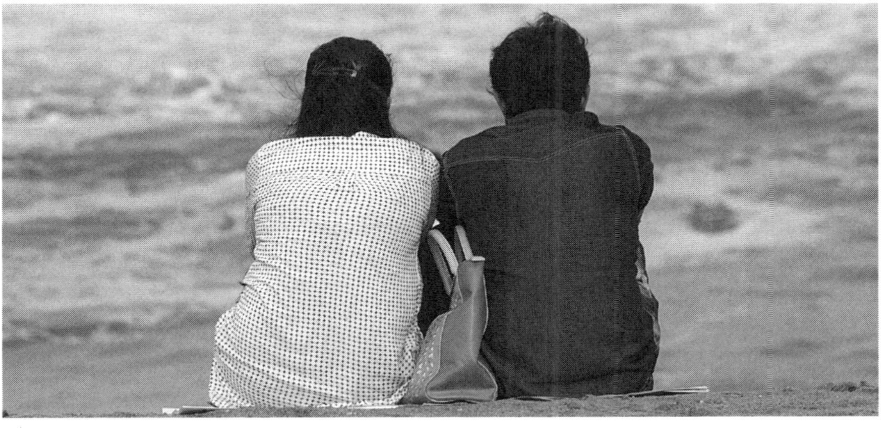

Emergency birth control (also called 'morning-after' contraception, emergency birth control or backup birth control) prevents pregnancy by stopping ovulation or fertilization.

Reasons for using emergency contraception

Emergency contraception is used in the following situations:

- No contraception used during intercourse
- Condom breakage, slippage or incorrect use
- 3 or more combination birth control pills missed in a row
- Progestin-only pill taken more than 3 hours late
- Expulsion of IUD

Methods of emergency contraception

The following options are available for emergency contraception:

- Levonorgestrel pills
- Birth control pills
- Mifepristone (RU-486)
- Copper-containing intrauterine device

Levonorgestrel tablets

These come in a package with two pills (containing the progestin levonorgestrel). You can take both tablets at the same time, or you can take one tablet and then take the other one after 12 hours. Levonorgestrel tablets are most effective when taken immediately after unprotected intercourse but can be taken within 5 days to be effective. These tablets are less likely to cause nausea.

Levorgestrel prevents pregnancy by stopping or delaying ovulation, blocking fertilization or keeping a fertilized embryo from implanting in the uterus.

Combined birth control pills

A packet of regular birth control pills containing 20 mcg of estrogen and 0.15 mg of levonorgestrel is used. Five pills must be taken orally within 72 hours (and no later than 5 days) of unprotected intercourse and 5 more pills must be repeated 12 hours after the first dose. The estrogen in the pill can cause severe nausea and vomiting so your doctor will prescribe tablets for that. Combined birth control pills prevent pregnancy by stopping or delaying ovulation.

Mifepristone (RU-486)

A 50 mg tablet of Mifepristone is 99–100 per cent effective in preventing a pregnancy if taken within 72 hours of unprotected intercourse. It can be effective up to 12–17 days of unprotected intercourse. The World Health Organization recommends this as the drug of choice for emergency contraception.

Mifepristone prevents pregnancy by keeping a fertilized embryo from implanting in the uterus or by preventing the further development of an implanted embryo. It may cause nausea and vomiting but to a lesser extent than birth control pills.

Copper-containing intrauterine device (IUD) for emergency contraception

A copper-containing IUD is the most effective form of emergency contraception available. When inserted within 5 days of unprotected intercourse, a copper-containing IUD is over 99 per cent effective in preventing pregnancy. The advantage of the IUD is that it can be left in place for the next five years and will continue to provide protection against pregnancy.

Has the emergency contraception worked?

Though emergency contraception can greatly reduce a woman's risk of getting pregnant after having unprotected sex, there is still a small chance of a pregnancy.

If you get your period at the expected time, EC has been effective. If you miss your period, it is wise to get a pregnancy test immediately.

Manasa asked: I took tablets for emergency contraception. I have now missed my period and my pregnancy test is positive. My husband and I have discussed this and we are okay with going ahead with the pregnancy. Is this safe? Will the baby have any birth defects?

My answer: You can go ahead with the pregnancy with a clear mind. The hormones estrogen and levonorgestrel have absolutely no harmful effect on the baby and are not associated with any birth defects. The rate of major birth defects after mifepristone is only slightly higher than the expected rate of 2–3 per cent in the general population. It is therefore safe to continue with the pregnancy.

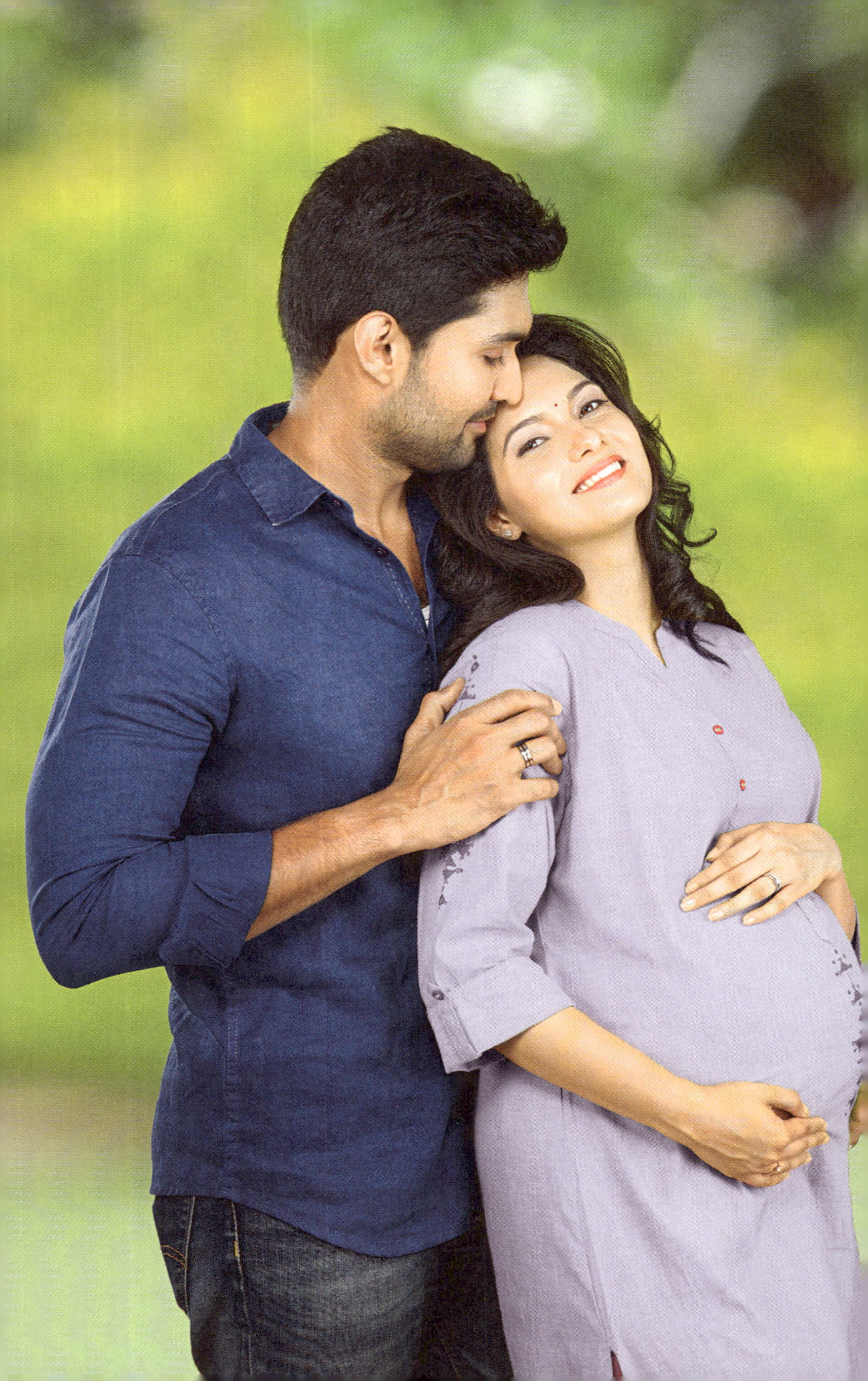

Congratulations on your pregnancy!

We hope this book helps you handle the anxieties and fears that all pregnant couples face. We also hope that this book makes it all real for you. Knowing what is happening with your little one at every stage, and understanding what is happening to you, will make it easier to cope with the enormous transformations that are occurring in your body, and in your life!

For you

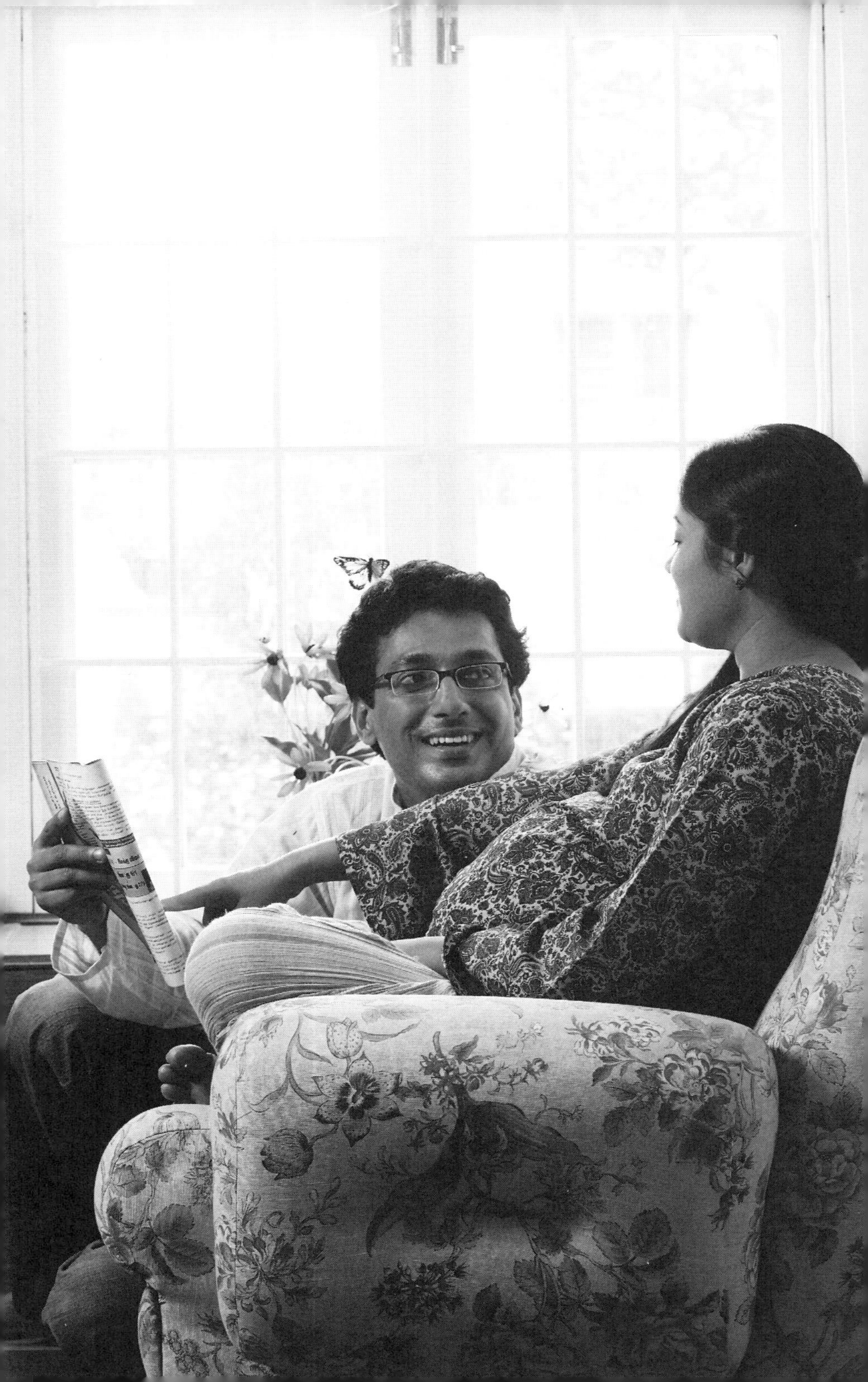

CHECKLIST FOR PREGNANCY

This is just a short checklist. Your obstetrician will guide you about everything else that is required especially for you.

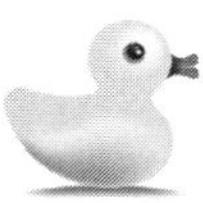

First trimester

- Blood tests
- Ultrasound scan to look for age, growth and number
- First trimester screening for Down syndrome (that includes ultrasound for nuchal translucency and special blood tests)
- Screening for diabetes in pregnancy

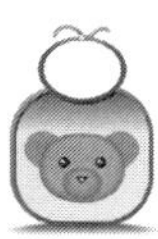

Second trimester

- Screening for diabetes in pregnancy
- Second trimester screening for Down syndrome (if not done in the first trimester)
- Ultrasound scan for foetal anomalies
- Immunization for tetanus

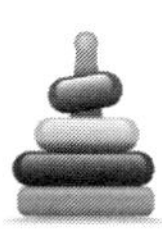

Third trimester

- Ultrasound scan, if recommended by obstetrician
- Labour preparation class
- Pack your hospital bag!

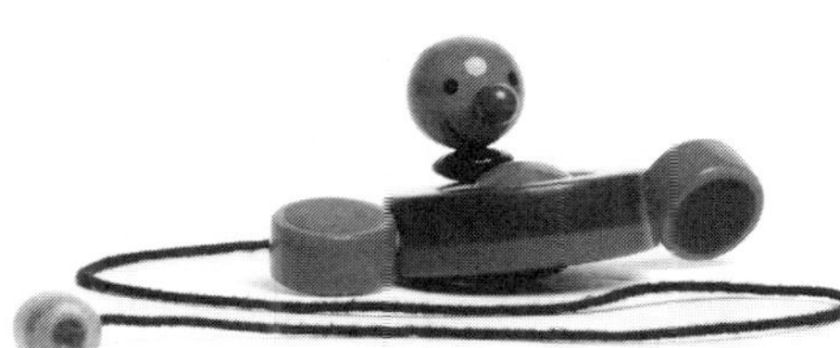

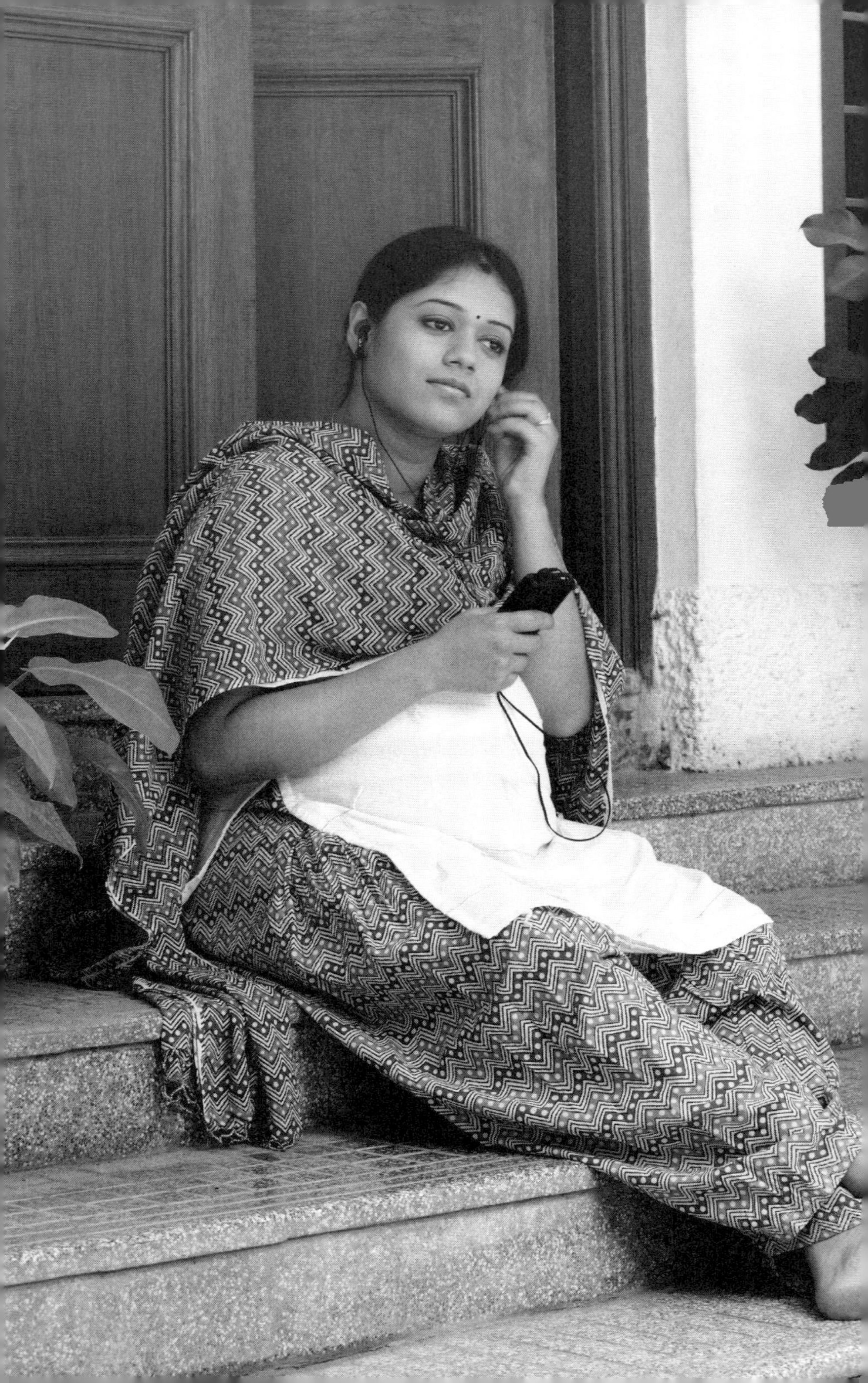

MY PERSONAL PREGNANCY CALENDAR

My pregnancy test was positive on: ____________________

My first visit to my obstetrician was on: ____________________

I felt the baby move on:

Mom: ____________________

Dad: ____________________

I had my first ultrasound scan on: ____________________

I had subsequent ultrasound scans on: ____________________

____

____

I first heard the baby's heartbeat on: ____________________

Shortlist of baby names:

Girl ____________________

____

____

Boy ____________________

____

____

QUESTIONS FOR YOUR OBSTETRICIAN

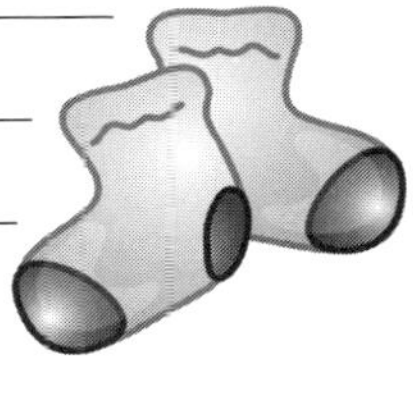

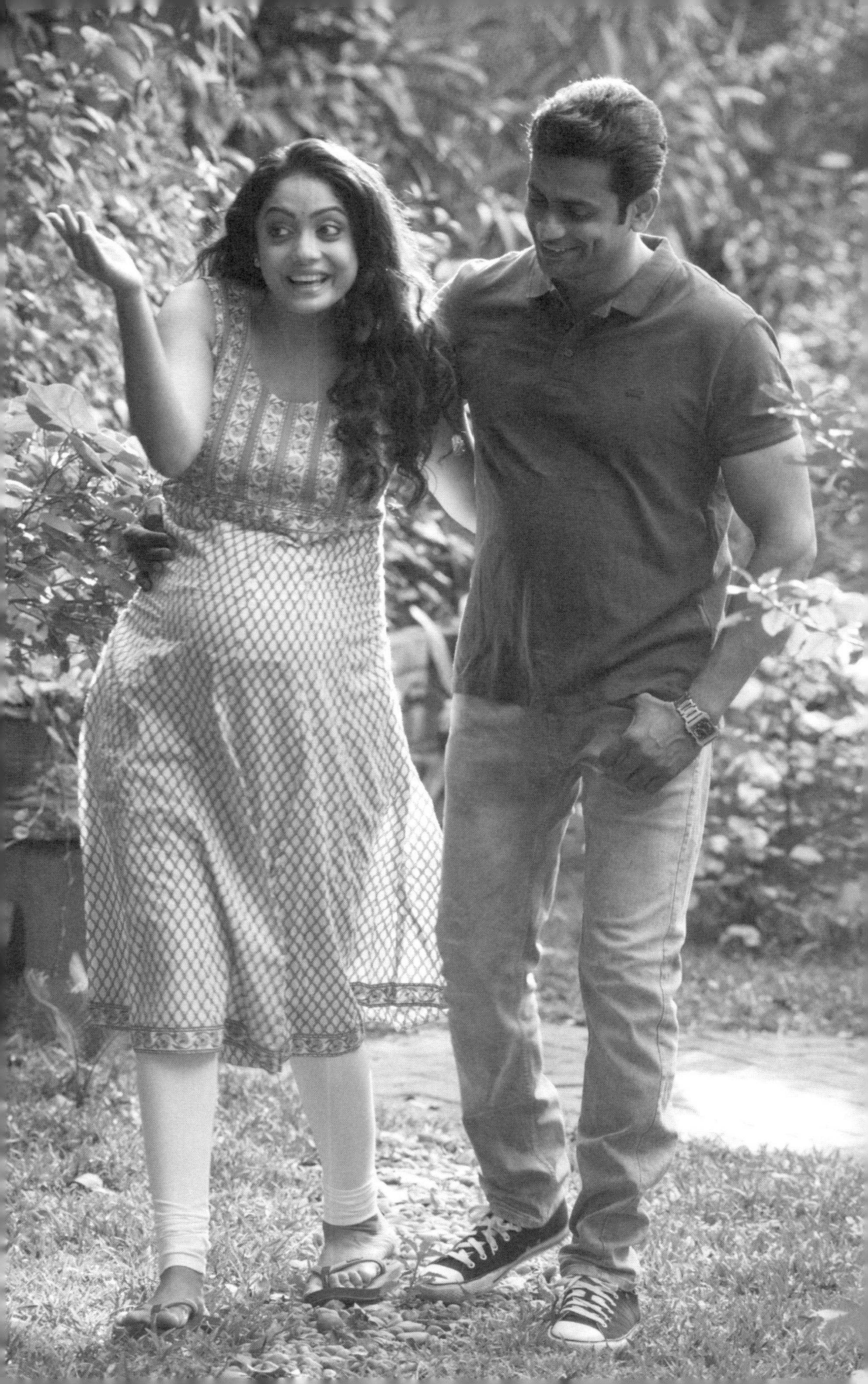

YOUR OBSERVATIONS DURING YOUR PREGNANCY

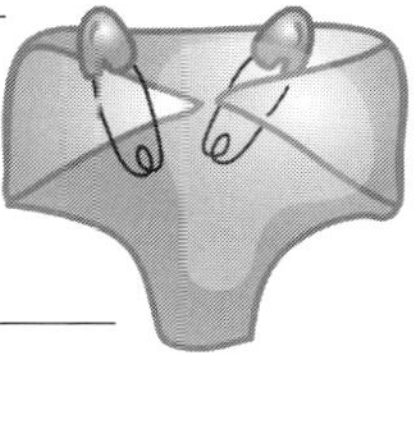

YOUR OBSERVATIONS DURING YOUR PREGNANCY

Acknowledgements

Over a career spanning more than four decades, I realized that couples needed to be armed with knowledge to go through pregnancy with a degree of confidence and mental comfort. It was also important to give Indian couples a book that was grounded in the realities and perspectives of our own cultural background. It was Gautam Padmanabhan of Westland, who encouraged me to bring out the first edition of this book. When I approached him with the idea of an updated and expanded second edition, he supported me with the same enthusiasm. For that, I will always be grateful to him.

It was the amazing response to the first edition of the book that persuaded me to embark on the second edition. I am so grateful to the hundreds of couples who have posted such positive online reviews of the book and have encouraged me with their enthusiastic words.

This book received a boost of youthful input from Amrtha Kasturi Rangan, a new mother who had used the first edition of this book to guide her through her pregnancy. Her sharp insights and focussed suggestions helped me enormously with this edition.

Sudha Sadhanand of Westland, gave me invaluable editorial guidance.

Malvika Mehra, and her able assistant Venu, of Art Works, Chennai, typeset the book. They are responsible for the pick-me-up-and-read-me quality of the book. Malvika's infectious enthusiasm carried me through the difficult final stages of putting this book together. If not for her, my energy would have floundered.

Arjun Dogra, a brilliant photographer (www.arjundogra.com) has made the book come alive with his images.

A big thanks to Dr S Suresh and Dr Sudarshan Suresh, Mediscan Systems, Chennai, for the ultrasound images.

Arjun has always been the 'wind beneath my wings'. Without his continued unconditional support and the unstinting love of Ashvin, Kavita and Sruti, I could never have delivered this.

Dr Gita Arjun

Index

D

E

F

G

H

I

R

S

T

U